Congenital Brain Malformations

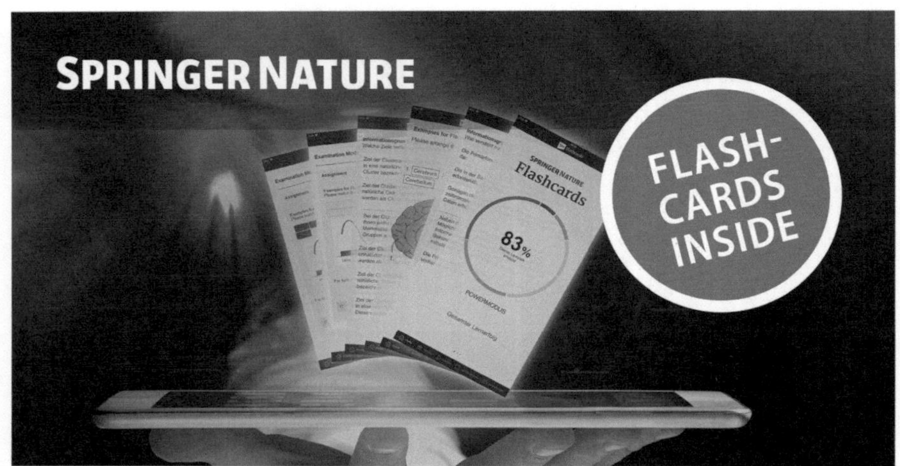

SN Flashcards Microlearning

Quick and efficient studying with digital flashcards – for work or school!

With SN Flashcards you can:

- **Learn** anytime and anywhere on your smartphone, tablet or computer
- **Master** the content of the book and test your knowledge
- **Get motivated** by using various question types enriched with multimedia components and choosing from three learning algorithms (long-term-memory mode, short-term-memory mode or exam mode)
- **Create** your own question sets to personalise your learning experience

How to access your SN Flashcards content:

1. Go to the **1st page of the 1st chapter** of this book and follow the instructions in the box to sign up for an SN Flashcards account and to access the flashcards content for this book.
2. Download the SN Flashcards mobile app from the Apple App Store or Google Play Store, open the app and follow the instructions in the app.
3. Within the mobile app or web app, select the flashcards content for this book and start learning!

If you have difficulties accessing the SN Flashcards content, please write an email to **customerservice@springernature.com** mentioning "**SN Flashcards**" and the book title in the subject line.

Khaled Fares AlAli • Hashim Talib Hashim
Editors

Congenital Brain Malformations

Clinical and Surgical Aspects

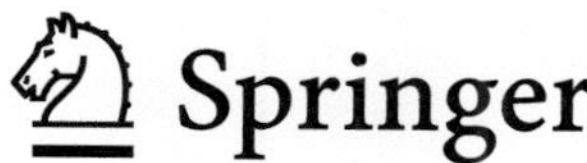 Springer

Editors
Khaled Fares AlAli
Department of Neurosurgery
Zayed Military Hospital
Abu Dhabi, Abu Dhabi
United Arab Emirates

Hashim Talib Hashim
Department of Research
University of Warith Al-Anbiyaa
College of Medicine
Karbala, Iraq

ISBN 978-3-031-58632-3   ISBN 978-3-031-58630-9   (eBook)
https://doi.org/10.1007/978-3-031-58630-9

This Springer imprint is published by the registered company Springer Nature Switzerland AG
The registered company address is: Gewerbestrasse 11, 6330 Cham, Switzerland

Paper in this product is recyclable.

To my Dearest Parents,

Your unwavering love, support, and sacrifices have been the guiding light on my scientific journey. Your belief in my potential has fueled my passion for discovery. This book is a tribute to your enduring faith in me.

To my Beloved Brothers and Sister,

Your encouragement, enthusiasm, and unending curiosity have been my constant source of inspiration. You have made every moment of this scientific exploration a shared adventure. This book is dedicated to the bond that has grown stronger through the years.

To my Loyal Friends,

Through laughter, challenges, and countless discussions, you have made this journey truly memorable. Your friendship has enriched my life, and your encouragement has fueled my determination. This book is a token of my gratitude for your unwavering support.

To my Respected Teachers,

You have imparted knowledge, nurtured curiosity, and ignited the spark of inquiry within me. Your guidance has shaped my scientific perspective, and your mentorship has been invaluable. This book is dedicated to the educators who have shaped my intellectual growth.

In this work, I strive to share the discoveries and insights that I have gained throughout my scientific career. Each page is a testament to the collective impact of those who have touched my life in various ways. With heartfelt gratitude, I present this book as a symbol of the profound influence you all have had on my journey.

May this book inspire others as you have inspired me, and may the spirit of discovery and learning continue to unite us.

With profound appreciation and love,

Hashim Talib Hashim
1-10-2023
H.T.H

Preface

In the complex tapestry of human biology, congenital brain malformations represent a profound enigma that has captured the fascination of scientists, clinicians, and individuals affected by these conditions. The pages of this scientific book are dedicated to unraveling the mysteries that shroud these malformations, to shedding light on their underlying causes, and to exploring the implications for diagnosis, treatment, and, ultimately, the lives of those who bear this burden.

As we embark on this journey through the intricate realm of congenital brain malformations, we are confronted by a profound sense of responsibility. This book is the result of years of tireless research, collaboration, and the collective wisdom of countless experts in the field. It seeks to bridge the gap between the scientific community and the wider world, offering a comprehensive overview of these conditions that are both rare and devastating in their consequences.

Throughout these pages, we will delve into the diverse array of congenital brain malformations, from the more common anomalies, such as neural tube defects and microcephaly, to the rare and intricate disorders that challenge our understanding of neural development. We will explore the genetic, environmental, and multifactorial determinants that contribute to their occurrence, as well as the mechanisms that underlie their pathogenesis. We will also discuss the latest diagnostic techniques, the potential for early intervention, and the ongoing quest for effective treatments.

This book is intended for a wide readership, from medical professionals and researchers to patients and their families. We hope that it will serve as a valuable resource for those seeking knowledge, understanding, and support in their journey through the labyrinth of congenital brain malformations. It is our aspiration that the information contained herein will foster collaboration and inspire new research endeavors, ultimately improving the lives of those affected by these conditions.

The study of congenital brain malformations is a testament to the resilience of the human spirit and the power of science to illuminate even the darkest corners of our existence. It is a journey of empathy and discovery, and as we delve into the intricacies of these malformations, we are reminded of the remarkable capacity of the human brain to adapt, evolve, and inspire.

We owe immense gratitude to the scientists, clinicians, patients, and families whose relentless dedication to understanding and confronting these conditions has made this book possible. It is our hope that the knowledge imparted here will pave the way for further breakthroughs and, ultimately, contribute to the well-being of those whose lives are touched by congenital brain malformations.

Abu Dhabi, Abu Dhabi, United Arab Emirates   Khaled Fares AlAli
Karbala, Iraq   Hashim Talib Hashim
1-10-2023

Contents

Contributors

Toufik Abdul-Rahman Sumy State University, Sumy, Ukraine

Usama Afzaal King Edward Medical University, Lahore, Pakistan

Mays Sufyan Ahmad College of Medicine, University of Baghdad, Baghdad, Iraq

Aymar Akilimali Faculty of Medicine, Official University of Bukavu, Bukavu, DR, Congo

Nooralhuda Sameer Alash College of Medicine, University of Baghdad, Baghdad, Iraq

Sajjad Ghanim Al-Badri College of Medicine, University of Baghdad, Baghdad, Iraq

Danish Ali Rawalpindi Medical University, Rawalpindi, Pakistan

Hossam Tharwat Ali MBBCH, Qena Faculty of Medicine, South Valley University, Qena, Egypt

Zahraa Hussein Ali College of Medicine, University of Baghdad, Baghdad, Iraq

May Saad Al-Jorani College of Medicine, Mustansiriyah University, Baghdad, Iraq

Muntadher H. Almufadhal College of Medicine, University of Baghdad, Baghdad, Iraq

Ahmed Dheyaa Al-Obaidi College of Medicine, University of Baghdad, Baghdad, Iraq

Mustafa Najah Al-Obaidi College of Medicine, University of Baghdad, Baghdad, Iraq

F. A. Ameer College of Medicine, Al-Qadisiyah University, Babil Governorate, Iraq

College of Medicine, University of Al-Qadisiyah, Al Diwaniyah, Iraq

Debrah Fosuah Anastasia Sumy State University, Sumy, Ukraine

Rayan Awada Faculty of Medical Sciences, Lebanese University, Beirut, Lebanon

Wireko Andrew Awuah Sumy State University, Sumy, Ukraine

Tulika Garg Government Medical College and Hospital, Chandigarh, India

Ibrahim Saeed Gataa Oral and Maxillofacial Surgery, University of Warith Al-Anbiyaa, Karbala, Iraq

Ali Qais Hasan College of Medicine, University of Baghdad, Baghdad, Iraq

Ali Talib Hashim Golestan University for Medical Sciences, Gorgan, Iran

Hashim Talib Hashim Department of Research, University of Warith Al-Anbiyaa, College of Medicine, Karbala, Iraq

Helen Huang Royal College of Surgeons in Ireland, University of Medicine and Health Sciences, Dublin, Ireland

Abbas Fadhil Abdul Hussein College of Medicine, Babylon University, Babil, Iraq

Mohammed Mohammed Hussein College of Medicine, University of Baghdad, Baghdad, Iraq

Karrar Ali Idan College of Medicine, University of Baghdad, Baghdad, Iraq

Hafiz Muhammad Iqbal King Edward Medical University, Lahore, Pakistan

Arda Isik Department of General Surgery, Istanbul Medeniyet University, Istanbul, Turkey

Riaz Jiffry Royal College of Surgeons in Ireland, University of Medicine and Health Sciences, Dublin, Ireland

Zaher Odai Khudher College of Medicine, University of Baghdad, Baghdad, Iraq

Mrinmoy Kundu Institute of Medical Sciences and SUM Hospital, Bhubaneswar, India

Moath Mohammed Madlool College of Medicine, University of Baghdad, Baghdad, Iraq

Ali Mahdi Mansoor College of Medicine, University of Baghdad, Baghdad, Iraq

Qasim Mehmood King Edward Medical University, Lahore, Pakistan

Abbas Mohammad College of Medicine, Thi Qar University, Al-Nassiryah, Iraq

Mohammed Qasim Mohammed College of Medicine, University of Baghdad, Baghdad, Iraq

Zahraa Qasim Mohammed Baghdad Medical City, Baghdad, Iraq

Hadi Mouslem Faculty of Medical Sciences, Lebanese University, Beirut, Lebanon

Hadi Mroueh Carol davila University of Medicine and Pharmacy, Bucharest, Romania

Ahraaf Munawar King Edward Medical University, Lahore, Pakistan

Abubakar Nazir King Edward Medical University, Lahore, Pakistan

Awais Nazir King Edward Medical University, Lahore, Pakistan

Saira Naz King Edward Medical University, Lahore, Pakistan

Jyi Cheng Ng Faculty of Medicine and Health Sciences, University of Putra Malaysia, Serdang, Malaysia

Hafiza Qurat ul ain CMH Multan Institute of Medical Sciences, Multan, Pakistan

Ahsan Rashid Rana CMH Multan Institute of Medical Sciences, Multan, Pakistan

Ali Abid Saadoon College of Medicine, University of Warith Al-anbiyaa, Karbala, Iraq

Faizan Saleem King Edward Medical University, Lahore, Pakistan

Aalaa Saleh Faculty of Medical Sciences, Lebanese University, Beirut, Lebanon

Hadiqa Shahid King Edward Medical University, Lahore, Pakistan

Farah Shibli Faculty of Medical Sciences, Lebanese University, Beirut, Lebanon

Moatamn Skuk al-Kindi Medical College, Baghdad, Iraq

Ta'ef Mohammed College of Medicine, University of Baghdad, Baghdad, Iraq

Shehroze Tabassum King Edward Medical University, Lahore, Pakistan

Rohan Yarlagadda Rowan University School of Osteopathic Medicine, Stratford, NJ, USA

Fatima Yasin King Edward Medical University, Lahore, Pakistan

Muhammad Zeeshan King Edward Medical University, Lahore, Pakistan

Chapter 1
General Introduction to the Congenital Brain Malformations

Hashim Talib Hashim, Mays Sufyan Ahmad, and Mohammed Qasim Mohammed

Test your learning and check your understanding of this book's contents: use the "Springer Nature Flashcards" app to access questions.
To use the app, please follow the instructions below:

1. Go to https://flashcards.springernature.com/login
2. Create a user account by entering your e-mail address and assigning a password.
3. Use the following link to access your SN Flashcards set: ▶ https://sn.pub/YnQHwS

If the link is missing or does not work, please send an e-mail with the subject "SN Flashcards" and the book title to customerservice@springer-nature.com

1.1 Introduction

The brain is the organ that is contained within the cranium and controls all the body's actions including memory, sensory, movement and emotions. Each part of it is dealing with action and exerts some work and it acts in a synergic way to keep the body moving [1].

H. T. Hashim (✉)
Department of Research, University of Warith Al-Anbiyaa, College of Medicine, Karbala, Iraq

M. S. Ahmad · M. Q. Mohammed
College of Medicine, University of Baghdad, Baghdad, Iraq

During the embryological development of the brain, there will be very complex processes happening to result in the final shape that we see for the brain, and these processes are affected by many factors in the womb and the most effective factor is the folic acid deficiency during pregnancy [2].

When a defect occurs in one or all of the processes, congenital brain malformations will occur. There is a wide list of malformations that each one of them will be discussed in an independent chapter in this book. Each defect will result from a different process and each defect has its own criteria and nature. Each one of them will have different features from the other.

The malformations that will be discussed in this book will be as follow:

1. Anencephaly
2. Cephalocele
3. Chiari malformation
4. Porencephalies
5. Septo-optic dysplasia
6. Pituitary maldevelopment
7. Posterior fossa malformations
8. Microcephaly
9. Megalencephaly and Hemimegalencephaly
10. Neurocutaneous syndrome
11. Schizencephaly
12. Lissencephaly
13. Heterotopias
14. Polymicrogyria
15. Encephaloclastic disorders

Those 15 malformations will be discussed in our book. Each one of them will be extensively discussed and managed either medically or surgically.

1.2 Epidemiology

A study between 1995–1999, conducted in several European countries registered 11 congenital defects,2075 cases with anencephalus, encephalocele, spina bifida, and hydrocephalus were detected. 141 cases had proven to be caused by chromosomal anomalies. The highest prenatal detection rate for malformation is for anencephalus, with a total number of cases 498 with a termination rate of 85%. There was a significant association between prenatal tests conduction and early diagnosis and termination of pregnancies with congenital diseases [3].

In a meta-analysis studying the prevalence of neural tube defects in Africa,' For 36 studies, "the median value of neural tube defects was 24.5 and the inter-quartile range was between 8.5 and 53 per 10, 000 birth" [4].

1.3   Diagnosis of These Malformations

The diagnosis of brain malformations can be divided into many stages:

1. Prenatal diagnosis by ultrasound or amniocentesis.
2. After delivery diagnosis by laboratory tests, imaging and general inspection and examination (Fig. 1.1).
3. Later one by neurological assessment for follow-up.

Genetic testing and karyotyping are also an important step of diagnosis either prenatally or after birth that can discover the genes defects and leads to the management protocol [5].

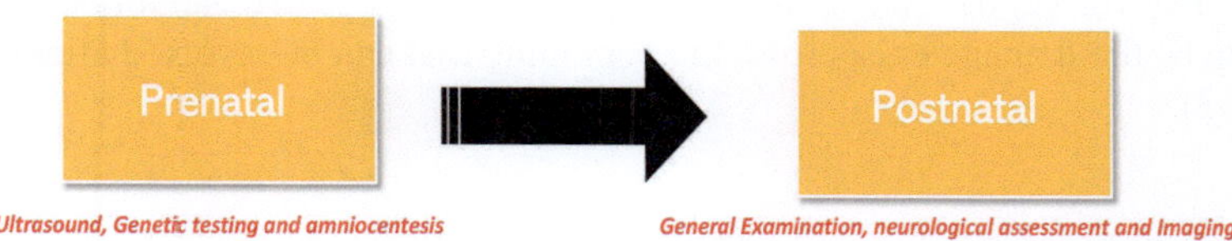

Fig. 1.1   The diagnosis map for brain malformations

1.4 The Management and the Prognosis

The management of the brain's malformations depends on the type and the severity of this malformation. Some of these malformations can be left without any intervention if they are not dangerous or affect the body's functions. Some of them must be operated on as quickly as possible to prevent their progression [6].

The prognosis of the malformations is also dependent on the type of malformation and the severity. And it depends also on the way of choice to treat it and of course, surgical interventions have a worse prognosis than medical management especially since the brain is the operable organ and many complications and consequences are encountered to happen [7].

1.5 The Complications of Congenital Brain Malformations

There are many complications encountered with these malformations starting from cosmetic effects to low IQ and finally to loss of movement or paralysis [8].

The most serious complications are muscle paralysis which can involve the respiratory muscles and cause respiratory failure and death.

The complications' extent and severity depend on the site of the malformations and the region of the brain involved and also the management ways. Some surgeries even if they correct the defect but leave permanent damage that cannot be corrected and maybe the damage exists from the beginning that can be reversed after surgery (Fig. 1.2).

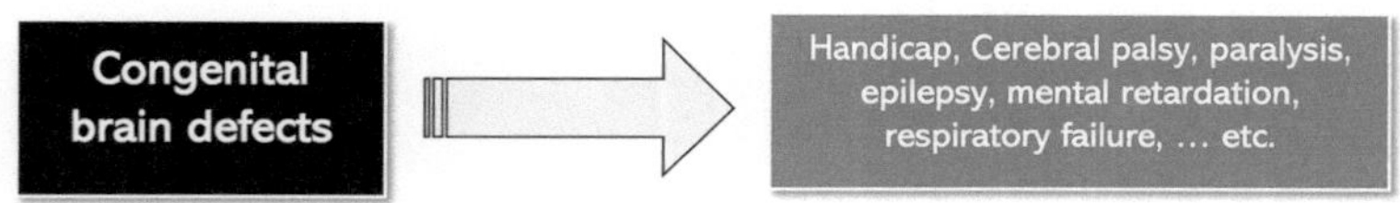

Fig. 1.2 The possible complication for the congenital brain malformations

Multiple Choice Questions

1. **Congenital brain malformations(CBM) are:**

   (a) Prenatally developed
   (b) Postnatally developed
   (c) Can be managed medically
   (d) Without any effects on life quality

   Answer: a

2. **The management of CBM depends on:**

   (a) The site of the defects
   (b) The extent of the defects
   (c) The severity of the defects
   (d) All the above

   Answer: d

3. **The complications of the CBM include:**

   (a) Heart failure
   (b) Respiratory failure
   (c) Autism
   (d) High IQ

   Answer: b

4. **The CBM can be diagnosed prenatally by:**

   (a) X-ray imaging
   (b) MRI imaging
   (c) Genetic studies
   (d) Cardiotocography

   Answer: c

5. **If the malformation involves the occipital region and the brainstem, then it has:**

   (a) Good prognosis
   (b) Bad prognosis
   (c) Can be managed surgically with high successive rate
   (d) Cannot be treated

   Answer: b

6. **The congenital brain malformations can be affected by folic acid deficiency:**

   (a) True
   (b) False

   Answer: a

7. **The CBM can be managed surgically without any complications:**

    (a) True
    (b) False
    (c) It depends on the malformation

    Answer: c

8. **The prognosis of the CBM s almost always good:**

    (a) True
    (b) False

    Answer: b

9. **The management of the CBM include:**

    (a) Surgeries
    (b) Medical therapy
    (c) No intervention
    (d) All the possibilities

    Answer: d

10. **Would you abort a fetus with CBM?**

    (a) Yes
    (b) No
    (c) It depends on the parents' choice
    (d) It depends on the country's law and the parents' choice

    Answer: d

References

1. Patel MM, et al. Getting into the brain. CNS Drugs. 2009;23(1):35–58.
2. Wald NJ. Folic acid and the prevention of neural-tube defects. N Engl J Med. 2004;350(2):101–3.
3. Garne E, Loane M, Dolk H, De Vigan C, Scarano G, Tucker D, Stoll C, Gener B, Pierini A, Nelen V, Rösch C. Prenatal diagnosis of severe structural congenital malformations in Europe. Ultrasound Obstetr Gynecol. 2005;25(1):6–11.
4. Oumer M, Tazebew A, Silamsaw M. Birth prevalence of neural tube defects and associated risk factors in Africa: a systematic review and meta-analysis. BMC Pediatr. 2021;21:190. https://doi.org/10.1186/s12887-021-02653-9.
5. Parrini E, et al. Genetic basis of brain malformations. Molecular syndromology. 2016;7(4):220–33.
6. Hervey-Jumper SL, Cohen-Gadol AA, Maher CO. Neurosurgical management of congenital malformations of the brain. Neuroimaging Clin. 2011;21(3):705–17.
7. Raymond J, et al. Assessing prognosis from nonrandomized studies: an example from brain arteriovenous malformations. Am J Neuroradiol. 2011;32(5):809–12.
8. Cannon M, Jones PB, Murray RM. Obstetric complications and schizophrenia: historical and meta-analytic review. Am J Psychiatry. 2002;159(7):1080–92.

Chapter 2
The Epidemiology of Congenital Brain Anomalies

Fatima Yasin, Qasim Mehmood, Hadiqa Shahid, Ahraaf Munawar, and Ali Abid Saadoon

Test your learning and check your understanding of this book's contents: use the "Springer Nature Flashcards" app to access questions using ▶ https://sn.pub/YnQHwS
To use the app, please follow the instructions in Chapter 1.

2.1 Introduction

Congenital brain anomalies are a group of brain tissue defects that result from abnormal developmental processes during fetal life. The exact cause of these defects is not known, but they are hypothesized to arise as a result of genetic mutations or defects during various stages of fetal and embryonic life. Brain development in the fetus starts at a very early stage, and any disruption in the normal development of neurons or nerve cells can give rise to congenital brain anomalies. They can also occur if the development of the skull and cranium is not proper. Furthermore, various environmental insults to the mother, like toxins, trauma, drugs, and infections, can predispose to the development of congenital brain lesions. The signs and symptoms of these anomalies are highly varied and can range from a delay in early

F. Yasin · Q. Mehmood (✉) · H. Shahid · A. Munawar
King Edward Medical University, Lahore, Pakistan

A. A. Saadoon
College of Medicine, University of Warith Al-anbiyaa, Karbala, Iraq
e-mail: ali.sa@uwoa.edu.iq

K. F. AlAli, H. T. Hashim (eds.), *Congenital Brain Malformations*,
https://doi.org/10.1007/978-3-031-58630-9_2

7

development to life-threatening seizures and epilepsy [1]. Various congenital brain lesions have been noted in children and the epidemiology of some of them is explained below.

2.2 Anencephaly

Anencephaly is the most widely recognized CNS problem. The general global estimation of the prevalence of anencephaly is approximately 5.1 per 10,000 births, with a 95% confidence interval between 4.7 and 5.5 per 10,000 births. Globally, the incidence of anencephaly is 8.3 per 10,000 births, with a 95% confidence interval between 5.5 and 9.9 per 10,000 births. Similarly, the worldwide attenuation value for anencephaly is 5.5 per 10,000 births, with a 95% confidence interval between 1.8 and 15 per 10,000 births. The most noteworthy of these values, according to the subgroup analysis, is on the Australian mainland, with 8.6 per 10,000 births and a 95% confidence interval between 7.7 and 9.5 per 10,000 births [2].

2.3 Cephalocele

Cephalocele is depicted as an inherent skull vault imperfection with related herniation of hidden intracranial contents, with prevalence changing from 1 out of 3500 to 1 of every 5000 live births [3]. Atretic cephalocele is an interesting and rarely diagnosed condition, with a prevalence of cephalocele assessed to be about 0.8–3.0 per 10,000 births. An atretic cephalocele alludes to a cephalocele that is arrested during the phase of development and addresses roughly 40% to half of all cephaloceles [4].

2.4 Chiari Malformations

Chiari malformations are an assortment of hindbrain and craniocervical intersection irregularities, of which the Chiari 1 malformation is the most commonly seen type in clinical practice with a prevalence of 0.56–0.75% on MRI [5]. Chiari malformation type 1 influences roughly one out of 1000 individuals, albeit one out of 100 meet radiological rules, making it a typical neurological issue [6]. Moreover, the rates of Chiari malformation don't vary based on gender in children. Chiari malformation is more common in grown-up women compared to men. Women are diagnosed 3–5 times more often with Chiari malformation than men [7].

2.5 Porencephaly

Porencephaly is a neurological condition that can develop previously or after birth and is characterized by cysts situated in any spot inside the brain parenchyma, which by and large is covered by plain walls and encompassed by an atrophic crust. Its inheritance is autosomal dominant [8]. Porencephaly is an uncommon disorder, assessed in 3.5 out of every 10,000 live births [9]. Moreover, porencephaly is rare in the elderly and is seen mostly in neonates because it is usually congenital [10].

2.6 Septo-Optic Dysplasia

Septo-optic dysplasia, also known as de Morsier's syndrome, is a rarely occurring congenital disorder. Its occurrence is about 1 in 10,000 live births [11]. A population-based study was done in Europe that tracked down a lower prevalence of 1.9–2.5 per 100,000 live births. One more review from Canada tracked down a prevalence from 53.3 per 100,000 to 113.3 per 100,000 live births showing an advancing rate with time. By and large, there is no preference for gender, with fundamentally the same affection for men and women [12]. The reported incidence for this rare disorder is 1.9–2.5 per 100,000 live births. Most of these cases were reported in childhood or early adolescence [13].

2.7 Pituitary Maldevelopement

Congenital hypopituitarism has an annual incidence of 4.2 cases per 100,000. It is more common in males, with a male-to-female ratio of 1.9:1. Mean age for congenital hypopituitarism is 12.8 years [14]. According to a study, 22 out of 37 patients with idiopathic hypopituitarism had congenital hypoplasia of the anterior pituitary with stalk agenesis and an ectopic posterior pituitary (group 1). 15 out of 37 showed isolated hypoplasia of the anterior pituitary (group 2). 81.81% of children in Group 1 had a history of adverse perinatal incidents, and 68.18% had a breach presentation. 54.54% of group 1 born via vaginal delivery developed multiple pituitary hormone deficiencies and 13.6 born via cesarean section had only isolated growth hormone deficiency. The incidence of breech delivery in group 2 was only 13.33 percent and only isolated growth hormone deficiency [15].

2.8 Posterior Fossa Malformation

Anomalies of the posterior fossa are relatively common, but limited data is available on their epidemiology [16]. The most commonly observed posterior fossa malformations include Dandy-Walker malformation, mega cisterna magna, Blake's pouch, and vermian hypoplasia [17]. According to a European population-based study, the prenatal diagnosis of Dandy-Walker malformation is 6.79 per 100,000 births (with a 95% confidence interval of 5.79–7.96). Live birth prevalence was 2.74 per 100,000 births (95% confidence interval: 2.08–3.61). The Dandy-Walker variant had a prevalence of 2.08 per 100,000 births (95% confidence interval between 1.39 and 3.13) [18]. The prevalence of chromosomal aberrations in Dandy-Walker malformation was 16.3% [17].

2.9 Microcephaly

Risk factors for isolated microcephaly include alcohol use, inadequate weight gain in pregnancy, and black ethnicity. Mothers with a previous live birth are protected against microcephaly as compared to nulliparous mothers [19]. There are limited population-based studies available on the epidemiology of microcephaly. The prevalence of total and total severe congenital microcephaly are 14.7 and 4.8 per 10,000 live births, respectively. Young maternal age, higher BMI, and multiparity reduced the risk of unexplained congenital microcephaly [20]. Epidemiological data shows a temporal association between the epidemic of the Zika virus and the incidence of microcephaly [21].

2.10 Megalencephaly and Hemimegalencephaly

Megalencephaly is more likely to be an isolated cerebral anomaly in almost 71 percent of cases. The adjusted prevalence of megalencephaly is 0.08 per 10,000 births, with a 95% confidence interval between 0.05 and 0.11. Published incidence figures for this anomaly are not available [22]. Often, hemimegalencephaly is found as an isolated cerebral anomaly or as an occasional finding in a large number of syndromes. A retrospective study showed that 53% of cases of HME were not syndromic, while 47% of cases were part of a known or suspected genetic syndrome [23].

2.11 Neurocutaneous Syndromes

Common neurocutaneous syndromes include neurofibromatosis, tuberous sclerosis, Sturge-Weber syndrome, von Hippel-Lindau disease, and Ehlers-Danlos syndrome. They are mostly genetically determined, except for Sturge-Weber syndrome, although sporadic cases may be present [24]. The prevalence of Sturge Weber syndrome is 1 in every 50,000 live births. Males and females are equally affected by it. The prevalence of tuberous sclerosis is 1 in 6000–9000 [25]. The prevalence of neurofibromatosis type 1 is 1 in every 3000 live births [26].

2.12 Schizencephaly

It is a rare disorder [27], which is why its exact prevalence has always been difficult to estimate [28]. A study in the UK has shown the prevalence of schizophrenia to be 1.48 in every 100,000 births [29]. A retrospective study, however, was done in southeast Hungary to estimate the prevalence of schizophrenia over the age of 14 years. Among 185,486, only 10 patients were suffering from Schizencephaly, among which 6 were boys and 4 were girls. This study concluded a prevalence of 0.54 per 10,000 births [30]. A study done in Japan concluded the incidence of schizophrenia to be 5.2 per 100,000 live births [31]. A study of more than four million people in California showed that the population prevalence of Schizencephaly was 1.54/100000 births from 1985 to 2001 [32]. Another study by Oxford University said that this rare malformation is associated with an estimated incidence of 1.5 per 100,000 live births and 1 in 650 to 1 in the 1650 children suffering from epilepsy [33].

2.13 Lissencephaly

Lissencephaly is a range of disorders that encompasses a wide variety of brain malformations. It includes agyria (that is, the absence of brain gyri), pachygyria (that is, the presence of broad brain gyri), and subcortical band heterotopia [34], but it is a very rare CNS malformation [35]. It consists of two types, type 1 and type 2 [36]. Type 1 Lissencephaly has an estimated prevalence of 11.2 per 10,000 live births according to a study in the Netherlands [37]. However, the prevalence of this type has not been described in any study to date [36].

2.14 Heterotopia

Heterotopias are of various types. The reported prevalence of gastric heterotopia of the cervical esophagus is 0.18–14%. The gastric heterotopias are also called inlet patches (IP). However, there is a motion that this prevalence is underestimated [38]. Because a study in the tertiary care hospital showed that the prevalence there is much lower, at 0.18% [39]. According to [40], the prevalence of gastric heterotopia was 1. 9% and 2.2% of these patients had associated H pylori gastritis. Another study reported it to b 4.3% [41] and comparable results were reported by [42], which is almost 3%.

2.15　Polymicrogyria

It is a disorder of late migration and then post-migratory organization of the cortex in a way that results in a malformation. This malformation is accompanied by many small but fused gyri [43]. It is a rare disease; however, it is more common as compared to other malformations. The prevalence of polymicrogyria is 1 in 2000 [44]. Another study showed that 10.37% of patients were found to have polymicrogyria [45].

2.16　Encephalopathy Disorders

Hashimoto encephalopathy (HE) is a common clinical manifestation that presents as an encephalopathy; however, a central nervous system infection or tumor is not associated with it. The HE is associated with low prevalence [46]. However, Wernicke encephalopathy has a prevalence between 0.4% and 2.8% [47, 48]. The highest prevalence was found in Austria (1.1–2.8%), as shown by [47, 49, 50]. However, the use of alcohol is associated with an increased prevalence of 12 percent, as reported by [47]. However, chronic traumatic encephalopathy is associated with 0.79% of them, and 60% of them were associated with a history of traumatic brain injury [51].

Multiple Choice Questions
1. **Q 1. A rare brain malformation accompanied by slits in the cerebral hemispheres is called:**

    (a) Schizencephaly
    (b) Lissencephaly
    (c) Hemimegalencephaly
    (d) Polymicrogyria
    (e) None of these

    Answer: a
    Explanation: Slits are observed n cerebral hemispheres of patients suffering from Schizencephaly.

2. **Q 2. How many types of Lissencephaly are there?**

    (a) One
    (b) Two
    (c) Three
    (d) Four
    (e) None of the Above

    Answer: b
    Explanation: There are two types of Lissencephaly, Type 1 and Type 2.

3. **Q 3. Polymicrogyria is a CNS malformation characterized by:**

   (a) Early migration
   (b) Late migration
   (c) Non migration
   (d) Excessive migration
   (e) None of the above

   Answer: b
   Explanation: Late migration leads to a new subcortical organization that results in small fused gyri known as Polymicrogyria.

4. **Q 4. Gastric heterotopias in the cervical esophagus are also known as:**

   (a) Inlet patch
   (b) Outlet patch
   (c) Cerebral Heterotopia
   (d) Both A and B
   (e) None of these

   Answer: a
   Explanation: Inlet patch is another term used for cervical gastric heterotopias.

5. **Q 5. Alcohol abuse is associated with the following encephalopathy:**

   (a) Hashimoto encephalopathy
   (b) Hepatic encephalopathy
   (c) Wernicke encephalopathy
   (d) Hypoxic Ischemic encephalopathy
   (e) Chronic traumatic encephalopathy

   Answer: c
   Explanation: Research has proved the association of alcohol with the increased prevalence of Wernicke encephalopathy.

6. **Q 6. Congenital hypopituitarism is more common in**

   (a) Males
   (b) Females
   (c) Equal distribution
   (d) Transgender
   (e) None of these

   Answer: a
   Explanation: Congenital hypopituitarism is more common in males having male to female ratio of 1.9: 1

7. **Q 7. Posterior fossa malformations include all except:**

    (a) Dandy Walker malformation
    (b) Mega cisterna magna
    (c) Porencephaly
    (d) Blake 's pouch cyst
    (e) Vermian hypoplasia

    Answer: c
    Explanation: Mostly observed posterior fossa malformations include Dandy Walker malformation, mega cisterna magna, Blake 's pouch and vermian hypoplasia.

8. **Q 8. Risk of congenital microcephaly is decreased by:**

    (a) Black ethnicity
    (b) Nulliparous mothers
    (c) Maternal alcohol use
    (d) Multiparity
    (e) Lower BMI

    Answer: d
    Explanation: Young maternal age,higher BMI and multiparity reduced the risk of unexplained congenital microcephaly.

9. **Q 9. Congenital brain malformation characterized by unilateral enlargement of cerebral hemisphere is called:**

    (a) Megalencephaly
    (b) Hemimegalencephaly
    (c) Archinencephaly
    (d) Holoprosencephaly
    (e) None of the above

    Answer: b
    Explanation: Congenital brain malformation characterized by unilateral enlargement of cerebral hemisphere is called hemimegalencephaly.

10. **Q 10. Which of the following neurocutaneous syndrome is not genetically determined?**

    (a) Neurofibromatosis
    (b) Tuberous Sclerosis
    (c) Sturge Weber syndrome
    (d) Von hippel Lindau disease
    (e) Ehlers Danlos syndrome

    Answer: c
    Explanation: neurocutaneous syndromes are mostly genetically determined except for sturge Weber syndrome.

11. **Q 11. What is an inherent skull vault imperfection with herniation of intra-cerebral contents?**

(a) Anencephaly
(b) Porencephaly
(c) Cephalocele
(d) Septo-optic dysplasia
(e) None

Answer: c

Explanation: Cephalocele is the skull vault imperfection that is assosiated to herniation of intracerebral contents.

12. **Q 12. What is the other name for Morsier's syndrome?**

(a) Anencephaly
(b) Chiari malformations
(c) Porencephaly
(d) Septo-optic dysplasia
(e) None

Answer: d

Explanation: Septo-optic dysplasia is the other name for Morsier's syndrome and is a rarely occuring congenital disorder.

13. **Q 13. Chiari malformation is more common in:**

(a) Women
(b) Men
(c) Equal incidence
(d) None
(e) Transgender

Answer: a

Explanation: Chiari malformation is more in grown up women as compared to men.

14. **Q 14. Which of these presents as cysts occuring anywhere inside the brain parenchyma?**

(a) Anencephaly
(b) Hemimegalencephaly
(c) Holoprosencephaly
(d) Porencephaly
(e) None of the above

Answer: d

Explanation: Porencephaly manifests itself as cysts that can be present at any part inside the mind parenchyma.

15. **Q 15. Septo-optic dysplasia affects more:**
    (a) Women
    (b) Men
    (c) No gender preferences
    (d) Equal distribution
    (e) Transgender

    Answer: c
    Explanation: Septo-optic dysplasia shows no gender preference for men or women.

References

1. Chaudhari BP, Ho ML. Congenital brain malformations: an integrated diagnostic approach. Semin Pediatr Neurol. 2022;42:100973. https://doi.org/10.1016/j.spen.2022.100973.
2. Salari N, Fatahi B, Fatahian R, Mohammadi P, Rahmani A, Darvishi N, Keivan M, Shohaimi S, Mohammadi M. Global prevalence of congenital anencephaly: a comprehensive systematic review and meta-analysis. Reprod Health. 2022;19(1):1–8.
3. Singh A, Devgan A, Kaur S. Atretic cephalocele: infrequent cause of cystic scalp swelling—a case report. AMEI's Curr Trends Diagn Treat. 2021;5(1):42–4.
4. Loyal JT, Farrell E, Pierson JC. Atretic cephalocele with hypertrichosis. Cutis. 2020;106(1):E7–8.
5. Bezuidenhout AF, Chang YM, Heilman CB, Bhadelia RA. Headache in chiari malformation. Neuroimaging Clin N Am. 2019;29(2):243–53.
6. Sadler B, Kuensting T, Strahle J, Park TS, Smyth M, Limbrick DD, Dobbs MB, Haller G, Gurnett CA. Prevalence and impact of underlying diagnosis and comorbidities on Chiari 1 malformation. Pediatr Neurol. 2020;106:32–7.
7. Garcia MA, Allen PA, Li X, Houston JR, Loth F, Labuda R, Delahanty DL. An examination of pain, disability, and the psychological correlates of Chiari malformation pre-and post-surgical correction. Disabil Health J. 2019;12(4):649–56.
8. Rodriguez LS, Barea MV, Solis MO. Behavioral disturbances in porencephaly. Report of a case. Eur Psychiatry. 2021;64(S1):S735–6.
9. Guerra MA, Araujo J, Staring G, Amorim F, Barracha I, Amorim R. Porencephaly in the adult age. Ann Clin Case Rep. 2021;6:1955.
10. Siddardha SS, Ghule A, Garikapati A, Kakade Y, Kumar S. Porencephaly presenting as status epilepticus in adult: a rare case report. Med Sci. 2020;24(106):4639–42.
11. Sataite I, Cudlip S, Jayamohan J, Ganau M. Septo-optic dysplasia. Handb Clin Neurol. 2021;181:51–64.
12. Lobo AR, Ocampo M. Septo-optic dysplasia a case presentation for revisiting this intriguing and uncommon condition. J Radiol Med Imaging. 2021;4(1):1044.
13. Leńska-Mieciek M, Wąsowski M, Nagańska E, Michałowska M, Fiszer U. Incidental diagnosis of septo-optic dysplasia in an adult: a case report. Neurol Neurochir Pol. 2022;57:219–21.
14. Omer A, Haddad D, Pisinski L, Krauthamer AV. The missing link: a case of absent pituitary infundibulum and ectopic neurohypophysis in a pediatric patient with heterotaxy syndrome. J Radiol Case Rep. 2017;11(9):28–34.
15. Maghnie M, Larizza D, Triulzi F, Sampaolo P, Scotti G, Seven F. Hypopituitarism and stalk agenesis: a congenital syndrome worsened by breech delivery? Horm Res Paediatr. 1991;35(3–4):104–8.

16. Long A, Moran P, Robson S. Outcome of fetal cerebral posterior fossa anomalies. Prenatal Diagnosis. 2006;26(8):707–10.
17. D'Antonio F, Khalil A, Garel C, Pilu G, Rizzo G, Lerman-Sagie T, Bhide A, Thilaganathan B, Manzoli L, Papageorghiou AT. Systematic review and meta-analysis of isolated posterior fossa malformations on prenatal ultrasound imaging (part 1): nomenclature, diagnostic accuracy and associated anomalies. Ultrasound Obstet Gynecol. 2016;47(6):690–7.
18. Santoro M, Coi A, Barišić I, Garne E, Addor MC, Bergman JE, Bianchi F, Boban L, Braz P, Cavero-Carbonell C, Gatt M. Epidemiology of Dandy-Walker malformation in Europe: a EUROCAT population-based registry study. Neuroepidemiology. 2019;53(3–4):169–79.
19. Krauss MJ, Morrissey AE, Winn HN, Amon E, Leet TL. Microcephaly: an epidemiologic analysis. Am J Obstet Gynecol. 2003;188(6):1484–90.
20. Hoyt AT, Canfield MA, Langlois PH, Waller DK, Agopian AJ, Shumate CJ, Hall NB, Marengo LK, Ethen MK, Scheuerle AE. Pre-Zika descriptive epidemiology of microcephaly in Texas, 2008–2012. Birth Defects Res. 2018;110(5):395–405.
21. Nunes ML, Carlni CR, Marinowic D, Kalil Neto F, Fiori HH, Scotta MC, Zanella PL, Soder RB, Costa JC. Microcephaly and Zika virus: a clinical and epidemiological analysis of the current outbreak in Brazil. J Pediatr. 2016;92:230–40.
22. Morris JK, Wellesley DG, Barisic I, Addor MC, Bergman JE, Braz P, Cavero-Carbonell C, Draper ES, Gatt M, Haeusler M, Klungsoyr K, Kurinczuk JJ, Lelong N, Luyt K, Lynch C, O'Mahony MT, Mokoroa O, Nelen V, Neville AJ, Garne E. Epidemiology of congenital cerebral anomalies in Europe: a multicentre, population-based EUROCAT study. 2019;104(12):1181–7.
23. Tinkle BT, Scherry EK, Franz DN, Crone KR, Saal HM. Epidemiology of hemimegalencephaly: a case series and review. Am J Med Genet A. 2005;139(3):204–11.
24. Dahan D, Fenichel GM, El-Said R. Neurocutaneous syndromes. Adolescent Med Clinics. 2002;13(3):495.
25. Zaroff CM, Isaacs K. Neurocutaneous syndromes: behavioral features. Epilepsy Behav. 2005;7(2):133–42.
26. Friedman JM. Epidemiology of neurofibromatosis type 1. Am J Med Genet. 1999;89(1):1–6.
27. Patwal R, Pai NM, Ganjekar S, Arshad F, Alladi S, Sharma MK, Desai G, Chaturvedi SK. Schizencephaly and the neurodevelopmental model of psychosis. Neurol India. 2022;70(2):740–3.
28. Siti BC, Zulkifli MM, Yusoff SS, Muhamad R, Ahmad TM. A rare case of an infant with left hemiparesis: a case report of bilateral open-lip Schizencephaly. Malaysian Fam Physician. 2020;15(3):90–4.
29. Howe DT, Rankin J, Draper ES. Schizencephaly prevalence, prenatal diagnosis and clues to etiology: a register-based study. Ultrasound Obstet Gynecol. 2012;39(1):75–82.
30. Szabó N, Gyurgyinka G, Kóbor J, Bereg E, Túri S, Sztriha L. Epidemiology and clinical spectrum of schizencephaly in South-Eastern Hungary. J Child Neurol. 2010;25(11):1335–9.
31. Hino-Fukuyo N, Togashi N, Takahashi R, Saito J, Inui T, Endo W, Sato R, Okubo Y, Saitsu H, Haginoya K. Neuroepidemiology of porencephaly, schizencephaly, and hydranencephaly in Miyagi prefecture. Japan Pediatric Neurol. 2016;54:39–42.
32. Curry CJ, Lammer EJ, Nelson V, Shaw GM. Schizencephaly: heterogeneous etiologies in a population of 4 million California births. Am J Med Genet A. 2005;137(2):181–9.
33. Stevenson RE, Hall JG, editors. Human malformations and related anomalies. Oxford: Oxford University Press; 2005. is associated with an estimated incidence of 1.5 per100,000 live births and 1 in 650 to 1 in the 1,650 among children suffering from epilepsy (7).
34. Das JM. Lissencephaly. In: StatPearls [Internet]. Treasure Island: StatPearls Publishing; 2021.
35. Di Donato N, Timms AE, Aldinger KA, Mirzaa GM, Bennett JT, Collins S, Olds C, Mei D, Chiari S, Carvill G, Myers CT. Analysis of 17 genes detects mutations in 81% of 811 patients with lissencephaly. Genet Med. 2018;20(11):1354–64.
36. Pilz DT, Quarrell OW. Syndromes with lissencephaly. J Med Genet. 1996;33(4):319–23.

37. De Rijk-van Andel JF, Arts WF, Hofman A, Staal A, Niermeijer MF. Epidemiology of lissencephaly type I. Neuroepidemiology. 1991;10(4):200–4.
38. Peitz U, Vieth M, Evert M, Arand J, Roessner A, Malfertheiner P. The prevalence of gastric heterotopia of the proximal esophagus is underestimated, but preneoplasia is rare-correlation with Barrett's esophagus. BMC Gastroenterol. 2017;17(1):1–8.
39. Neumann WL, Luján GM, Genta RM. Gastric heterotopia in the proximal oesophagus ("inlet patch"): association with adenocarcinomas arising in Barrett mucosa. Dig Liver Dis. 2012;44(4):292–6.
40. Genta RM, Kinsey RS, Singhal A, Suterwala S. Gastric foveolar metaplasia and gastric heterotopia in the duodenum: no evidence of an etiologic role for helicobacter pylori. Hum Pathol. 2010;41(11):1593–600.
41. Trigo L, Eixarch E, Bottura I, Dalaqua M, Barbosa AA, De Catte L, Demaerel P, Dymarkowski S, Deprest J, Lapa DA, Aertsen M. Prevalence of supratentorial anomalies assessed by magnetic resonance imaging in fetuses with open spina bifida. Ultrasound Obstet Gynecol. 2022;59(6):804–12.
42. Sanz Cortes M, Guimaraes C, Yepez M, Torres P, Shetty AN, Davila I, Zarutskie A, Sharhan D, Pyarali M, Hsiao A, Nassr A. OC14.04: brain abnormalities in fetuses and infants that underwent a prenatal neural tube defect (NTD) repair using a fetoscopic and open approach. Ultrasound Obstet Gynecol. 2018;52:33–4.
43. Quelin C, Saillour Y, Poirier K, Roubertie A, Boddaert N, Desguerre I, Letourneur F, Beldjord C, Chelly J, Bahi-Buisson N. Focal polymicrogyria are associated with submicroscopic chromosomal rearrangements detected by CGH microarray analysis. Eur J Med Genet. 2012;55(10):527–30.
44. Golden JA. Polymicrogyria. Developmental. Neuropathology. 2018;20:85–90.
45. Palagallo GJ, McWilliams SR, Sekarski LA, Sharma A, Goyal MS, White AJ. The prevalence of malformations of cortical development in a pediatric hereditary hemorrhagic telangiectasia population. Am J Neuroradiol. 2017;38(2):383–6.
46. Zhou JY, Xu B, Lopes J, Blamoun J, Li L. Hashimoto encephalopathy: literature review. Acta Neurol Scand. 2017;135(3):285–90.
47. Galvin R, Brathen G, Ivashynka A, Hillbom M, Tanasescu R, Leone MA. EFNS guidelines for diagnosis, therapy and prevention of Wernicke encephalopathy. Eur J Neurol. 2010;17:1408–18.
48. Torvik A. Wernicke encephalopathy: prevalence and clinical spectrum. Alcohol Alcohol. 1991;Suppl 1:381–4.
49. Harper CG, Giles M, Finlay-Jones R. Clinical signs in Wernicke Korsakoff complex: a retrospective analysis of 131 cases diagnosed at autopsy. J Neurol Neurosurg Psychiatry. 1986;49:341–5.
50. Harper CG, Sheedy DL, Lara AI, Garrick TM, Hilton JM, Raisanen J. Prevalence of Wernicke-Korsakoff syndrome in Australia: has thiamine fortification made a difference? Med J Aust. 1998;168:542–5.
51. McCann H, Bahar AY, Burkhardt K, Gardner AJ, Halliday GM, Iverson GL, Shepherd CE. Prevalence of chronic traumatic encephalopathy in the Sydney brain Bank. Brain Commun. 2022;4(4):fcac189.

Chapter 3
Diagnosis of Congenital Brain Anomalies

Zahraa Hussein Ali and Sajjad Ghanim Al-Badri

Test your learning and check your understanding of this book's contents: use the "Springer Nature Flashcards" app to access questions using ▶ https://sn.pub/YnQHwS
To use the app, please follow the instructions in Chapter 1.

3.1 Introduction

The accurate diagnosis of congenital central nervous system (CNS) anomalies is complex due to overlapping symptoms and variability in presentation. Such anomalies stem from disruptions in fetal neurodevelopmental processes in uteru, ranking an advanced position among other congenital anomalies. Early detection and evaluation of these structural or functional aberrations are crucial.

Diagnosing CNS anomalies requires a multidisciplinary approach, considering prenatal and postnatal aspects, the postnatal conformation is being required whenever such anomalies in a suspected child were prenatally detected.

While neurosonography offers initial benefits, its effectiveness is further enhanced by integrating magnetic resonance imaging (MRI) and computed tomography (CT). Both MRI and CT have demonstrated significant contributions in visualizing complex structural defects within the central nervous system (CNS). Particularly noteworthy is the application of cranial ultrasound (US) examinations in neonates during their earliest days of life, capitalizing on ultrasound's proficiency in routine pregnancy assessments.

Z. H. Ali (✉) · S. G. Al-Badri
College of Medicine, University of Baghdad, Baghdad, Iraq

© The Author(s), under exclusive license to Springer Nature Switzerland AG 2024
K. F. AlAli, H. T. Hashim (eds.), *Congenital Brain Malformations*,
https://doi.org/10.1007/978-3-031-58630-9_3

As gestational age progresses, the utilization of more advanced imaging techniques becomes paramount. In the case of identified abnormalities, the inclusion of MRI scans provides an additional layer of precision. Genetic work-up plays a pivotal role, employing techniques such as amniocentesis with chromosomal microarray (CMA) and karyotyping to investigate potential associations between congenital brain anomalies and genetic aberrations. The prominence of genetic considerations within the prenatal diagnosis of CNS structural abnormalities is evidenced by their status as recommended first-line tests.

A noteworthy study has sought to compare the diagnostic accuracy of MRI and ultrasound, yielding insights that underscore the complementary nature of these imaging modalities. This study highlights that, following ultrasound examinations during the neonatal period, MRI serves as an indispensable follow-up for cases where ultrasound may have provided suboptimal visualizations. The mutual reinforcement between these imaging techniques is evident in their ability to compensate for each other's limitations [1, 2].

The diagnostic accuracy itself is intricately linked to fetal age, as the developmental stage imparts critical context to the interpretation of structural appearances. It's important to recognize that the absence or presence of certain structures can be misconstrued as normal or anomalous, respectively, if developmental considerations are overlooked [3].

In situations where warranting. sign and symptoms are noticed, Family history and thorough neonatal examinations provide valuable leads for identifying CNS anomalies [4].

Furthermore, the imperative for timely and precise diagnosis cannot be overstated, given its pivotal role in enabling appropriate medical intervention and control strategies for these conditions.

Upon discharge, it's prudent to advocate for a neurodevelopmental follow-up, acknowledging the enduring impact of congenital CNS anomalies.

In the realm of addressing congenital brain anomalies, the triad of early detection, meticulous evaluation, and subsequent comprehensive care assumes paramount significance. This collective effort stands as the cornerstone for facilitating efficacious medical interventions, refined management approaches, and ultimately, positive and optimistic outcomes.

3.2 Prenatal Diagnosis: Limitations and Risks Associated with Each Method

3.2.1 Routine Ultrasounds Screening: Timings and Indications

Earlier detection of several congenital anomalies that causing severe morbidity or mortality is provided by the routinely screening methods in each pregnancy thereby an effective management to the emerging defect is applied.

Ultrasound is one of the effective prenatal screening techniques that provide early detection of birth defects with a precise depiction of intrauterine brain development, depending on a deep knowledge of embryology and anatomy of the CNS.

Since the majority of pregnant females undergo at least one prenatal ultrasonographic assessment, meanwhile in many times, more than once is also admissible, Bedside performance is feasible with minimal disruption to the infant with The possibility of early stage Initiation even directly after birth reported the major advantages of ultrasound applications [5].

Trimester gestational age determines the will chosen by Many patients, as many of them persuaded applying second-trimester transabdominal ultrasonography only for assessing any defect arised, on the other hand, first-trimester transvaginal or transabdominal ultrasonography is being taken to determine first trimester major anomalies as well as pregnancy number, given the continued development of fetal brain throughout pregnancy, with the resulting impact of exogenous factors, such as infection, trauma, and hemorrhage. some features are susceptible to altered throughout gestation, the importance of visualizing and evaluating the fetal brain at any gestational stage arises, in the first trimester, the anomalies such as the most severe one (e.g., acrania and alobar holoprosencephaly).can be visualized as well as diagnosed using abdominal and transvaginal approaches through multiplanar analysis the classical three axial planes, adding to that coronal and sagittal planes, transabdominal visualization provides a classical approach for fetal brain evaluation through three different axial planes: the transthalamic, transventricular, and transcerebellar planes. Given The significance of assessing the morphological characteristics of skulls for instance, or the, the cerebral parenchymal tissues, adding to this the lateral ventricles which should be measured for any considerable dilation (ventriculomegaly), the choroid plexus, the interhemispheric fissure, the cavum septum pellucidum (CSP), the thalami, the cerebellum, and lastly cisterna magna, thus the adequate evaluation of the deformed area is determined, With considering the occurrence of most CNS malformations in the second trimester, thus excluding any fetal alterations during pregnancy should not be considered if the result of CNS assessment was normal, the timing provided a clear elucidation for the emergence of different malformations hence on the various processes that might be disrupted, adding to that the late development of a specific congenital or acquired pathology.

Thus for example might be illustrated in the cavum septum pellucidum which it's absence might indicate a sign of abnormality if the the ultrasound was performed between 17 and 37 weeks of gestation. Another point to be noticed is that uncovered fourth ventricle by the cerebellar vermis may suggests malformation in the posterior fossa particularly a defect in the cerebellar vermis if this finding was obtained After week 20 of gestation.

However the multi planes showed some limitations, as this seems to be issues associated with proximity to the transducer such as the impairment of the result obtained of the cerebral hemisphere (in acoustic shadowing beams by The skull). Or The midline structures that are improperly evaluated, such as the corpus callosum, the brainstem, the cerebellar vermis, and the cerebral cortex, because the of the three-dimensional nature of the brain.

Fetal presentation determines which appropriate approach of the multiplanar analysis is used for fetal brain visualization as if it was normal(cephalic) presentation, a transabdominal or transvaginal approach could be applied given the transvaginal approach the higher image resolution through the vaginal transducer mainly if fetuses in a vertex presentation, with using transfundal approach in breech(oblique) presentation, thus showed a degree of accuracy in diagnosing many congenital CNS anomalies [6, 7] .

So appropriate counseling regarding the prenatal follow-up, treatment, and prognosis can be given to these suspected patients.

3.2.2 Maternal Blood Tests for Risk Assessment

Early identification of congenital issues in the central nervous system (CNS) is critical for a child's long-term health, making prenatal diagnostic tests essential for timely medical intervention. Typically between the 18th and 22nd weeks of pregnancy, ultrasounds are performed to assess the fetus's structural development, pinpointing potential irregularities like hydrocephalus, anencephaly, and spina bifida.

Beyond ultrasound evaluations, the Maternal Serum Alpha-Fetoprotein (MSAFP) test is usually carried out between the 15th and 20th weeks. This blood test measures alpha-fetoprotein levels in the expecting mother, and heightened levels may signify neural tube defects in the fetus [8].

Furthermore, the quad screen is another important evaluation tool that is generally conducted between the 15th and 22nd weeks of gestation. This test measures a combination of proteins in the maternal serum, including hCG, alpha-fetoprotein (AFP), inhibin A, and unconjugated estriol. The measurements are then analyzed alongside factors like the mother's age, ethnicity, weight, the number of fetuses, diabetes status, and the pregnancy's gestational age to assess risk. While its detection rate is somewhat lower than the first-trimester screen, the quad screen still has a detection rate of 81% based on a 5% positive rate [9].

If any of these screenings—whether it's the MSAFP test, ultrasound, or the quad screen—indicate potential abnormalities, additional diagnostic procedures like amniocentesis are usually advised. Administered around the same gestational window as the MSAFP and quad screen tests, amniocentesis evaluates amniotic fluid for chromosomal irregularities and open neural tube defects. This layered approach to prenatal screening offers clinicians a more precise diagnostic picture, which in turn enables the development of targeted treatment and management plans for those affected.

3.2.3   Fetal MRI: Benefits and Limitations

It is worth noting that given the importance of the diversity of contrast options with the being of superior upon sonography in soft tissues imaging adding the absence of ionizing radiation,. MR imaging developed an ideal technique for fetal and neonatal imaging, aside from this, decreasing in imaging quality due to the presence of motion artifacts or anesthetized neonate with given the fact of the slow modality using MR imaging leaves the necessity of repeating the process much more required. In certain medical establishments, maternal sedation is employed in an attempt to suppress fetal motion which exhibits in unpredictable and uncontrollable three-dimensional nature that declines with advancing gestational age.

Influenced by multiple factors including maternal chemical exposure (e.g., alcohol or caffeine ingestion, steroids or other pharmaceuticals)administration, the quality and quantity of pre-scan meals, and maternal emotional stress.

Which, as a result, could impair the quality of imaging modality.

However, even in instances when the fetus remains motionless, cranial movement could be noted, depending on the fetal gestational period.

As direct transmission of maternal respiratory motion to the fetal cranium wherein the fetal head is proximate to the maternal diaphragm in breech presentation occurred.

the quality of fetal brain magnetic resonance imaging (MRI) assessments could also be impaired by Maternal motion Which could be involuntary or voluntary, spanning from maternal bowel and diaphragmatic activity to bodily shifts induced by discomfort, ineffective communication with the imaging team, or maternal stress.

Maternal diaphragmatic movements played a common source in motion artifacts during incomplete or unsuccessful maternal breath-holding. Due to the proximity of chest and cranial anatomy in neonates, respiratory motion is often transmitted from the neck to the cranium. Given that the average resting neonatal respiratory rate is 40 breaths per minute comparing to adults which approximate 12 breaths per minute, leading to minimal stationary time between breaths., Artifacts stemming from substantial cranial motion are deleterious, impeding accurate diagnosis and timely intervention, necessitating costly repeat scans. While various motion compensation methods are available for adults, a dearth of techniques tailored to neonates and fetuses are available.

Efforts to customize these methods are driven by increasing clinical interest in fetal and neonatal MRI, along with its use as a biomarker and surrogate outcome measure in clinical trials. The use of parallel imaging and motion-correction techniques using rapid navigator echoes and fast reconstruction is essential for improving motion correction between views. Compensating for motion within views is also crucial for enabling diffusion tensor imaging and functional MRI studies., These efforts are supported by advances in hardware, including high-field imaging, more powerful gradients, advanced coil design, and transmit coil technology. Additionally, new mathematical theories like compressed sensing have the potential to enhance postprocessing techniques, making them applicable in clinical settings [10].

3.2.4 *Amniocentesis and Genetic Testing*

Research has highlighted an association between the growing importance of genetic counseling with the possibility of emergence of brain anomalies. Given the significance of neurodevelopmental anomalies and genetic defects in medical literature, therefore it's believed that mutated dominant or X-linked genes could impact neuronal migration and cortical configuration. This is exemplified by the X-linked doublecortin gene which associated with conditions such as epilepsy and mental retardation [11].

The early the suspected genetic defect is detected through prenatal genetic counseling, the more time remained to decide whether terminating the pregnancy or providing adequate prenatal care for the affected child after birth is more suitable to approach [12]. The first trimester diagnostic options covered under a range of techniques including fluorescence in situ hybridization (FISH), karyotyping, microarray analysis, molecular testing, and gene sequencing. These tests facilitate in-depth diagnostic analyses.

While fluorescence in situ hybridization (FISH) remains a valuable method in detection of specific chromosomal aneuploidies and deletions/duplications, a more refined molecular approach is often necessary for single-gene disorders. Microarray analysis alongside FISH.has emerged as a recommended initial testing strategy for structural abnormalities capable of detecting both aneuploidy and smaller chromosomal abnormalities, However, it's important to verify these preliminary outcomes through karyotype analysis due to the occasional occurrence of false-positive and false-negative results.

The potential identification of uncertain clinical significance detected through microarray testing should be considered in patients Approaching amniocentesis with normal anatomical survey.

Chorionic villus sampling (CVS) considered a crucial method for genetic evaluation with distinctive advantage of enabling early prenatal diagnosis without invasion the amniotic sac and carefully applied under ultrasound guidance, through either the transcervical or transabdominal approach, typically scheduled between the tenth and 14th weeks of gestation, thereby curtailing the period of uncertainty and a safer manner in .expediting pregnancy termination, if required, in cases where false-negative results occur in CVS or amniocentesis, the early diagnosis could be approached using In vitro fertilization (IVF) with preimplantation genetic diagnosis (PGD) [8, 13, 14]. Different phenotypic presentations clarify themselves as a result of loss or gain of-function mutations As well as Mosaicism can occur, In a case of periventricular nodular heterotopia, lissencephaly, or cobble stone malformations where a specific genetic disorder is considered to be the cause, Sanger sequencing for that particular gene is considered the most straightforward diagnostic method while chromosomal study or chromosomal microarray if an associated anomalies are present, in contrast, The best approach for diagnosing a multiple genes For broader genetic conditions as in case of microcephaly, targeted gene panel testing utilizing next-generation sequencing is recommended, And If the detection was done with absence of the causative gene, trio whole-exome sequencing involving the proband and parental elements should be considered [15].

Furthermore, given the established association between such brain anomalies and chromosomal abnormalities and particularly when dealing with severe forms that are incompatible with sustaining life the significance of early detection of these anomalies should not be undervalued. With necessitates the significance of chromosomal analysis in such expected cases [16].

3.3 Postnatal Diagnosis

3.3.1 *The Significance of Neonatal Examinations and Clinical Presentation*

Since a huge part in achieving diagnosis of many diseases could be reached through an informative speech from the patient or the relative, a history taking plays an integral component in the diagnostic process, thus, obtaining some clinical manifestations could be a clear indication of having congenital brain defects which might be observed as having epilepsy,developmental retardation intellectual disability which pervasive across patients, though its severity spans a wide spectrum. The stridor, apnea, cyanotic spells, and dysphagia. Liver and renal involvement can also occur and other unmentioned problems varying according to the defect itself a thorough assessment during the second trimester of gestation, typically around the 18th week of the craniofacial and cervical regions, constituting an integral aspect of the fetal anatomical survey in any pregnant women with suspected fetal anomalies.

Furthermore, The measurements like biparietal diameter and head circumference, under the cranial biometric evaluation highlighted the importance of establishing a prenatal examination.

Postnatal evaluations of Such anomalies may elucidate themselves through detecting of the exhibiting somatic alteration, for instance impairment in suck, swallowing or ocular movements, or might be Hypopigmented macules which serve an indicator of tuberous sclerosis-associated cortical tubers or subependymal nodules or might be manifested as limited limb mobility and contractures that concomitantly with brain malformations.

Hydrocephalus is recognized as the most prevalent manifestation observed in cases of Dandy Walker malformation, cerebellar involvement in term of ataxia enables an early diagnostic opportunity in emphasizing Joubert syndrome with the majority exhibit varying degrees of hypotonia with An array of craniofacial dysmorphic traits can be identified, including a prominent forehead, high rounded eyebrows, epicanthal folds, and an open mouth. During the neonatal period, systemic abnormalities like colobomas, retinal dystrophy, and polydactyly are also observable. With time progression, ataxia, ocular motor apraxia, and intellectual disability commonly emerge as features of this syndrome cerebellum and brainstem as observed in in chiari malformation such as abnormalities in central or obstructive ventilation, dysphagia, vocal cord paralysis accompanied by laryngeal stridor.

Thus whenever a suspected anomaly is detected, a more exhaustive examination should be performed [4, 17, 18].

3.3.2   *MRI and CT: Benefits and Limitations*

CT scans utilize X-ray technology to create sectional images of the brain and spinal cord. They are especially proficient in providing intricate details about bone structures, which makes them highly valuable for revealing defects in the cranial bones associated with CNS abnormalities. Conditions like hydrocephalus, where there is an excessive build-up of fluid in the ventricles, can also be effectively diagnosed through CT. Furthermore, CT scans excel in identifying calcifications often seen in congenital infections. However, there are limitations, one of which is the use of ionizing radiation, making CT scans less ideal for pediatric cases unless the bone structures are the main focus of the examination.

On the other hand, MRI uses magnetic fields and radiofrequency waves to produce high-definition images, excelling in the delineation of soft tissues. This makes it highly effective for detecting a range of birth defects like the absence of the corpus callosum, Chiari deformities, and neural tube issues such as spina bifida. One of MRI's unique advantages is its ability to distinguish between gray and white matter, crucial for identifying cortical structure malformations. Since it lacks ionizing radiation, MRI is more suitable for repeat imaging, particularly in young patients. However, the MRI process is generally longer than CT, which may require sedation for younger patients. Also, MRI is not as proficient in bone imaging as is CT.

Both CT and MRI play vital roles in diagnosing congenital CNS anomalies. The choice between them often depends on the specific clinical needs. While MRI is more commonly preferred due to its high-quality soft tissue images and absence of ionizing radiation, CT remains crucial for focusing on bone structures and calcifications.

In a study conducted in southern Iran, MRI was found to be more effective than ultrasound and live birth examinations in identifying CNS anomalies. The most commonly observed anomalies in this single-referral study were Dandy-Walker variants and Arnold-Chiari II malformations. Less commonly observed were conditions like the complete and partial absence of the corpus callosum, blockage of the cerebral aqueduct, frontal spina bifida, schizencephaly, arachnoid cysts, lissencephaly, and isolated enlargement of the cisterna magna [19].

In summary, while both imaging modalities have their benefits and limitations, the choice often comes down to the specific needs of the diagnostic investigation.

3.3.3 *Postnatal Genetic Testing*

As mentioned above in section (exa)the possibility of the emergence of neurodevelopmental disorders in patients with chromosomal aberration, which in turn highlights the importance of genetic counseling whether it was prenatally or after birth, the primary recommendation for evaluating individuals presenting with developmental delay (DD), intellectual disabilities (ID), and congenital anomalies is the assessment of copy number variations (CNVs) at the genomic level. Over the past decade, chromosomal microarray analysis (CMA) has gained widespread adoption in clinical settings as a preferred method for identifying genomic imbalances of intermediate size. This approach encompasses a range of array-based genomic analyses, including comparative genome hybridization (CGH) and single nucleotide polymorphism (SNP) microarrays.

On other hand, Postnatal assessments could be done depending on the manifestation that attained such as epilepsy, autism spectrum disorder (ASD), and various behavioral anomalies, as well as specific impairments in communication, learning, and motor skills [7, 20].

3.3.4 *Electrophysiological Tests Electrocardiography (ECG)*

Given a glimpse to the possibility of emerging multiple congenital anomalies at once, with multiple organs to be affected, brain malformations should not be excluded whenever a congenital heart disease is detected, hence some studies have shown a high prevalence of emergence of structural brain anomalies in patients with congenital heart disease like ventriculomegaly, agenesis of the corpus callosum, white matter abnormalities, neurodevelopmental delay and others, in other words, elevated extra-axial cerebrospinal fluid (CSF) compartments were predominantly identified in fetuses exhibiting acyanotic congenital heart disease (7 out of 10), whereas unilateral ventriculomegaly demonstrated a threefold higher incidence in fetuses with cyanotic congenital heart disease., MR imaging findings related to fetus with congenital heart disease revealed a reduction in brain growth mainly in the third trimester this association has been mentioned in multiple studies whether these abnormalities were postnatal or even present before birth,. thus the potential of using Echocardiogram arises even in CNS-specific syndrome [18, 21].

3.4 Conclusion

Diagnosing congenital central nervous system (CNS) anomalies is a complex and multi-faceted endeavor, necessitating a spectrum of methods that involve both imaging and genetic screening to ensure accuracy and timely intervention. Owing to the intricacies of fetal neurodevelopment, symptoms often overlap and may present variably, making accurate diagnosis is challenging task. Advances in neuroimaging, such as neurosonography, MRI, and CT, have revolutionized our ability to detect and characterize these anomalies early on. Ultrasound remains the first-line modality for prenatal screening, but its utility is complemented by the precision offered by MRI, especially in cases where ultrasound fails to offer clear visualization.

The role of genetic testing cannot be understated, with techniques such as amniocentesis coupled with chromosomal microarray (CMA) and karyotyping offering essential information. These tests are particularly invaluable in cases where a family history of congenital anomalies or other risk factors are present, allowing for a more targeted and comprehensive diagnostic approach.

However, it is crucial to acknowledge the limitations and risks associated with each method. While ultrasound is minimally invasive and widely accessible, its diagnostic efficacy can be compromised by factors such as fetal positioning and gestational age. MRI, although highly detailed, is susceptible to motion artifacts and may require maternal sedation, complicating its execution. Genetic testing carries its own set of risks, including miscarriage in the case of amniocentesis.

In instances where potential anomalies are detected, a more detailed assessment of the fetal neuroanatomy is strongly recommended. Moreover, post-discharge neurodevelopmental follow-ups are essential to ascertain the long-term impact of any diagnosed anomalies. This is critical for formulating effective intervention and management strategies aimed at optimizing the quality of life for affected individuals.

Therefore, a multidisciplinary approach that combines multiple screening tools, timely genetic work-up, and continuous follow-up is indispensable for the comprehensive diagnosis and management of congenital CNS anomalies. Such an integrated approach maximizes the chances for early intervention, thereby improving the prognosis and enhancing the long-term outcomes for affected individuals and their families.

The early detection of congenital central nervous system (CNS) anomalies is of paramount importance for both pre- and postnatal management. Prenatal diagnosis has evolved with techniques such as chorionic villus sampling (CVS), amniocentesis, and in vitro fertilization coupled with preimplantation genetic diagnosis (IVF-PGD). These techniques offer the advantage of reducing the period of uncertainty and enabling early interventions. However, each method has its drawbacks, including false-negative results, highlighting the need for comprehensive genetic counseling and confirmatory testing.

Postnatally, the diagnostic process is equally intricate, involving a multi-modality approach that includes MRI and CT scans, each with their specific strengths and limitations. Genetic testing in the postnatal period, particularly chromosomal microarray analysis (CMA), is increasingly becoming a standard of care, especially for children presenting with developmental delays, intellectual disabilities, and other neurodevelopmental disorders. Electrophysiological tests like ECG are also pivotal when congenital heart disease is detected, as it may indicate concurrent structural brain anomalies.

Early detection not only provides an opportunity for timely therapeutic intervention but also allows parents and healthcare providers more time for decision-making concerning the future management and quality of life for the affected individual. The role of accurate family history and detailed neonatal examinations cannot be overemphasized, as they often provide the initial leads for suspecting a CNS anomaly.

Multiple Choice Questions
1. **Elevated extra-axial cerebrospinal fluid (CSF) compartments were predominantly identified in fetuses with which type of congenital heart disease?**

   (a) A cyanotic congenital heart disease
   (b) An acyanotic congenital heart disease
   (c) A combined cyanotic and acyanotic congenital heart disease
   (d) A complex congenital heart disease

2. **What is the primary reason for utilizing both imaging and genetic screening in diagnosing congenital CNS anomalies?**

   (a) To minimize the need for early interventions
   (b) To simplify the diagnostic process
   (c) To enhance accuracy and timely intervention
   (d) To rely solely on genetic testing

3. **What are the limitations of using ultrasound for diagnosing CNS anomalies?**

   (a) Motion artifacts
   (b) Maternal sedation
   (c) Gestational age
   (d) All of the above

4. **What is one advantage of using MRI for fetal and neonatal imaging?**

   (a) Reduced exposure to ionizing radiation
   (b) No chance of motion artifacts
   (c) Low cost
   (d) Quick modality

5. **What is a primary benefit of using Fluorescence In Situ Hybridization (FISH) in prenatal testing?**

   (a) Detection of specific chromosomal abnormalities
   (b) No risk of false-negative or false-positive results
   (c) Cheap and easily accessible
   (d) Can detect all types of genetic abnormalities

6. **In which trimester is the reduction in brain growth mainly observed in fetuses with congenital heart disease?**

   (a) First trimester
   (b) Second trimester
   (c) Third trimester
   (d) It's evenly distributed across all trimesters

7. **brain malformations should not be excluded when a patient is diagnosed with:**

   (a) Neurodevelopmental delay
   (b) Cyanotic congenital heart disease
   (c) Acyanotic congenital heart disease
   (d) Ventriculomegaly

8. **What type of genetic testing is recommended for diagnosing multiple genes in broader genetic conditions like microcephaly?**

   (a) Sanger sequencing
   (b) Targeted gene panel testing
   (c) Fluorescence In Situ Hybridization (FISH)
   (d) Karyotyping

9. **Which of the following diagnostic procedures is most likely to be recommended for additional assessment in the same gestational timeframe as the Maternal Serum Alpha-fetoprotein (MSAFP) and quad screen tests if there are concerns about fetal abnormalities?**

   (a) Fetal MRI with gadolinium contrast
   (b) High-resolution computed tomography (CT) scan of the fetal head
   (c) Amniocentesis for chromosomal and biochemical analysis
   (d) Fetal electrocardiogram (ECG) to assess cardiac function
   (e) Umbilical artery Doppler ultrasound

10. **What is often the timing for thorough assessments during the second trimester of gestation?**

    (a) tenth week
    (b) 14th week
    (c) C18th week
    (d) 24th week

11. **What is the limitation of the three-dimensional nature of the brain in ultrasound imaging?**

    (a) Provides less detail
    (b) Improperly evaluates structures like the corpus callosum
    (c) Cannot detect any anomalies
    (d) Requires more time

12. **What technique has gained widespread adoption for identifying genomic imbalances?**

    (a) Ultrasound
    (b) Chromosomal Microarray Analysis (CMA)
    (c) Karyotyping
    (d) Amniocentesis

13. **Which technique provides essential information in cases where a family history of congenital anomalies is present?**

    (a) ECG
    (b) Ultrasound
    (c) Amniocentesis coupled with CMA
    (d) MRI

14. **How does magnetic resonance imaging (MRI) complement other imaging modalities?**

    (a) MRI entirely supersedes ultrasound in both spatial and temporal resolution for all CNS structures.
    (b) MRI is primarily utilized as a second-line modality when ultrasound provides inconclusive or suboptimal results.
    (c) MRI is generally contraindicated due to the risks outweighing any diagnostic benefit.
    (d) MRI is the first-line modality due to its superior sensitivity and specificity compared to ultrasound.
    (e) MRI and ultrasound offer identical benefits and either can be used interchangeably.

15. **What is the key factor that makes accurate diagnosis challenging?**

    (a) Equipment malfunction
    (b) Lack of expert radiologists
    (c) Symptoms often overlap and present variably
    (d) Absence of family history

16. **What unique advantage does MRI have over CT in terms of identifying brain structures?**

    (a) Ability to image bones effectively
    (b) Shorter scanning time
    (c) Distinguishing between gray and white matter
    (d) Lower cost

Answers
  1. **1-Ans/b**

     Explanation: Elevated extra-axial cerebrospinal fluid (CSF) compartments were predominantly identified in fetuses with An acyanotic congenital heart disease

2. **2-Ans/c**

   Explanation: The primary reason for using both imaging and genetic screening in diagnosing congenital CNS (Central Nervous System) anomalies is to enhance accuracy and timely intervention. Combining these methods provides a more comprehensive view of potential anomalies, allowing for more accurate diagnoses and the opportunity for early, targeted treatment.

3. **3-ans/d**

   Explanation: The limitations of using ultrasound for diagnosing CNS anomalies include motion artifacts, maternal sedation, and gestational age. Motion artifacts can distort images, maternal sedation may affect the quality of the ultrasound, and the fetus's gestational age can limit the clarity and detail of what can be seen. Therefore, the answer is "All of the above" because each of these factors can pose limitations to ultrasound's diagnostic accuracy for CNS anomalies.

4. **4-Answer: A) Reduced exposure to ionizing radiation**

   Explanation: The text mentions that one advantage of MRI is the absence of ionizing radiation, making it ideal for fetal and neonatal imaging.

5. **5-Answer: A) Detection of specific chromosomal abnormalities**

   Explanation: The text mentions that FISH is valuable for the detection of specific chromosomal aneuploidies and deletions/duplications.

6. **6-Ans/c**

   Explanation: The reduction in brain growth is mainly observed in the third trimester for fetuses with congenital heart disease. This suggests that these fetuses are especially vulnerable to slower brain development later in pregnancy, which could be crucial for planning prenatal care and interventions.

7. **7-Answer: C)**

   Explanation: Elevated extra-axial cerebrospinal fluid (CSF) compartments were predominantly identified in fetuses exhibiting acyanotic congenital heart disease

8. **8-Answer: B) Targeted gene panel testing**

   Explanation: The text recommends targeted gene panel testing utilizing next-generation sequencing for broader genetic conditions like microcephaly.

9. **9-Answer: C) Amniocentesis for chromosomal and biochemical analysis**

   Explanation: Amniocentesis is often advised around the same gestational window as the MSAFP and quad screen tests when there are concerns about potential fetal abnormalities. It allows for chromosomal and biochemical analysis to gain more information regarding the health of the fetus.

10. **10-Answer: C) 18th week**

    Explanation: The text states that a thorough assessment is typically conducted around the 18th week of gestation.

11. **I1-Answer: B) Improperly evaluates structures like the corpus callosum**
    Explanation: The text says that some midline structures like the corpus callosum are improperly evaluated due to the three-dimensional nature of the brain.
12. **12-Answer: B) Chromosomal Microarray Analysis (CMA)**
    Explanation: CMA has gained widespread adoption for identifying genomic imbalances of intermediate size.
13. **13-Answer: C) Amniocentesis coupled with CMA**
    Explanation: Amniocentesis coupled with chromosomal microarray (CMA) offers essential information, especially in cases where a family history of congenital anomalies is present.
14. **14-Answer: B) MRI is primarily utilized as a second-line modality when ultrasound provides inconclusive or suboptimal results.**
    Explanation: While MRI offers excellent spatial resolution for assessing CNS structures, it typically acts as a follow-up modality when ultrasound, which is often the first-line imaging technique, yields suboptimal or inconclusive findings. MRI does not replace ultrasound but rather complements it in providing a more comprehensive diagnostic picture.
15. **15-Answer: C) Symptoms often overlap and present variably**
    Explanation: Owing to the intricacies of fetal neurodevelopment, symptoms often overlap and may present variably, making accurate diagnosis a challenging task.
16. **16-Answer: c) Distinguishing between gray and white matter.**
    Explanation:MRI has the unique advantage of distinguishing between gray and white matter in the brain more effectively than CT scans. This capability allows for a more detailed and nuanced understanding of brain structures, making MRI superior for certain types of neurological assessments.

References

1. Van den Veyver IB. Prenatally diagnosed developmental abnormalities of the central nervous system and genetic syndromes: a practical review. Prenat Diagn. 2019;39(9):666–78. https://doi.org/10.1002/pd.5520. Epub 2019 Jul 28.
2. Kołak M, Herman-Sucharska I, Radoń-Pokracka M, Stolarek M, Horbaczewska A, Huras H. The assessment of the usefulness of prenatal magnetic resonance imaging in the diagnosis of central nervous system defects. Diagnostics. 2021;11:1723. https://doi.org/10.3390/diagnostics11091723.
3. Kohlenberg C, Lumley J, Yates J, Bell R. A prospective population-based study of CNS abnormality detection at 16 to 20 weeks by ultrasonography. J Ultrasound Med. 1996;15:29.
4. Anon. AIUM-ACR-ACOG-SMFM-SRU practice parameter for the performance of standard diagnostic obstetric ultrasound examinations. J Ultrasound Med. 2018;37(11):E13–24.
5. Anon. Cranial ultrasonography: advantages and aims. In: Neonatal cranial ultrasonography. Berlin: Springer; 2007. https://doi.org/10.1007/978-3-540-69908-8_1.
6. Milani HJF, Barreto EQS, Araujo Júnior E, Peixoto AB, Nardozza LMM, Moron AF. Ultrasonographic evaluation of the fetal central nervous system: review of guidelines. Radiol Bras. 2019;52(3):176–81. https://doi.org/10.1590/0100-3984.2018.0056. PMID: 31210692; PMCID: PMC6561375.

7. Malinger G, Lev D, Lerman-Sagie T. Normal and abnormal fetal brain development during the third trimester as demonstrated by neurosonography. Eur J Radiol. 2006;57(2):226–32.

8. Baffero GM, Somigliana E, Crovetto F, et al. Confined placental mosaicism at chorionic villous sampling: risk factors and pregnancy outcome. Prenat Diagn. 2012;32(11):1102–8.

9. Dugoff L, Hobbins JC, Malone FD, Vidaver J, Sullivan L, Canick JA, Lambert-Messerlian GM, Porter TF, Luthy DA, Comstock CH, Saade G. Quad screen as a predictor of adverse pregnancy outcome. Obstet Gynecol. 2005;106(2):260–7.

10. Malamateniou C, Malik SJ, Counsell SJ, Allsop JM, McGuinness AK, Hayat T, Broadhouse K, Nunes RG, Ederies AM, Hajnal JV, Rutherford MA. Motion-compensation techniques in neonatal and fetal MR imaging. AJNR Am J Neuroradiol. 2013;34(6):1124–36. https://doi.org/10.3174/ajnr.A3128. Epub 2012 May 10. PMID: 22576885; PMCID: PMC7964586.

11. Gleeson JG, Luo RF, Grant PE, Guerrini R, Huttenlocher PR, Berg MJ, Ricci S, Cusmai R, Wheless JW, Berkovic S, Scheffer I. Genetic and neuroradiological heterogeneity of double cortex syndrome. Ann Neurology. 2000;47(2):265–9.

12. Adzick NS, Thom EA, Spong CY, et al. A randomized trial of prenatal versus post- natal repair of myelomeningocele. N Engl J Med. 2011;364(11):993–1004.

13. Audibert F, Wilson RD, Allen V, et al. Preimplantation genetic testing. J Obstet Gynaecol Can. 2009;31(8):761–75.

14. Practice bulletin No. 162: prenatal diagnostic testing for genetic disorders. Obstet Gynecol. 2016;127(5):e108–22.

15. Lee J. Malformations of cortical development: genetic mechanisms and diagnostic approach. Korean J Pediatr. 2017;60(1):1–9. https://doi.org/10.3345/kjp.2017.60.1.1. Epub 2017 Jan 31. PMID: 28203254; PMCID: PMC5309318.

16. Bronshtein M, Wiener Z. Early transvaginal sonographic diagnosis of alobar holoprosencephaly. Prenat Diagn. 1991;11(7):459–62. https://doi.org/10.1002/pd.1970110708. PMID: 1754562

17. Klein JL, Lemmon ME, Northington FJ, et al. Clinical and neuroimaging features as diagnostic guides in neonatal neurology diseases with cerebellar involvement. Cerebellum Ataxias. 2016;3:1. https://doi.org/10.1186/s40673-016-0039-1.

18. Barañano K, Burd I. CNS Malformations in the Newborn. Matern Health Neonatol Perinatol. 2022;8:1. https://doi.org/10.1186/s40748-021-00136-4.

19. BoAli AY, Alfadhel M, Tabarki B. Neurometabolic disorders and congenital malformations of the central nervous system. Neurosciences (Riyadh). 2018;23(2):97–103. https://doi.org/10.17712/nsj.2018.2.20170481. PMID: 29664449; PMCID: PMC8015440.

20. Perovic D, Damnjanovic T, Jekic B, Dusanovic-Pjevic M, Grk M, Djuranovic A, Rasic M, Novakovic I, Maksimovic N. Chromosomal microarray in postnatal diagnosis of congenital anomalies and neurodevelopmental disorders in Serbian patients. J Clin Lab Anal. 2022;36(6):e24441. https://doi.org/10.1002/jcla.24441. Epub 2022 Apr 20. PMID: 35441737; PMCID: PMC9169173.

21. Khalil A, Bennet S, Thilaganathan B, Paladini D, Griffiths P, Carvalho JS. Prevalence of prenatal brain abnormalities in fetuses with congenital heart disease: a systematic review. Ultrasound Obstet Gynecol. 2016;48(3):296–307.

Chapter 4
Anencephaly

Muntadher H. Almufadhal and Zahraa Qasim Mohammed

Test your learning and check your understanding of this book's contents: use the "Springer Nature Flashcards" app to access questions using ▶ https://sn.pub/YnQHwS
To use the app, please follow the instructions in Chapter 1.

4.1 Introduction

Anencephaly is a developmental disorder defined by a fetus lacking the calvarium and most or all of its brain tissue [1]. Anencephaly, which is a member of a group of conditions known as neural tube defects (NTD) results during fetal development by failure of the neural tube to shut in its rostral end [2]. The neural tube is formed by folding and fusing the neural plate, as the central nervous system (CNS) develops in a fetus. Any interference with the neural tube closure process might result in structural malformations known as neural tube defects. Anencephaly is one of the two main types of neural tube closure failure [3]. The second main kind, known as spina bifida, results from the caudal end's failure to close. Anencephaly is thought to develop for a variety of reasons, including environmental and dietary factors, and is not thought to have a single cause [2].

M. H. Almufadhal (✉)
College of Medicine, University of Baghdad, Baghdad, Iraq

Z. Q. Mohammed
Baghdad Medical City, Baghdad, Iraq

© The Author(s), under exclusive license to Springer Nature Switzerland AG 2024
K. F. AlAli, H. T. Hashim (eds.), *Congenital Brain Malformations*,
https://doi.org/10.1007/978-3-031-58630-9_4

4.2 Pathophysiology

Anencephaly's pathogenesis and etiology are still poorly understood, but several environmental and dietary factors are believed to play a role in the illness [2].

4.2.1 Nutritional Factors

Folate is a coenzyme that makes it easier for one-carbon units to move between reactions, such as the synthesis of purines and pyrimidines and reaction of methylation [4]. A key nutritional risk component is folic acid deficiency that has been linked to the development of the disease [5]. There are several potential causes of a folate deficiency, including the following:

- Drugs that prevent the absorption of folate
- Folate malabsorption
- Increased need for folate from the body
- Dietary folate consumption that is insufficient

Cytosine and homocysteine are methylated with the help of folate. Additionally, it aids in the synthesis of pyrimidines and purines. As a result, a lack of folate interferes with the expression of specific genes and the appropriate DNA and protein synthesis [4]. Reproductive-age women are urged to add a folate supplement to their diets even though it is unclear how much of a role folate plays in lowering the incidence of NTD [4, 6].

4.2.2 Dietary Factors

NTDs have been linked to anti-epileptic medicines (AEDs). AED use changes the absorption of folate, resulting in reduced folate levels in the blood. Examples of these AEDs include valproate, carbamazepine, and phenytoin. It should be noted that valproate, particularly when paired with lamotrigine, is thought to be the most teratogenic AED [5]. Aspirin, triamterene, and trimethoprim are additional antagonists of folic acid. Trimethoprim is a type of antibiotic that is used to treat infections like malaria (an over-the-counter anti-coagulant) [5, 7].

4.3 Diagnosis

4.3.1 History and Physical Examination

Due to the lack of the cranial vault and some of the cerebrum and cerebellum, anencephaly is easily visible at birth. A positive diagnosis requires the following criteria; There is no calvarium present; the lack of a scalp; the presence of a hemorrhagic, fibrous mass or tissue; the absence of cerebral hemispheres [8]. Facial structures are present and seem rather normal. There are times when the skin covers the cranial lesion, but this is uncommon. Maternal serum alpha-fetoprotein (MSAFP) prenatal screening is ineffective when the lesion is concealed by skin. Stillbirths are prevalent, and pregnancies end spontaneously frequently. Although anencephaly symptoms are easily visible, a physical examination to look for anomalies unrelated to anencephaly is advised to determine whether cytogenetic testing is required. Cytogenetic abnormalities are more likely to occur when there are other anomalies.

4.3.2 Lab Studies

The great majority of cases of anencephaly can be detected by maternal serum alpha-fetoprotein (MSAFP) testing during pregnancy's second trimester in women with or without a positive family history of neural tube abnormalities or other risk factors [9].

Testing for anencephaly throughout the second and late first trimesters of pregnancy using amniotic alpha-fetoprotein (AFAFP) is a diagnostic biochemical procedure. False positives from AFAFP can be ignored depending on the results of acetylcholinesterase (ACHE) testing, which should be clearly positive for open anencephaly. In the majority of cases of solitary anencephaly, postnatal laboratory tests are not done. Testing for cytogenetic abnormalities can rule out trisomy 13 and imbalanced structural chromosome abnormalities [10].

4.3.3 Imaging Studies

The screening method of maternal serum alpha-fetoprotein readings has been replaced by prenatal 2-dimensional ultrasound, which has steadily improved over time. Anencephaly should not be detected by ultrasonography until the pregnancy's 12th week because cranial vault ossification is rarely visible before then.

Anencephaly is characterized in the first trimester by the absence of the calvarium, a shorter distance between the crown and the rump, absence or exposure of neural tissue with a lobular appearance (exencephaly), as well as a lack of the typical head contour geometry with the orbits defining the face upper border (coronal view). Polyhydramnios may develop later in pregnancy as a result of decreased amniotic fluid swallowing.

Postnatal MRI scans have revealed the cerebellum, supratentorial structures, and lack of the cranial vault [11].

4.4 Management

Life is incompatible with anencephaly. Preventive care is the most crucial component of this condition's management. Recommending supplements of folic acid to reproductive age women is the simplest strategy to lower the prevalence of anencephaly. Any dosage of 0.4 mg or higher per day is useful; this is critical for any woman taking anticonvulsant medication. Counseling about the dangers of teratogenicity and the dangers of seizures during pregnancy are crucial for a young female patient with epilepsy. Before the patient has children, a plan should be created with the provider. With as few anti-epileptic medications as feasible administered at the lowest effective dose, the seizures should be as well controlled as possible. Avoiding valproate is advised. Lamotrigine is the anticonvulsant with the lowest teratogenicity record [8].

During pregnancy, maternal serum and fetal ultrasound are recommended for the diagnosis of any neural tube defect, including anencephaly. Upon receiving a diagnosis of anencephaly, an early pregnancy termination may be an option [8].

Multiple Choice Questions
1. **Which of the following congenital malformations can be detected during the first trimester of pregnancy?**

    (a) Anencephaly
    (b) Meningocele
    (c) Encephalocele
    (d) Microcephaly

    Answer: a

2. **The most severe form of "cranial" NTD characterized by: major portions of the cranium and intracranial structures being absent, orbits and face are present (bulging eyes), polyhydramnios, macroglossia, very short neck, is?**

    (a) Encephalocele
    (b) Iniencephaly
    (c) Acrania
    (d) Anencephaly

    Answer: d

3. **Anencephaly is a condition in which a large portion of the brain, skull, and scalp do not develop normally. Which of the following structures would most likely result from improper development?**

   (a) Caudal neuropore
   (b) Neural groove
   (c) Neural crest
   (d) Rostral neuropore

   Answer: d

4. **Which of the following conditions is caused by the anterior neuropore failing to close?**

   (a) Anencephaly
   (b) Craniosynostosis
   (c) Mongolism
   (d) Hydrocephalus

   Answers: a

5. **The screening method of maternal serum alpha-fetoprotein readings has been replaced by prenatal 2-dimensional ultrasound.**

   (a) True
   (b) False

   Answer: a

6. **Anencephaly is not clearly obvious at birth.**

   (a) True
   (b) False

   Answer: b

7. **Anencephaly is characterized in the first trimester by the presence of the calvarium.**

   (a) True
   (b) False

   Answer: b

8. **Anencephaly's pathogenesis and etiology are still poorly understood, but it is thought that only environmental factors cause this condition.**

   (a) True
   (b) False

   Answer: b

9. **The great majority of cases of anencephaly can be detected by maternal serum alpha-fetoprotein (MSAFP) testing during the third trimester of pregnancy.**

   (a) True
   (b) False

   Answer: b

10. **Folate deficiency is a significant nutritional risk factor that has been linked to the development of the disease.**

    (a) True
    (b) False

    Answer: a.

References

1. Naidich TP, Altman NR, Braffman BH, McLone DG, Zimmerman RA. Cephaloceles and related malformations. AJNR. Am J Neuroradiol. 1992;13(2):655.
2. Padmanabhan R. Etiology, pathogenesis and prevention of neural tube defects. Congenit Anom (Kyoto). 2006;46(2):55–67.
3. Yamaguchi Y, Miyazawa H, Miura M. Neural tube closure and embryonic metabolism. Congenit Anom. 2017;57(5):134–7.
4. Ebara S. Nutritional role of folate. Congenit Anom. 2017;57(5):138–41.
5. Kondo A, Matsuo T, Morota N, Kondo AS, Okai I, Fukuda H. Neural tube defects: risk factors and preventive measures. Congenit Anom. 2017;57(5):150–6.
6. Doležálková E, Unzeitig V. Kyselina listová a prevence rozštěpových vad centrálního nervového systému [Folic acid and prevention of the neural tube defects]. Ceska Gynekol. 2014;79(2):134–9.
7. Hernández-Díaz S, Werler MM, Walker AM, Mitchell AA. Folic acid antagonists during pregnancy and the risk of birth defects. N Engl J Med. 2000;343(22):1608–14.
8. Tafuri SM, Lui F. Embryology, anencephaly. Treasure Island: Stat Pearls Publishing; 2019.
9. Cameron M, Moran P. Prenatal screening and diagnosis of neural tube defects. Int Soc Prenatal Diag. 2009;29(4):402–11.
10. Philipp T, Philipp K, Reiner A, Beer F, Kalousek DK. Embryoscopic and cytogenetic analysis of 233 missed abortions: factors involved in the pathogenesis of developmental defects of early failed pregnancies. Hum Reprod. 2003;18(8):1724–32.
11. Poretti A, Meoded A, Ceritoglu E, Boltshauser E, Huisman TA. Postnatal in-vivo MRI findings in anencephaly. Neuropediatrics. 2010;41(06):264–6.

Chapter 5
Encephalocele

Ali Mahdi Mansoor and F. A. Ameer

Test your learning and check your understanding of this book's contents: use the "Springer Nature Flashcards" app to access questions using ▶ https://sn.pub/YnQHwS
To use the app, please follow the instructions in Chapter 1.

5.1 Introduction

Encephalocele is a prolapsed sac outside of the skull through a bone defect, as the sac may contain brain tissue, meninges, and cerebrospinal fluid (CSF). Congenital encephalocele is considered a type of neural tube defect, It is an embryonic anomaly caused by a defect in the separation of the ectoderm from the neuroectoderm [1] Acquired encephalocele may result from tumors, trauma, or post-surgical defect (iatrogenic injury) [2].

Encephaloceles are either pedunculated or sessile [3, 4], generally, the size of the encephalocele is an indication of its content, Usually, the size of the head is small [5, 6], it depends on the amount of herniated neural tissue, the larger the herniated tissue the smaller is the head size, usually, the encephalocele is transilluminated on examination and the degree of translumination depend on the amount of gliosed brain tissue inside the herniated sac [5].

A. M. Mansoor (✉)
College of Medicine, University of Baghdad, Baghdad, Iraq

F. A. Ameer
College of Medicine, Al-Qadisiyah University, Babil Governorate, Iraq

© The Author(s), under exclusive license to Springer Nature Switzerland AG 2024
K. F. AlAli, H. T. Hashim (eds.), *Congenital Brain Malformations*,
https://doi.org/10.1007/978-3-031-58630-9_5

Encephaloceles are considered less common than other neural tube defects. Their prevalence is between 0.8–5 per 10,000 live births [7]. In North America and Western Europe, Occipital encephalocele is the most frequent type, approximately 85 percent of all encephaloceles are occipital [8], their incidence is 1 to 3.33 per 10,000 live births [1], and Females account for 70% of cases of occipital encephaloceles [9]. while in Southeast Asia countries such as India, Thailand, Cambodia, Burma, Indonesia and Malaysia, central Africa, and parts of Russia, the most common type is anterior encephalocele, the incidence is 1–1.42 per 5000 live births [7] The reason behind this specific geographical distribution is unclear [10].

Ten percentage to twenty percentage of all craniospinal dysraphisms are encephaloceles [8]. There is a 60–80% risk of associated structural anomalies in the presence of encephalocele like retinal, choroidal, and optical dysplasia, severe ocular alterations, CNS anomalies, tectocerebellar dysraphia, dermoid cyst, and necrosis [11].

Usually, the protrusion is covered with normal skin, but it may be covered with dysplastic skin or thin malformed meningeal membrane [1, 12] Unless the presence of CSF leakage or skin ulceration of encephalocele which may lead to meningitis, surgical treatment of encephalocele is not an emergency. Due to the small amount of total blood volume of infants, the surgery is usually delayed until 4 months to several years. The goals of surgical repair are the closure of the skull defect and dural defect with watertight sutures to prevent CSF leakage and the reconstruction of the bony defect [13].

5.1.1 Classification

According to the anatomical location of the herniated sac, encephalocele is divided into four major types including [14, 15]:

1. ***Occipital encephalocele***(Fig. 5.1): typically in the midline, between the lambda and foramen magnum.
2. ***Sincipital encephalocele***:

    (a) Frontoethmoidal encephalocele and most of them herniates anterior to crista galli through the foramen cecum (further subdivisions: Nasofrontal, Nasoorbital, and Nasoethmoidal)
    (b) Interfrontal encephalocele: between bregma and nasal bone, often locates in the midline, in the metopic suture.

3. ***Basal encephalocele:***

    (a) transethmoidal
    (b) sphenoethmoidal
    (c) sphenoorbital (usually, this type results in unilateral exophthalmos because it passes through the superior orbital fissure)
    (d) transsphenoidal (passes through the sella turcica)

Fig. 5.1 Classical occipital encephalocele. (Image attributes to Centers for Disease Control and Prevention)

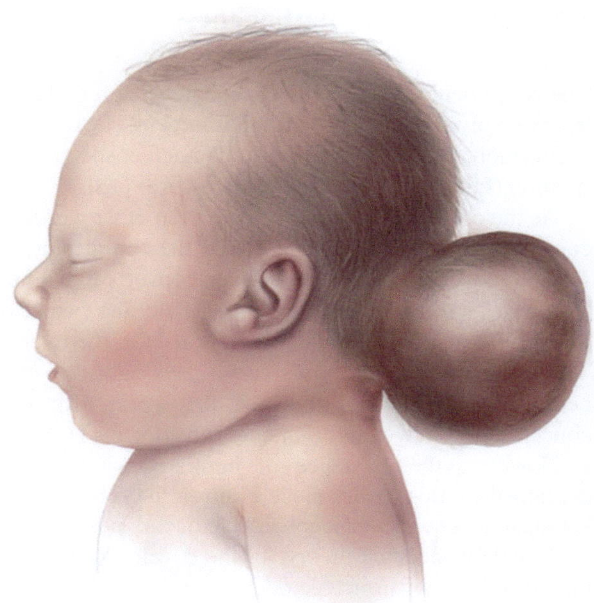

4. *Convexity encephalocele:*

   (a) Parietal (it locates between bregma and lambda)
   (b) Anterior fontanelle
   (c) Posterior fontanelle
   (d) Temporal

However, there are primarily four types of encephaloceles, based on their content [16]:

1. meningo-encephalocele: the sac contains neuroparenchyma, meninges, and CSF and the neuroparenchyma is usually gliotic [15].
2. meningocele: the sac contains meninges and CSF.
3. atretic encephalocele: the herniated sac consists of the dura, degenerated brain tissue, and fibrous tissue, It is commonly seen in the parieto-occipital area.
4. gliocele: consist of a glial-lined cyst with CSF.

Occasionally In specific situations, if there is a herniation of the ventricle into an encephalocele, it is referred to as a meningo-encephalo-cystocele [17].

5.2 Etiology and Pathogenesis

The cause behind congenital encephaloceles formation is not completely clear and it may involve both genetic and environmental factors (multifactorial). Encephalocele is considered a part of the neural tube defect spectrum caused due to failure of neurulation (failure of the neural tube closure) [18].

As the origin of the neural tube (in the other words the origin of CNS) is a thickened ectoderm plate which is called the neural plate at the beginning of the third week of conception, the neural plate converts into a neural tube after elevation and fusion of lateral edges of the neural plate, the fusion begins in the cervical region toward the rostral and caudal directions. On the twenty-fifth day after conception, The rostral neuropore closes and 2 days later, the caudal neuropore closes If the neural tube fails to close between the twenty-fifth day and twenty-seventh day of conception, it may result in neural tube defects [19].

However, the existence of herniated well-formed neural structures is not explained by this theory since brain tissue forms after the neural tube closure, so, some authors suggest encephalocele occurs post-neurulation [14].

A widely accepted theory for the development of a congenital encephalocele is the failure of the surface ectoderm to completely separate from the neuroectoderm after the closure of the neural folds, If the two layers adhere together, the paraxial mesoderm is unable to normally migrate and form an adequate skull bone and meninges [20, 21].

This theory explains the stretched, distorted appearance of the neuroparenchyma near the calvarial defect since there are many observations in a lot of cases in which, the brain near the cranial vault defect appeared stretched and distorted, so some authors consider this supporting evidence for the post-neurulation theory [14].

Another theory suggests that the amniotic band syndrome develops the encephalocele [13].

On the other hand, Some encephaloceles are acquired and may occur due to post-traumatic injury, post-surgical injury (iatrogenic), erosion caused by infection or tumors, or idiopathic [14].

5.2.1 Genetic Etiologies of Primary Encephalocele

Genetic factors play a role in the development of Encephalocele. Encephalocele May be caused by chromosomal abnormalities like Trisomies 13, 18, and 21.

encephalocele associated with more than 30 different syndromes, such as Meckel-Gruber syndrome(Table 5.1), Walker-Warburg syndrome, Knobloch syndrome, Fraser syndrome, morning glory syndrome, Roberts syndrome, and amniotic band syndrome [13, 22, 23].

Table 5.1 Pattern of inheritance and responsible genes for some associated syndromes with encephalocele

Associated syndrome	Pattern of inheritance	Responsible genes
Meckel-Gruber syndrome	Autosomal recessive	8q24, 11q13, 17q23
Walker-Warburg syndrome	Autosomal recessive	POM1, POM2 9q34.1, 9q3.1, 14q24.3, FCMD
Knobloch syndrome	Autosomal recessive	COL18A1
Fraser syndrome	Autosomal recessive	FRAS1, FREM2 4q21 and 13q13.3

5.2.2 Environmental Etiologies of Primary Encephalocele

Many environmental factors have been linked to the formation of encephalocele. TORCH infections (toxoplasmosis, rubella, cytomegalovirus, herpes simplex), Consanguinity, and prior NTD pregnancy have been implicated in the development of encephalocele. The impact of maternal folate use on encephalocele is unclear [24].

5.3 Clinical Presentation

Clinical presentation of encephalocele may vary significantly depending on factors such as the size and location of the defect, the amount and type of brain tissue that herniates, related conditions affecting cerebrospinal fluid circulation, and other anomalies which are commonly associated with cases of encephalocele.

5.3.1 Occipital Encephalocele

Occipital encephaloceles usually are noticeable at birth and the neural tissue usually is covered by skin, relatively large size encephalocele may lead to cranial nerve deficits, difficulty with sucking and feeding, spasticity, quadriplegia, blindness, seizures, learning disabilities, ataxia or delays in reaching developmental milestones.

Occipital encephalocele may associate with Chiari III malformation (a hindbrain anomaly) where the occipital and cerebellar tissues protrude and distort structures in the posterior fossa structures [1, 25].

5.3.2 *Sincipital Encephalocele*

Sincipital Encephalocele (Frontoethmoidal encephalocele) presents with a facial mass at birth but in some cases, it may be unnoticeable in inspection (occult lesion), sincipital encephalocele may be characterized by palpable cerebral pulsation, enlargement on crying, impulse on coughing, positive Furstenberg sign (enlargement of the mass after compression of the jugular vein), the patient may develop other associated abnormalities like mental retardation, hydrocephalus, squint, decreased visual acuity, epiphoria, and anosmia. in some conditions, it may be associated with marked craniofacial deformities (telecanthus, hypertelorism, unilateral micro/anophthalmos, or orbital dystopia) [25, 26].

5.3.3 *Basal Encephalocele*

Basal encephalocele may be occult and not visible at birth but there may be signs of facial deformities like hypertelorism and broadened nasal bridge.

Patients affected by basal encephalocele may present as an epipharyngeal or nasal mass, repeated upper respiratory infections, nasal discharge, difficulty breathing, cerebrospinal fluid leaks, and recurrent meningitis [25, 27].

5.3.4 *Associated Anomalies*

Encephaloceles may be caused by chromosomal abnormalities like Trisomies 13, 18, and 21, A study of 134 cases of encephalocele showed that 9 (6.7%) were due to chromosomal abnormalities [28].

Encephalocele may be part of a Mendelian disorder. Many syndromes have been associated with encephalocele. Meckel-Gruber syndrome (also known as Meckel syndrome) is the most common syndrome associated with encephalocele, this syndrome is characterized by occipital encephalocele, polycystic kidneys, cleft lip and palate, polydactyly, microcephaly, microphthalmia, ambiguous genitalia and other malformations [29]. Other syndromes like Walker-Warburg syndrome (it may include lissencephaly, retinal dysplasia, cerebellar malformations, microphthalmia congenital muscular dystrophy), Fraser syndrome (is characterized by abnormal ears, eyelid fusion, laryngeal anomalies, syndactyly, abnormal genitalia, renal agenesis/dysgenesis, mental retardation), Knobloch syndrome (It may include stereotyped ocular abnormalities, Occipital encephalocele, occipital bone defect, and cutis aplasia), Roberts syndrome, morning glory syndrome, and amniotic band syndrome. [22, 30]

5.4 Diagnosis

5.4.1 Neuroimaging

Radiologists aim to accurately define the type, contents, extension, and size of encephalocele, and also identify if there are associated anomalies [31].

Diagnosis of encephalocele by imaging is mainly made using a combination of ultrasound, CT scans, MRI with MR venography, and MR angiography.

Ultrasonography

for detecting prenatal CNS anomalies US scanning remains the modality of choice [32] ultrasound diagnosis of encephalocele in the prenatal period depend on the demonstration of cranial defect plus the varying degree of brain herniation [33]. Encephalocele diagnosis is considered when a skull defect accompanied by the protrusion of brain tissue or meninges is observed in both axial and sagittal sections during a routine ultrasound examination of the fetal head [33]. the classic appearance is a mass in the midline of the skull mostly in the occipital region. The mass may be either cystic or contain echoes from brain tissue. During the second trimester, the diagnosis of encephalocele can be confidently and easily determined through ultrasound results and also can be established in the first trimester [34] Approximately 80% of encephaloceles are detected by prenatal ultrasonography [34]. There are difficulties in detecting encephalocele by us due to the small size of the defect or artifacts caused by shadowing which may mimic a skull defect [35].

MRI

MRI is The best choice of imaging modality for identifying the contents of encephalocele [31, 36] as it is the best for defining intracranial extension [31]. MRI aids in prognosis and surgical planning as it defines if there is an extension of cerebral tissue(extent of neural herniation) in an encephalocele [31]. Fetal MRI has higher sensitivity for encephaloceles if the ultrasonography result is uncertain [37].

MR venography and MR angiography are important to evaluate the presence of dural sinuses and vessels in the herniated sac and to identify any associated venous anomalies. Venous anomalies usually accompany atretic conditions and the most frequent is the presence of the falcine sinus [38].

CT Scan

Using computed tomography (CT) for fetal imaging is not recommended due to radiation risks, especially in the first two trimesters [1] After birth, CT is useful for its clear visualization of the bony defect as the CT scan is recommended to reveal the correct dimensions of the calvarial defect for proper surgical planning [39], however, it is less effective than magnetic resonance imaging (MRI) in showing soft tissue in the herniated sac. Using water-soluble contrast material can provide a clearer assessment. CT cisternography scanning is useful for identifying connections between the encephalocele and the intracranial subarachnoid space [1]. A CT scan of the head with three-dimensional reconstruction could be done for better-making decision [13].

5.4.2 Multimaterial 3D Printing Modeling

This relatively new technique relies on using multi-material tissues with different consistencies and resistances to allow a detailed discussion about the proper management of encephalocele. The 3D model is considered a valuable tool in the planning of surgical management of encephalocele especially sincipital encephaloceles in which there is a craniofacial deformity, 3D model allows precise surgical measurements and location of osteotomies like in bilateral orbitotomy, the 3D model facilitated the reduction of surgery time [40].

5.4.3 Genetic Studies and Counseling

When encephalocele is detected, diagnostic tests such as amniocentesis or chorionic villus sampling with chromosomal microarray analysis (CMA) should be offered. It's recommended to start with karyotype analysis or fluorescence in situ hybridization and move to CMA if the results are normal. If there are other anomalies, a family history of a specific condition, or consanguinity, gene panel testing or exome sequencing might be helpful as CMA doesn't detect single-gene disorders [28].

For infants who don't survive, autopsy strongly recommended to search for specific signs such as cystic kidneys which could indicate Meckel-Gruber syndrome and this syndrome is autosomal recessive, so there is a 25% risk of recurrence in future pregnancies [22].

5.5 Differential Diagnosis

Table 5.2 this table below summarize the main differential diagnosis of encephalocele [14, 25, 41].

Table 5.2 A comparison between occipital encephalocele and sincipital encephalocele

Occipital encephalocele	Sincipital encephalocele
Hemangioma, cystic hygroma, dermoid cyst, vascular malformations of the scalp, and neurofibroma.	Nasal glioma, dermoid/epidermoid cyst, hemangioma, frontal sinus mucocele, dacryocystocele, sinus pericranii and neurinoma.
Basal encephalocele	**Convexity encephalocele**
Nasal polyp, nasal glioma, neoplasms of the pharynx and nasal cavity, mucocele of the paranasal sinuses, and dermoid cyst.	Sinus pericranii, hemangioma, aplasia cutis, congenital parietal foramina and dermoid cysts.

5.6   Management

After prenatal diagnosis, the type of delivery should be determined and it mainly depends on the size of the encephalocele, vaginal delivery may be safe if the encephalocele is relatively small but in case of a large encephalocele, cesarean section is required due to the risk of uncontrolled bleeding inside the sac which may lead to a rapid expansion in the size and raised intracranial pressure [25, 42].

Surgical treatment is the appropriate choice in most cases unless there are lethal anomalies such as massive encephalocele and severe microcephaly [25]. There are many conditions considered as surgical indications like if there is a risk of rupture of the sac, leakage of the CSF from the defect, meningitis, hydrocephalous and brain anomalies associated with encephalocele. The presence of venous sinus in the prolapsed brain tissue indicates a surgical intervention, lastly, surgery is also indicated for cosmetic issues [1, 42]. the surgeon generally removes the overlying sac and herniated neuroparenchyma and repairs the cranial defect including the dural defect without causing neurological deficits [14]. the closure must be performed as soon as possible to reduce the risk of infection in a patient with CSF leakage or basal encephalocele [43], hydrocephalus is commonly developed with encephalocele, especially with occipital type as 60% of occipital encephalocele associated with hydrocephalous [44, 45]. a ventriculoperitoneal shunt is inserted in these patients before the management of encephalocele, or another option is a third ventriculostomy [46].

5.6.1   Occipital Encephalocele

The type of herniated neural tissue determines the surgical management method of patients with occipital encephalocele. Occipital encephalocele rarely contains the cerebellum, brainstem, and torcula. The herniated sac may contain an occipital lobe [45] .frequently neuroparenchyma of the sac is gliotic [14], Generally gliosed, ischemic, Dysplastic, non-functional brain tissue should be excised, but herniated essential vascular and brain structures are handled carefully [42, 45, 47, 48], wrong handling of essential vessels may lead to brain infarction [48]. there is a risk of cerebral deep venous thrombosis if the herniated brain tissue contains the torcula [45]. During the surgery, the preferred position of the patient is prone, some conditions should be considered and avoided by monitoring such as hypothermia, blood loss, and electrolytes disturbance [42]. In specific conditions, intrauterine surgical intervention of occipital encephalocele may be performed to stop the progression of sac prolapsing but it is a reversal in microcephaly, this intervention may lead to a better cognitive outcome than those without intervention [49].

If the occipital encephalocele is larger than the head, it is described as giant and it is riskier [47]. In cases of giant occipital encephalocele with a herniated functional visual cortex, the visual evoked response is often required to avoid the development of hemianopia and cortical blindness [42]. the surgeon should attempt to preserve the viable functional neural tissue which herniated in the sac, there are many techniques are used to accommodate large amounts of herniated neural tissues, one of them expansion cranioplasty, by this technique the surgeon creates an extracranial space for herniating contents of the sac, tantalum mesh may be used as a technique of cranioplasty, alongside with expansion of calvarium due to increased intracranial pressure, the mesh gradually imbricated into calvarium by daily digital compression [50], in addition to expansion cranioplasty, Ventricular volume reduction and incision of tentorium also considered as options to create a space for the preservation of herniated neural tissues [51, 52].

Generally, neonates with giant occipital encephalocele have a poor prognosis [1] also the Cases of occipital encephalocele with microcephaly have a poor prognosis if the sac contains the cerebrum, cerebellum, and brain stem structures [5].

Sincipital Encephalocele

This type of encephalocele causes deformities in frontal, orbital, and nasal regions [53] In a frontoethmoidal encephalocele, the internal skull defect is situated in the midline, however, the location of the external skull defect can vary within the facial bony structure [10].

In all classical cases of the frontoethmoidal encephalocele, the swelling is over the bridge of the nose or inner canthus of the eye, with hypertelorism in varying degrees [54]. The nasal encephalocele is a subclass of basal and frontoethmoidal encephalocele based on the encephalocele herniates from the skull base or ethmoid bone [15]. Surgery is the primary treatment option for this type of encephalocele [15]. Surgical Treatment for frontoethmoidal encephalocele is usually not necessary immediately after birth, as they are typically covered with normal skin or an epidermal layer [41, 55]. It is widely agreed among authors that early surgical intervention for encephaloceles is preferable to achieve a more comprehensive and effective repair of the dural defect and also to avoid progressive facial distortion during growth [56, 57]. Some authors recommend surgery to be performed at 8–10 months of age [58, 59]. Different surgical approaches have been employed such as the Endoscopic transnasal approaches, transfacial incision, and coronal flap approach [56]. The transnasal endoscopic approach is commonly used in many cases of nasal encephalocele as it has been very successful in these cases [56]. In cases that require facial reconstruction, the combined procedure (transfacial and coronal flap approach) with facial reconstruction is recommended by most authors [60] although some authors recommend using only one approach of the three common types [15] a study by Oucheng et al. recommends combined procedure because three main advantages of this technique: better closure of the meningoencephalocele, reduction of facial scars, better telecanthus correction [60].

Basal Encephalocele

For the management of encephalocele, there are many surgical approaches such as the endoscopic transnasal approach, transcranial approach, the transoral transpalatal approach, and other extracranial approaches.

The traditional approach for basal encephalocele is the transcranial approach, but it associates with many morbidities such as anosmia, cerebral oedema, postoperative intracranial haemorrhage, epilepsy, osteomyelitis of the frontal bone flap, frontal lobe dysfunction, hair loss along the incision line, and 5–7 days in hospital [61], so the transcranial approach is reserved for large basal encephalocele with other anomalies [62]. In some cases, the transcranial approach is combined with the extracranial approach [61].

When a cleft palate is absent, the Endoscopic transnasal approach is considered by many authors the preferred choice for treating the majority of basal encephalocele, even in children less than 1 year of age this approach remains safe and effective [63].

For successful repairing of basal encephalocele, some authors recommend circumferential dissection of the basal encephalocele plus a proper reconstruction of basal skull bone defect with a titanium plate or mesh [62].

5.7 Complications

Postoperative follow-up is paramount due to the risk of CSF leakage and meningitis. There are other complications like wound infection, severe post-operative emesis, hydrocephalus, developmental delay, developmental impairment, neurological lesions, seizures, convulsions, diabetes insipidus, panhypopituitarism, rhabdomyolysis, epiphora, recurrent meningitis, and endoscopic recurrence [13, 15, 63].

5.8 Prognosis

There are two important factors affecting patient outcome: the location of the herniated sac and its content, also there are other factors such as the size of the sac, amount of herniated brain tissue, presence of hydrocephalous, associated infections, associated anomalies (especially microcephaly) [14]. approximately, 15% of cases with encephalocele have intrauterine demise, 30% is the overall mortality rate, and 76% of them occur on the first day of life [64]. Preterm delivery and fetal growth restriction increase the risk of mortality in cases with encephalocele [64].

Usually, death occurs due to the inability to repair the defect or the severity of associated malformations [28]. Encephaloceles associated with other anomalies increase the mortality three-fold in comparison with cases of isolated encephalocele [28].

Disabilities are commonly seen in surviving children [28]. Many surviving children may develop neurologic problems such as seizures, ataxia intellectual disability, growth restriction, and visual impairment [65]. In 1 study of 85 cases with cephaloceles follow the development, found that 48% of them developed normally, 11% developed with mild delay, 16% developed with moderate delay, and 25% developed with severe delay [66]. As a general comparison between the two major types of encephalocele, the sincipital encephaloceles have a good prognosis while the prognosis of occipital encephaloceles is poor [14].

Multiple Choice Questions
  1. **The most common syndrome associated with occipital encephalocele is**

    (a) Fraser syndrome
    (b) Knobloch syndrome
    (c) Meckel-Gruber syndrome
    (d) Roberts syndrome
    (e) Morning glory syndrome

  2. **In North America and Western Europe, the most common type of encephalocele is:**

    (a) Occipital encephalocele
    (b) Sincipital encephalocele
    (c) Basal encephalocele
    (d) Parietal encephalocele
    (e) Temporal encephalocele

  3. **In Southeast Asia countries such as India, Thailand, Cambodia, Burma, Indonesia and Malaysia, central Africa, and parts of Russia, the most common type of encephalocele is:**

    (a) Occipital encephalocele
    (b) Sincipital encephalocele
    (c) Basal encephalocele
    (d) Parietal encephalocele
    (e) Temporal encephalocele

4. **The sac contains neuroparenchyma, meninges, and CSF is called**

   (a) Gliocele
   (b) Meningocele
   (c) Atretic encephalocele
   (d) Meningo-encephalocele
   (e) Meningo-encephalo-cystocele

5. **One of the following trisomies is not associated with encephalocele:**

   (a) Klinefelter syndrome
   (b) Trisomy 13
   (c) Trisomy 18
   (d) Trisomy 21
   (e) All of the above

6. **Which one of the following is considered a risk factor for the formation of encephalocele:**

   (a) Consanguinity
   (b) Prior NTD pregnancy
   (c) Cytomegalovirus
   (d) Herpes simplex
   (e) All of the above

7. **Which one of the following is the best choice of imaging modality for identifying the contents of encephalocele is:**

   (a) X-ray
   (b) Ultrasonography
   (c) CT scan
   (d) CT cisternography scanning
   (e) MRI

8. **The most common postoperative complication in sincipital encephalocele is:**

   (a) Seizures
   (b) CSF leakage
   (c) Hydrocephalus
   (d) Endoscopic recurrence
   (e) Developmental delay

9. **Which one of the following percentages represents the detected encephaloceles by prenatal ultrasonography:**

   (a) 10%
   (b) 20%
   (c) 40%
   (d) 60%
   (e) 80%

10. **which one of the following is considered a differential diagnosis for occipital encephalocele:**

    (a) Hemangioma
    (b) Cystic hygroma
    (c) Vascular malformations of the scalp
    (d) Dermoid cyst
    (e) All of the above

Answers and Explanation

1. **The answer is (c)** all the mentioned syndromes in the question are associated with encephalocele but the most common syndrome associated with occipital encephalocele is Meckel-Gruber syndrome, it is a Mendelian disorder and its pattern of inheritance is autosomal recessive.

2. **The answer is (a)** the most common type of encephalocele depends on geographical region. In North America and Western Europe, the most common location of the herniated sac is the occiput.

3. **The answer is (b)** geographical regions play a role in determining the most common type, sincipital encephalocele is the most common type in these regions mentioned in the question.

4. **The answer is (d)** [explained in the above paragraph 5.1.2 classification].

5. **The answer is (a)** there is an association between encephalocele and 13,18 and 21 trisomies but no association is found between encephalocele and Klinefelter syndrome.

6. **The Answer is (e)** encephalocele is a multi-factorial anomaly both environmental and genetic factors have a role in the formation of encephalocele.

7. **The answer is (e)** [explained in the above paragraph 5.4 diagnosis].

8. **The answer is (b)** follow-up after surgery is mandatory because of the risk of CSF leakage which may lead to meningitis, CSF leaks under the skin or through the wound, and other complications also may occur after the surgery but are not common as like the CSF leakage.

9. **The answer is (e)** approximately 80% of encephalocele is detected in the prenatal period by ultrasound, encephalocele may be detected in the first trimester and easily detected in the second and third trimesters.

10. **The answer is (e)** all the anomalies mentioned in the question are congenital and may present in the occipital region.

References

1. Markovic I, Bosnjakovic P, Milenkovic Z. Occipital encephalocele: cause, incidence, neuroimaging and surgical management. Curr Pediatr Rev. 2020;16(3):200–5.
2. Gump WC. Endoscopic endonasal repair of congenital defects of the anterior skull base: developmental considerations and surgical outcomes. J Neurol Surg Part B: Skull Base. 2015;76(04):291–5.

3. Jacob OJ, Rosenfeld JV, Waiters DA. The repair of frontal encephaloceles in Papua New Guinea. Aust N Z J Surg. 1994;64(12):856–60.
4. Leong AS, Shaw CM. The pathology of occipital encephalocoele and a discussion of the pathogenesis. Pathology. 1979;11(2):223–34.
5. Nath H, Mahapatra A, Borkar S. A giant occipital encephalocele with spontaneous hemorrhage into the sac: a rare case report. Asian J Neurosurg. 2014;9(03):158–60.
6. French BN. Midline fusion defects and defects of formation. Neurol Surg. 1982:1236–380.
7. Canaz H, Ayçiçek E, Akçetin MA, Akdemir O, Alataş I, Özdemir B. Supra-and infra-torcular double occipital encephalocele. Neurocirugia. 2015;26(1):43–7.
8. Chapman PH, Swearingen B, Caviness VS. Subtorcular occipital encephaloceles: anatomical considerations relevant to operative management. J Neurosurg. 1989;71(3):375–81.
9. Shokunbi T, Adeloye A, Olumide A. Occipital encephalocoeles in 57 Nigerian children: a retrospective analysis. Childs Nerv Syst. 1990;6(2):99–102.
10. Arifin M, Suryaningtyas W, Bajamal AH. Frontoethmoidal encephalocele: clinical presentation, diagnosis, treatment, and complications in 400 cases. Childs Nerv Syst. 2018;34(6):1161–8.
11. Ugras M, Kavak O, Alpay F, Bicer S. New born children with encephalocele. J Neurol Neurosci. 2016;7(1):1.
12. Agarwal A, Chandak AV, Kakani A, Reddy S. A giant occipital encephalocele. APSP J Case Rep. 2010;1(2):16.
13. Cruz AJ, De Jesus O. Encephalocele. In: StatPearls [Internet]. Treasure Island: StatPearls Publishing; 2021.
14. Pal NL, Juwarkar AS, Viswamitra S. Encephalocele: know it to deal with it. Egypt J Radiol Nucl Med. 2021;52:1–2.
15. Tirumandas M, Sharma A, Gbenimacho I, Shoja MM, Tubbs RS, Oakes WJ, Loukas M. Nasal encephaloceles: a review of etiology, pathophysiology, clinical presentations, diagnosis, treatment, and complications. Childs Nerv Syst. 2013;29(5):739–44.
16. Naidich TP, Altman NR, Braffman BH, McLone DG, Zimmerman RA. Cephaloceles and related malformations. AJNR Am J Neuroradiol. 1992;13(2):655.
17. Suwanwela C, Suwanwela N. A morphological classification of sincipital encephalomeningoceles. J Neurosurg. 1972;36(2):201–11.
18. Van Allen MI, Kalousek DK, Chernoff GF, Juriloff D, Harris M, McGillivray BC, Yong SL, Langlois S, Macleod PM, Chitayat D, Friedman JM. Evidence for multi-site closure of the neural tube in humans. Am J Med Genet. 1993;47(5):723–43.
19. Sadler TW. Langman's medical embryology. Philadelphia: Lippincott Williams & Wilkins; 2022 Dec 29.
20. Martínez-Lage JF, Poza M, Sola J, Soler CL, Montalvo CG, Domingo R, Puche A, Ramón FH, Azorín P, Lasso R. The child with a cephalocele: etiology, neuroimaging, and outcome. Childs Nerv Syst. 1996;12:540–50.
21. Gluckman TJ, George TM, McLone DG. Postneurulation rapid brain growth represents a critical time for encephalocele formation: a chick model. Pediatr Neurosurg. 1996;25(3):130–6.
22. Kumar P, Burton BK. Congenital malformations: evidence-based evaluation and management. New York: McGraw-Hill; 2007.
23. Suzuki OT, Sertié AL, Der Kaloustian VM, Kok F, Carpenter M, Murray J, Czeizel AE, Kliemann SE, Rosemberg S, Monteiro MB, Olsen BR. Molecular analysis of collagen XVIII reveals novel mutations, presence of a third isoform, and possible genetic heterogeneity in Knobloch syndrome. Am J Hum Genet. 2002;71(6):1320–9.
24. Yucetas SC, Uçler N. A retrospective analysis of neonatal encephalocele predisposing factors and outcomes. Pediatr Neurosurg. 2017;52(2):73–6.
25. Tomita T, Ogiwara H, Weisman LE. Primary (congenital) encephalocele. Waltham, MA: UpToDate; 2013.
26. Singh AK, Upadhyaya DN. Sincipital encephaloceles. J Craniofac Surg. 2009;20(8):1851–5.
27. Jimenez DF, Barone CM. Encephaloceles, meningoceles, and dermal sinuses. Principles and practice of pediatric neurosurgery, vol. 189. New York: Thieme; 1999.

28. Monteagudo A. Posterior encephalocele. Am J Obstetr Gynecol. 2020;223(6):B9–12.
29. Poduri A, Volpe JJ. Neuronal proliferation. Volpe's Neurol Newborn. 2018;1:100–19.
30. Caglayan AO, Baranoski JF, Aktar F, Han W, Tuysuz B, Guzel A, Guclu B, Kaymakcalan H, Aktekin B, Akgumus GT, Murray PB. Brain malformations associated with Knobloch syndrome—review of literature, expanding clinical spectrum, and identification of novel mutations. Pediatr Neurol. 2014;51(6):806–13.
31. Achar SV, Dutta HK. Sincipital encephaloceles: a study of associated brain malformations. J Clin Imaging Sci. 2016;6:20.
32. Chougule S, Desai S, Aironi V. Antenatal ultrasound diagnosis of occipital meningoencephalocele-a case report. Indian J Radiol Imaging. 2006;16(4):1.
33. Sepulveda W, Wong AE, Andreeva E, Odegova N, Martinez-Ten P, Meagher S. Sonographic spectrum of first-trimester fetal cephalocele: review of 35 cases. Ultrasound Obstet Gynecol. 2015;46(1):29–33.
34. Liao SL, Tsai PY, Cheng YC, Chang CH, Ko HC, Chang FM. Prenatal diagnosis of fetal encephalocele using three-dimensional ultrasound. J Med Ultrasound. 2012;20(3):150–4.
35. Carvalho MH, Brizot ML, Lopes LM, Chiba CH, Miyadahira S, Zugaib M. Detection of fetal structural abnormalities at the 11–14 week ultrasound scan. Prenatal Diagnosis. 2002;22(1):1–4.
36. Morón FE, Morriss MC, Jones JJ, Hunter JV. Lumps and bumps on the head in children: use of CT and MR imaging in solving the clinical diagnostic dilemma. Radiographics. 2004;24(6):1655–74.
37. Sefidbakht S, Iranpour P, Keshavarz P, Bijan B, Haseli S. Fetal MRI in prenatal diagnosis of encephalocele. J Obstet Gynaecol Can. 2020;42(3):304–7.
38. Brunelle F, Baraton J, Renier D, Teillac D, Simon I, Sonigo P, Hertz-Pannier L, Emond S, Boddaert N, Chigot V, Lellouch-Tubiana A. Intracranial venous anomalies associated with atretic cephalocoeles. Pediatr Radiol. 2000 Oct;30:743–7.
39. Franco A, Jo SY, Mehta AS, Pandya DJ, Yang CW. A rare triad of giant occipital encephalocele with lipomyelomeningocele, tetralogy of fallot, and situs inversus. J Radiol Case Rep. 2016;10(3):36–46.
40. Coelho G, Chaves TM, Goes AF, Del Massa EC, Moraes O, Yoshida M. Multimaterial 3D printing preoperative planning for frontoethmoidal meningoencephalocele surgery. Childs Nerv Syst. 2018;34:749–56.
41. Hoving EW. Nasal encephaloceles. Childs Nerv Syst. 2000;16:702–6.
42. Satyarthee GD, Moscote-Salazar LR, Escobar-Hernandez N, Aquino-Matus J, Puac-Polanco PC, Hoz SS, Calderon-Miranda WG. A giant occipital encephalocele in neonate with spontaneous hemorrhage into the encephalocele sac: surgical management. J Pediatr Neurosci. 2017;12(3):268.
43. Hammam E, Chaisrisawadisuk S, Moore MH, Santoreneos S. Encephaloceles. In: Pediatric neurosurgery for clinicians. Champions: Springer; 2022. p. 119–34.
44. Andarabi Y, Nejat F, El-Khashab M. Progressive skin necrosis of a huge occipital encephalocele. Indian J Plastic Surg. 2008;41(01):82–4.
45. Verma SK, Satyarthee GD, Singh PK, Sharma BS. Torcular occipital encephalocele in infant: report of two cases and review of literature. J Pediatr Neurosci. 2013;8(3):207–9.
46. Raja RA, Qureshi AA, Memon AR, Ali H, Dev V. Pattern of encephaloceles: a case series. J Ayub Med Coll Abbottabad. 2008;20(1):125–8.
47. Kanesen D, Rosman AK, Kandasamy R. Giant occipital encephalocele with Chiari malformation type 3. Journal Neurosci Rural Pract. 2018;9(04):619–21.
48. Rehman L, Farooq G, Bukhari I. Neurosurgical interventions for occipital encephalocele. Asian J Neurosurg. 2018;13(02):233–7.
49. Cavalheiro S, da Costa MD, Nicácio JM, Dastoli PA, Suriano IC, Barbosa MM, Milani HJ, Sarmento SG, de Faria TC, Moron AF. Fetal surgery for occipital encephalocele. J Neurosurg Pediatr. 2020;26(6):605–12.

50. Gallo AE. Repair of giant occipital encephaloceles with microcephaly secondary to massive brain herniation. Childs Nerv Syst. 1992;8(4):229–30.
51. Oi S, Saito M, Tamaki N, Matsumoto S. Ventricular volume reduction technique–a new surgical concept for the intracranial transposition of encephalocele. Neurosurgery. 1994;34(3):443–8.
52. Bozinov O, Tirakotai W, Sure U, Bertalanffy H. Surgical closure and reconstruction of a large occipital encephalocele without parenchymal excision. Childs Nerv Syst. 2005;21(2):144–7.
53. Songür E, Mutluer S, Gürler T, Bilkay U, Görken C, Güner U, Çelik N. Management of frontoethmoidal (sincipital) encephalocele. J Craniofac Surg. 1999;10(2):135–9.
54. Dhirawani RB, Gupta R, Pathak S, Lalwani G. Frontoethmoidal encephalocele: case report and review on management. Annals Maxillofac Surg. 2014;4(2):195–7.
55. Rapport RL, Dunn RC, Alhady F. Anterior encephalocele. J Neurosurg. 1981;54(2):213–9.
56. Abdel-Aziz M, El-Bosraty H, Qotb M, El-Hamamsy M, El-Sonbaty M, Abdel-Badie H, Zynabdeen M. Nasal encephalocele: endoscopic excision with anesthetic consideration. Int J Pediatr Otorhinolaryngol. 2010;74(8):869–73.
57. Horcajadas A, Palma A, Khalon BM. Frontoethmoidal encephalocele. Report Case Neurocirugía. 2019;30(2):94–9.
58. Mahapatra AK, Tandon PN, Dhawan IK, Khazanchi RK. Anterior encephaloceles: a report of 30 cases. Childs Nerv Syst. 1994;10(8):501–4.
59. Mahapatra AK, Agrawal D. Anterior encephaloceles: a series of 103 cases over 32 years. J Clin Neurosci. 2006;13(5):536–9.
60. Oucheng N, Lauwers F, Gollogly J, Draper L, Joly B, Roux FE. Frontoethmoidal meningoencephalocele: appraisal of 200 operated cases. J Neurosurg Pediatr. 2010;6(6):541–9.
61. Marshall AH, Jones NS, Robertson IJ. Endoscopic management of basal encephaloceles. J Laryngol Otol. 2001;115(7):545–7.
62. Morota N, Ihara S, Ogiwara H, Usami K, Tamada I, Kaneko T. Basal encephalocele: surgical strategy and functional outcomes in the Tokyo experience. J Neurosurg Pediatr. 2020;27(1):69–78.
63. Thompson HM, Schlosser RJ, Walsh EM, Cho DY, Grayson JW, Karnezis TT, Miller PL, Woodworth BA. Current management of congenital anterior cranial base encephaloceles. Int J Pediatr Otorhinolaryngol. 2020;131:109868.
64. Siffel C, Wong LY, Olney RS, Correa A. Survival of infants diagnosed with encephalocele in Atlanta, 1979–98. Paediatr Perinat Epidemiol. 2003;17(1):40–8.
65. Da Silva SL, Jeelani Y, Dang H, Krieger MD, McComb JG. Risk factors for hydrocephalus and neurological deficit in children born with an encephalocele. J Neurosurg Pediatr. 2015;15(4):392–8.
66. Lo BW, Kulkarni AV, Rutka JT, Jea A, Drake JM, Lamberti-Pasculli M, Dirks PB, Thabane L. Clinical predictors of developmental outcome in patients with cephaloceles. J Neurosurg Pediatr. 2008;2(4):254–7.

Chapter 6
Chiari Malformation

Mohammed Mohammed Hussein, Ahmed Dheyaa Al-Obaidi,
and Mustafa Najah Al-Obaidi

Abbreviations

PCF	Posterior Cranial Fossa
FM	Foramen Magnum
CSF	Cerebrospinal Fluid
CM	Chiari malformation
CIM	Chiari malformation type I
CIIM	Chiari malformation type II
CIIIM	Chiari malformation type III
MRI	Magnetic Resonance Imaging
CT	Computed Tomography

Test your learning and check your understanding of this book's contents: use the "Springer Nature Flashcards" app to access questions using ▶ https://sn.pub/YnQHwS
To use the app, please follow the instructions in Chapter 1.

6.1 Introduction

The malformation of Chiari, which is also known as "Arnold-Chiari Malformations" consist of congenital abnormalities affecting multiple anatomical structure such as the central nervous system specifically on the hindbrain in regards to the posterior

M. M. Hussein (✉) · A. D. Al-Obaidi · M. N. Al-Obaidi
College of Medicine, University of Baghdad, Baghdad, Iraq
e-mail: Mohammed.Mohammed1700d@comed.uobaghdad.edu.iq

© The Author(s), under exclusive license to Springer Nature
Switzerland AG 2024
K. F. AlAli, H. T. Hashim (eds.), *Congenital Brain Malformations*,
https://doi.org/10.1007/978-3-031-58630-9_6

fossa and the junction between the cranium and the cervical skeleton involving a range of malformation starting from herniation of the tonsils of cerebellum to the cerebellar agenesis [1, 2]. Chiari malformations have four types classified according to the severity of abnormality of cerebellum. The disorder is particularized with wide variability regarding clinical presentation in which can vary from asymptomatic state to severe and unrelenting symptoms according to the severity [1]. It also has variability in the treatment options and operative solutions and technicalities that are available to manage the anatomical abnormalities and ceasing or decreasing the symptoms [1, 2]. Chiari Malformations are also known for their frequency to have associated defects or congenital malformations for instance hydrocephalus, encephalocele, syrinx and others [3].

6.2   Anatomical Basis of the Disease

The posterior cranial fossa is the most sizeable part of the cranial cavity's floor, contributed by four bones, mostly by the temporal and occipital bones with less contributions by the sphenoid and parietal bones [4]. The main purpose of PCF is to hold and contain rhombencephalon (the hindbrain) involving pons, medulla and the cerebellum [5]. The PCF bounded anteromedially by dorsum sellae and the clivus, anterolaterally by the temporal bone, specifically petromastoid part and posteriorly the squamous part of the occipital bone [4, 5].

The main details in the architecture of PCF can be discussed in relation to the most noticeable element which is the foramen magnum, the largest foramen in the skull and assemble as key entrance for the spinal cord to cranial cavity in addition to vertebral arteries, the meninges, and the spinal roots of the accessory nerve [5]. The key bony prominence consists of the sloping surface of the clivus anterior to the FM, the jugular tubercles anterior to the FM, the internal occipital crest which traverses in the sagittal plane posterior to the FM, then the internal occipital protuberance [6]. Other foramina and canals include internal acoustic meatus contains the facial nerve, vestibulocochlear nerve, and the labyrinthine artery, the jugular foramen in which glossopharyngeal nerve, the vagus nerve and accessory nerve pass through, the hypoglossal canal in which the hypoglossal nerve passes, condylar canal which contains an emissary vain [6].

The PCF contains the hindbrain, which consists of brainstem and cerebellum. The midbrain is the most superior part of the brainstem which connects the cerebrum and the thalamus to pons and cerebellum [4]. Midbrain is a confined portion, its length shorter than 2 cm [7]. Regarding the anterior surface of the midbrain, the cerebral peduncles are situated, divided by the interpeduncular fossa. The cerebral peduncle are two bulky connections of fibers bilaterally [7]. In addition, it is separated into crus cerebri anteriorly and tegmentum mesencephali posteriorly. Regarding the dorsal surface of the midbrain, there are four prominent rounded elevations, the superior and inferior colliculi one on each side [7]. The midbrain is connected to the cerebellum by superior cerebellar peduncles [7].

Pons, when viewed externally, the anterior surface of the pons is curved and shows transverse fibers that cross from side to side. These fibers join on each side from the middle cerebellar peduncles [6]. A shallow groove is present in the middle of these fibers, called the basilar groove. The basilar groove lodges the basilar artery, which is the main artery for the blood supply of the entire brain. The posterior surface of pons contributes to the upper half of the roof of the fourth ventricle. It is divided into symmetrical halves by median sulcus [7]. The pons is connected to the cerebellum by middle cerebellar peduncles [7].

Medulla oblongata contains two parts: the ventral portion contains four main structures, a pair of triangular shaped bodies situated medially known as pyramid which encompasses the corticospinal and corticobulbar tracts [8]. Also, the ventral portion contains the olivary bodies, which are located laterally. The dorsal medulla forms the lower segment of floor of the fourth ventricle [7].

Cerebellum comprises of two lobes, known as cerebellar hemispheres. The cerebellar hemispheres attached to each other by a median structure called the vermis [8]. There are two surfaces of cerebellum, superior and inferior surfaces [7]. The cerebellum contains also two notches, the anterior notch encompasses the brainstem and the posterior one holds the falx cerebelli [9]. The inferior parts of the cerebellar hemispheres which are rounded in shape are known as cerebellar tonsils. The cerebellar tonsils are connected medially with inferior part of the vermis which is called uvula. Cerebellum is connected to the brainstem parts by the cerebellar peduncles [10].

6.3 The Classification of Chiari Malformation

In pursuit to make the followed chapters more comprehensible to be discussed, it is necessary to understand the classifications of Chiari malformations. The Chiari malformation can be classified depending on the level of herniation of the nervous tissue through the FM accompanied by the associated anomalies. Type 1 involves cerebellar tonsils herniation only through the FM with 5 mm or more displacement caudally [11]. In type 2, the herniation includes the cerebellar vermis, the brainstem and fourth ventricle in addition to non-nervous tissue might be herniated like related choroid plexus, the basilar artery and posterior inferior cerebellar arteries [12]. The severity is highly increased in type III, where the herniation is contained within encephalocele posteriorly with same herniated structures in type II [12]. In type IV, the pathology is changed from herniation to absence or agenesis of the cerebellar structure involving also the tentorium cerebelli. Some authors regard type IV is more centered as posterior fossa cyst rather than ordinary Chiari malformations which are concerned with the nervous tissue herniation [12].

There are some irregular types less ordinary, including type 0 and type 1.5. Type 0 is involving another different anomaly which is syringomyelia but with similar pathophysiology and therapeutic responsiveness to the regular Chiari malformations [13]. Type 1.5 is midway station between type I and II, encompassing herniation anomalies more severe than type I regrading brainstem descent but not severe as type II [14]. These two types are not regarded significant in regards to classifications [15]. The following chapter will concentrate on the main types which include CIM, CIIM and briefly CIIIM.

6.4　Chiari Type I

Type 1 involves cerebellar tonsils herniation with 5 mm or more Inferiorly [16]. CIM is the most common type of Chiari malformations. The associated pathologies include cervical syringomyelia then hydrocephalus and other congenital anomalies [16]. The main concept pathophysiologically is concerned with the balance in CSF pressure rather than hydrocephalus as the primary etiology because most cases of Chiari malformations are not associated with hydrocephalus and presented without ventricular dilation [17]. Not achieving the balance in CSF flow is a leading cause to produce force in the direction out the intracranial cavity forcing the cerebellar tonsils to herniate into the craniocervical junction compressing the brainstem and the cervical part of spinal cord [17]. It has been proposed that the symptoms and the development of other congenital anomaly like syringomyelia in the case of CIM are associated with dynamic imbalance in the FM (Fig. 6.1). The theories that explain

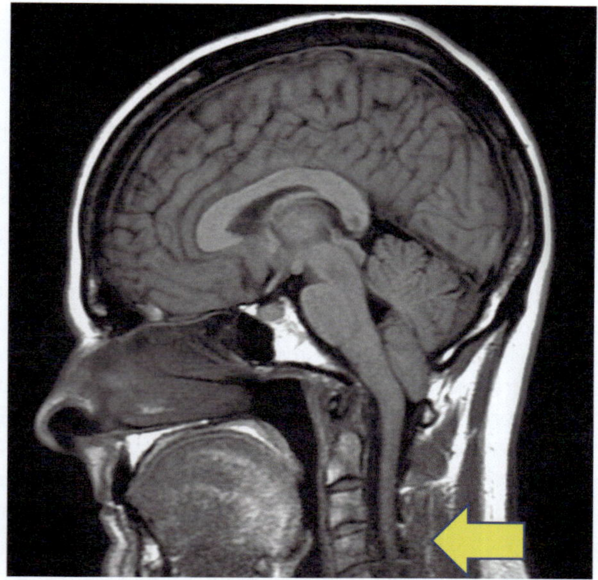

Fig. 6.1 Sagittal MRI scan of Chiari malformation type I in T1 image showing tonsillar herniation of the cerebellum through the foramen magnum. (Source: Radiopedia. Link: https://radiopaedia. org/articles/chiari-i-malformation?lang=us#image_list_item_3601)

CIM pathophysiology are concerned with the instability in craniocervical area, CSF pressure disturbances and possibly other craniocervical junction abnormalities [17].

The clinical presentation is very variable regarding CIM, the commonest presenting symptoms are occipital and cervical pain [18]. The pain is aggravated by Valsalva maneuver. In pediatric population, the symptoms usually are crying and irritability. The pain can also be manifested in the areas of back, shoulder and limbs but in non-radicular distribution. Other symptoms and clinical signs can be grouped as syndromes according to the part affected by herniation and compressions. The compression of cerebellar tissue can result in unsteadiness and ataxia with abnormal cerebellar neurological examination [19]. Brainstem compression can result in respiratory difficulties, frequent aspirations and the cranial nerves pathologies like facial sensory loss or trigeminal neuralgia. When the spinal cord is compressed, this could result in loss in the motor and sensory activity particularly in the hand due to that the nerves supplying this area have their roots arising from the cervical spinal cord [20]. On examination, the results are inconstant between hyporeflexia or hyperreflexia but with positive Babinski sign. Less frequents clinical findings include nystagmus, scoliosis, bradycardia, hoarseness, hiccups, tinnitus and others [21].

6.5 Chiari Type II

Type 2 defined as the herniation of the cerebellar vermis in addition to the brainstem, fourth ventricle and non-neurological tissue such as basilar artery and related meninges [22]. In contrast to CIM, CIIM has very high likelihood of associated anomalies such as hydrocephalus, syringomyelia, myelomeningocele and others.

CIIM is less common than CIM, but it is known for its serious prognosis. The Associated anomalies like myelomeningocele is the accountable cause of death in this population of patients with CIIM [23].

Pathologically, the vermis is the part that displaced not the tonsils, that is explained by some theories that suggest that the difference in CSF pressure that associated with fluid leakage from other abnormalities such as myelomeningocele. In other words, the assumption suggests that Chiari malformation is a consequent anomaly caused by primary neural defect [24]. Syringomyelia is common abnormality in CIIM population characterized as elongated CSF-filled cavity inside the spinal cord that extends across multiple spinal segments [25].

Newborns with CIIM frequently tend to be asymptomatic. The symptoms Brainstem compression usually manifest in the first year of life [26]. These symptoms involve irritability, aspiration with consequent recurrent chest infections, stridor and difficulties in breathing and feeding which are leading to loss of consciousness, breathing-hold spells and failure to thrive (Fig. 6.2), the physical examination may reveal hypotonia [26]. During older age groups, other manifestations take place like the clinical presentations of compressing the spinal cord including motor impairment in the upper limbs particularly the hand dysfunction and muscle atrophy [27]. Involvement of cerebellar vermis can result in ataxia. Other

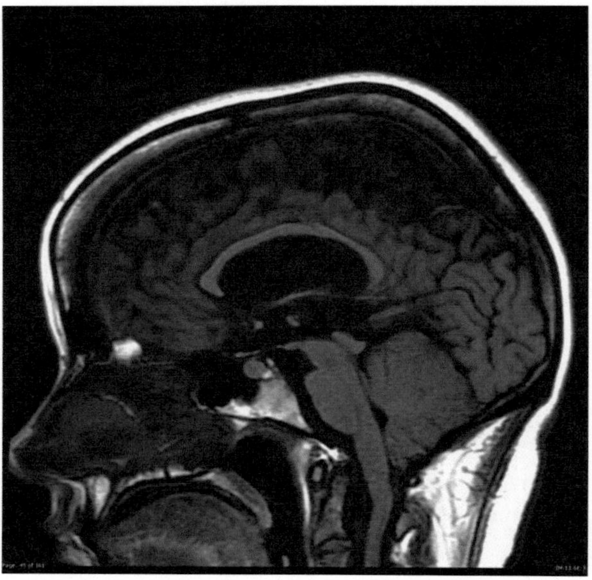

Fig. 6.2 Sagittal MRI scan of Chiari malformation type II. (Source: Radiopedia. Link: https:// radiopaedia.org/articles/ chiari-ii-malformation?lan g=us)

clinical consequences encompass nystagmus, strabismus and dysarthria [26]. CIIM can be presented as acute life-threatening condition as high as fifth of the patients particularly in the first two years of life as acute case of vocal cords impairment such as stridor, apnea and severe impairment of the brainstem [28].

6.6 Chiari Malformation Type III

CIIIM is the type that not only characterized by neural tissue herniation, but also formation of encephalocele encompasses it in the occipital and high cervical area. CIIIM known as very rare type of Chiari malformation and also the worst in regards to prognosis [29]. It carries high risk in mortality rate and neurological impairment and disabilities [30]. The pathogenesis is mostly ununderstood but there few theories try to explain it, mainly concerned about defective formation, abnormal neurulation and osseous defect in the occipital area leading to the herniation of PCF contents [31].

Patients with CIIIM are usually presented with occipital mass increasing in size with age (Fig. 6.3). The occipital mass is mainly encephalocele, this could be accompanied with occipital bone defect, small size of PCF, hydrocephalus, syringomyelia and other congenital abnormalities [31, 32]. Sometimes the mass is located in the upper cervical area posteriorly usually as meningoencephalocele. Meningoencephalocele is usually associated with cervical bone defect, herniation of PCF contents in addition to systemic manifestations such as respiratory failure [31, 32].

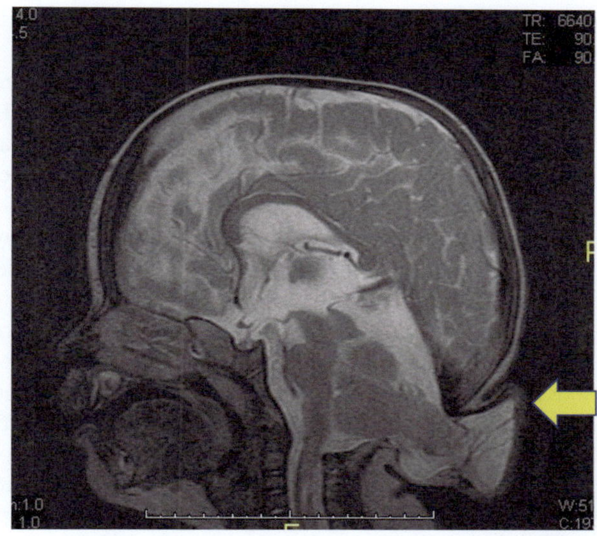

Fig. 6.3 Sagittal MRI scan of Chiari malformation type II in T2 image. (Source: Radiopedia. Link: https://radiopaedia.org/articles/chiari-iii-malformation?lang=us)

6.7   Diagnosis of Chiari Malformation

Regarding the diagnostics, there several available options to reach the diagnosis of Chiari malformations. The diagnostic of choice is the magnetic resonance imaging [33]. The goal of the MRI scan is to identify the herniation and caudal displacement of the cerebellar tonsils in CIM diagnosis. It should be kept in mind that the cerebellar tonsils can be displaced up to 3 mm and can be considered as normal or asymptomatic state of the disease [34]. The cerebellar tonsils in CIM are low-lying and pointed in peg-like shape in the sagittal plane. Nevertheless, the herniation is considered pathological when exceed the 5 mm displacement with unclear differentiation in the case of displacement between 3 to 5 mm [34, 35]. The MRI scan can detect also other associated pathologies including atlanto-occipital assimilation, basilar invagination and fused cervical vertebrae which are frequently associated with Chiari malformation [36]. It is also important to rule out other pathologies that can increase intracranial pressure and induce tonsillar herniation such as mass lesions, hydrocephalus and other anomalies.

In CIIM, MRI scan shows the displacement of cerebellar tonsils and vermis inferiorly across the FM and the brainstem is also caudally displaced [37]. MRI scan can also detect PCF abnormalities in CIIM such as the small size and low position of torcula herophili [38, 39]. CIIM is usually also associated with hydrocephalus in addition to other ventricular anomalies such as dilation of the third ventricle and shrinking of the fourth ventricle with elongation and extension through the cervical canal, Irregular dilation of the lateral ventricles and medullary kinking [40, 41]. Other radiological findings include, beaking of the tectal plate, elongation of inferior colliculus and aqueduct angulation and stenosis [41, 42]. Associated anomalies can also be detected in MRI scan of the spine which are myelomeningocele and tethering of the spinal cord [38].

MRI can be used in another different sequence in Chiari malformation, the cine-mode MRI which is helpful in such case. Cine-mode MRI can detect the CSF flow patterns and disturbances in CIM [43]. This technique can be very helpful preoperatively in the surgical decision making and postoperatively in the follow-up evaluations [43].

Computed tomography can be used to assess the bony defects and abnormalities in Chiari malformation [44]. Plain radiographs can used to identify the issues of instability. Ultrasonography can detect the frontal bone indentation known as lemon signs and abnormal configuration of cerebellum enveloping around the brainstem known as banana signing addition to detecting associated hydrocephalus [45].

Electrophysiological studies can be performed preoperatively to identify the syringomyelia that is associated with Chiari malformation and distinguish it from hydromyelia [46]. Electrophysiological tests including brainstem auditory evoked potentials can be considered as addition to the clinical data, but the surgical decision cannot be subject to it alone [47]. Intraoperative neurophysiological monitoring is applied during the surgical decompression of PCF to reduce the complications rate of the procedure [48].

6.8 Management of Chiari Malformation

Unfortunately, medical treatment is not suitable option for Chiari malformation. In patients with CIM, the decision of applying the surgical management is controversial [49]. The decision depends on multiple factors which are mainly can be collected in two categories, the severity of the clinical presentation and presence of associated anomalies such as syringomyelia and hydrocephalus. These factors affect the decision and timing of the surgery either early as possible or being delayed. Asymptomatic patients or patients with CIM with mild symptoms without major debilities in routine lifestyle, non-significant neurological signs or mild displacement of cerebellar tonsils radiologically can benefit from the conservative approach and waiting until the clinical situation is worsened [50]. The symptomatic patients who suffer from interactable symptoms such as severe headache or deformity like scoliosis, considerable neurological findings such as cranial nerve impairment, systemic complications such as respiratory difficulties and significant radiological findings can candidate the patient for earlier surgical approach and intervention [51].

The other critical factor is the presence of associated syringomyelia or syrinx with CIM. Patients with syringomyelia are indicated for surgical treatment [52]. However, the decision in some asymptomatic cases is difficult to make [52]. This approach is aiming at preserving and protecting spinal cord structure and function from further or permanent injury from the compressing pathologies. Some studies suggest ongoing examinations and radiological imaging with observative approach only indicated for small and asymptomatic cases of syringomyelia [53].

Hydrocephalus should be treated and resolved first before any surgical intervention directed to Chiari malformation or syringomyelia, this also applied for any condition that causing increased intracranial pressure. This step can enhance the clinical presentation without further surgical decompression [54]. If the clinical presentation is worsened or persist after the surgery, surgical intervention should be concerned with Chiari malformation.

Proper preoperative planning is mandatory for the posterior fossa decompression. This approach involves MRI scans for the PCF, cervical spine and in some cases the thoracic and lumbar spine also are involved in the scan. Plain radiographs of the cervical spine are also important regarding the instability, the radiographs should be in flexion-extension position. Brain MRI, CT scans and ultrasonography through the anterior fontanelle in infants is beneficial for evaluating and ruling out hydrocephalus.

Firstly, the patient is placed in prone position with head put in the flexion position [55]. The skin incision is made in the midline vertically from midocciput toward the skin overlying the second vertebra. Then, the underlying soft tissues are separated, then the exposure of posterior side of the FM and the first cervical vertebra with the dura matter. The decompression involves removing part of the occipital bone first with size of 2.2 wide and 2.5 cm long, the procedure is done with craniotome. Exposing and removing of occipital part firstly with posterior arch of C1 still intact in purpose of protecting the cervical spinal cord in case that there is an accident with craniotome. After that, a part of the posterior arch is removed with size of 2.2 cm, this can be done with bone rongeur. In some conditions, it is necessary to remove the upper surface of second cervical vertebra to expose the tonsillar herniation caudally, but that is limited to certain conditions rather than a usual procedure. If the anomaly is associated with syringomyelia which is commonly causes dural problem such as arachnoid webs that may alter the CSF flow decreasing the benefit of PCF decompression, opening the dura is required with mild separation of the cerebellar tonsils restoring the movement of CSF through the median aperture which connects the fourth ventricle and the cisterna magna. Shrinking of the cerebellar tonsils to restore the CSF flow can be achieved by performing extrapial coagulation of the tips of tonsils unilaterally or bilaterally. The option of dural graft is controversial but recommended by some surgeons to augment the decompression, avoiding the adhesions postoperatively and decrease the possibility for reoperation [55, 56]. After the surgery, the patient is transferred to the intensive care unit.

The initial step in managing CIIM is establishing normal and physiological level of intracranial pressure. In some instances, normalizing the intracranial pressure can reduce the necessity for the surgical decompression. This can be done by revision and inspection of the shunt. Significant or enlarging syringomyelia, progressive or fatal symptoms such as stridor, recurrent chest infections, severe dysphagia and regurgitant, apnea, cyanosis, spasticity and ataxia are all considerable indications to the surgical approach [55].

CIIM patients need more preoperative investigations than CIM particularly regarding the functions of brainstem and the cranial nerves such as swallow study, vocal cord examination and pulmonary functions tests and other related tests performed by specialists [22]. Type II Chiari malformation has more difficulties surgically and technically in the management that require specific experience of the surgeon in that field.

If the surgical decompression is indicated, there some differences between the decompression procedure performed in CIIM and the one in CIM. Some authors recommends leaving the FM and occipital bone intact [57, 58]. This difference might be attributed to the fact that is FM is usually larger in size in CIIM and reducing the risk for futural cervical instability due to the bony excision. In the decompression of CIIM, only the posterior arch of the vertebra that are overlying the cerebellar vermis are removed [55]. The main aim of the procedure is visualizing the fourth ventricle, this aim can be achieved by identifying the choroid plexus particularly in its embryological site, the choroid plexus is a key marker to reach the fourth ventricle.

Coagulation of the cerebellar vermis tip can help preserving the connection between the fourth ventricle and the subarachnoid space. Stenting is also available option if there is suspicion that the median aperture or the foramen of Magendie could be occluded [59, 60].

Multiple Choice Questions
1. **Newborn baby is suffering from occipital mass, the pediatric department sent for neurosurgical consult. The baby is born by cesarian section crying with no complications. MRI scan is done and showing cerebellar herniation into low occipital encephalocele. According to Arnold classification, the defect is:**

    (a) Chiari malformation Type I
    (b) Chiari malformation Type II
    (c) Chiari malformation Type III
    (d) Chiari malformation Type IV

2. **14 years old male is brought to the hospital for episodes of persistent mild headaches after failed medical therapy, the GP recommended performing brain MRI scan, incidentally the radiologist found descending of cerebellar tonsils into the foramen magnum with 4 mm displacement, The defect is classified as:**

    (a) Chiari malformation Type I
    (b) Chiari malformation Type II
    (c) Chiari malformation Type III
    (d) Chiari malformation Type IV

3. **5 years old female preschool girl presented to the emergency department with severe stridor and dyspnea. After stabilizing the patient, the family reports history of progressive unsteadiness in movement and difficulty in walking. The ER department send the patient for brain MRI scan and it**

showed small PCF, crowded foramen magnum with the cerebellar tonsils and vermis seen displaced inferiorly, displaced brainstem with low lying fourth ventricle. The patient is diagnosed with Chiari malformation. Regarding the classification, the MRI findings resemble:

(a) Chiari malformation Type I
(b) Chiari malformation Type II
(c) Chiari malformation Type III
(d) Chiari malformation Type IV

4. **Syringomyelia is associated with Chiari malformation, it has more common prevalence in the population of patients that diagnosed with:**

(a) Chiari malformation Type I
(b) Chiari malformation Type II
(c) Chiari malformation Type III
(d) Chiari malformation Type IV

5. **Chiari malformation has variable clinical presentations, the most common symptom that brings the patient to seek healthcare is:**

(a) Occipital and Cervical pain due to compression effect
(b) Loss of consciousness
(c) Loss of hand dexterity and muscle atrophy
(d) Acute respiratory symptoms due to brainstem involvement

6. **Regarding the types of Chiari malformation, which sentence below is true:**

(a) Tonsillar herniation with 3 mm displacement is always considered pathological in type I
(b) Type II has better prognosis than type I
(c) There is no cervical bone defect in type III that associated with meningoencephalocele.
(d) Type III is the rarest type in comparison to type I and II

7. **Regarding the types of Chiari malformation, which sentence below is true:**

(a) Hydrocephalus is more common with type I Chiari malformation
(b) Syringomyelia is relatively rare within patients of Chiari malformation
(c) Type II has more likelihood of associated hydrocephalus than type I
(d) None of the above

8. **Cerebellar aplasia or agenesis is classified as:**

(a) Chiari malformation Type I
(b) Chiari malformation Type II
(c) Chiari malformation Type 0
(d) Chiari malformation Type IV

9. **If the MRI scan findings indicates the presence of syringomyelia only with any neural tissue herniation through the foramen magnum, this is usually a case of:**

   (a) Chiari malformation Type I
   (b) Chiari malformation Type II
   (c) Chiari malformation Type 0
   (d) Chiari malformation Type IV

10. **Involvement of brainstem with the cerebellar tonsils displacement without the vermis is usually asymptomatic, this situation is classified as:**

   (a) Chiari malformation Type I
   (b) Chiari malformation Type II
   (c) Chiari malformation Type 0
   (d) Chiari malformation Type 1.5

11. **17 years old male patient is suffering from progressive symptoms of headache, upper cervical pain. The physical examination revealed nystagmus, bilateral upper limb weakness, tremor and sensory loss in the upper limbs also bilaterally. The MRI scan findings suggest the diagnosis of Chiari malformation type I. Regarding the management of this patient, which statement is true:**

   (a) Medical therapy is available approach in that situation
   (b) Conservative approach is preferred with lifestyle modifications
   (c) The patient's condition necessitates the surgical treatment by PCF decompression mainly.
   (d) None of the above.

12. **2 years old patient presented with Chiari malformation type I and hydrocephalus. Regarding the management, the best approach is:**

   (a) Normalizing intracranial pressure and managing the hydrocephalus is mandatory.
   (b) Shunting of the ventricular system is not necessary in this case.
   (c) Immediate decompression of the PCF without prior shunting is the best option.
   (d) None of the above.

Multiple Choice Questions Answers
   1. C
   2. A
   3. B
   4. B
   5. A
   6. D
   7. C

8. D
9. C
10. D
11. C
12. A

References

1. Holly LT, Batzdorf U. Chiari malformation and syringomyelia: JNSPG 75th anniversary invited review article. J Neurosurg Spine. 2019;31(5):619–28.
2. Alexandrou M, Politi M, Papanagiotou P. Chiari-malformation. Radiologe. 2018;58(7):626–8.
3. Hidalgo JA, Tork CA, Varacallo M. Arnold-Chiari malformation. Treasure Island: Stat Pearls Publishing; 2022.
4. Özek M, Cinalli G, Maixner W, Sainte-Rose C. Posterior fossa tumors in children. Cham: Springer International Publishing; 2015.
5. Moore K, Agur A, Dalley A, Moore K. Moore's essential clinical anatomy. 6th ed. Philadelphia: Wolters Kluwer; 2019.
6. Stranding S. Gray" anatomy international edition. 42nd ed. Elsevier Health Sciences; 2020.
7. Blumenfeld H. Neuroanatomy through clinical cases. Yale J Bio Med. 2010;83:165–6.
8. Waxman S. Clinical neuroanatomy. 29th ed. New York: McGraw-Hill Education; 2020.
9. Jacobson S, Marcus T, Pugsley S. Neuroanatomy for the neuroscientist. 3rd ed. New York: Springer International Publishing; 2018.
10. Splittgerber R. Snell's clinical neuroanatomy. 8th ed. Wolters Kluwer; 2019.
11. Fric R, Ringstad G, Eide P. Chiari-malformasjon type 1—diagnostikk og behandling. Tidsskrift for Den norske legeforening. 2019;
12. Fons K, Jnah A. Arnold-Chiari malformation: core concepts. Neonatal Netw. 2021;40(5):313–20.
13. Bogdanov E, Faizutdinova A, Heiss J. Posterior cranial fossa and cervical spine morphometric abnormalities in symptomatic Chiari type 0 and Chiari type 1 malformation patients with and without syringomyelia. Acta Neurochir. 2021;163(11):3051–64.
14. Giallongo A, Pavone P, Tomarchio S, Filosco F, Falsaperla R, Testa G, et al. Clinicoradiographic data and management of children with Chiari malformation type 1 and 1.5: an Italian case series. Acta Neurol Belg. 2020;121(6):1547–54.
15. Liu W, Wu H, Aikebaier Y, Wulabieke M, Paerhati R, Yang X. No significant difference between Chiari malformation type 1.5 and type I. Clin Neurol Neurosurg. 2017;157:34–9.
16. Sarnat H. Disorders of segmentation of the neural tube: Chiari malformations. Handb Clin Neurol. 2007;87:89–103.
17. Ellenbogen R, Sekhar L, Kitchen N. Principles of neurological surgery. Amsterdam: Elsevier; 2018.
18. Joseph Levy W, Mason L, Hahn J. Chiari malformation presenting in adults: a surgical experience in 127 cases. Neurosurgery. 1983;12(4):377–90.
19. Holly L, Batzdorf U. Chiari malformation and syringomyelia. J Neurosurg Spine. 2019;31(5):619–28.
20. Kalangu K, Katou Y, Dechambenoit G. Essential practice of neurosurgery. 1st ed. Nagoya: Access Publishing; 2009.
21. McClugage S, Oakes W. The Chiari I malformation. J Neurosurg Pediatr. 2019;24(3):217–26.
22. Talamonti G, Marcati E, Mastino L, Meccariello G, Picano M, D'Aliberti G. Surgical management of Chiari malformation type II. Childs Nerv Syst. 2020;36(8):1621–34.

23. McDowell M, Blatt J, Deibert C, Zwagerman N, Tempel Z, Greene S. Predictors of mortality in children with myelomeningocele and symptomatic Chiari type II malformation. J Neurosurg Pediatr. 2018;21(6):587–96.
24. McLone D, Knepper P. The cause of Chiari II malformation: a unified theory. Pediatr Neurosurg. 1989;15(1):1–12.
25. Flint G. Syringomyelia: diagnosis and management. Pract Neurol. 2021;21(5):403–11.
26. Winn H, Youmans J. Youman's neurological surgery. Philadelphia: Saunders; 2004. p. 3347–61.
27. Shane Tubbs R, Jerry OW. The Chiari malformations. 1st ed. New York: Springer; 2013. p. 430–1.
28. Bell W, Charney E, Bruce D, Sutton L, Schut L. Symptomatic Arnold-Chiari malformation: review of experience with 22 cases. J Neurosurg. 1987;66(6):812–6.
29. Ivashchuk G, Loukas M, Blount J, Tubbs R, Oakes W. Chiari III malformation: a comprehensive review of this enigmatic anomaly. Childs Nerv Syst. 2015;31(11):2035–40.
30. Elbaroody M, Mostafa H, Alsawy M, Elhawary M, Atallah A, Gabr M. Outcomes of Chiari malformation III: a review of literature. J Pediatr Neurosci. 2020;15(4):358.
31. Jeong D, Kim C, Kim M, Chung H, Kim T, Jung H. Arnold-Chiari malformation type iii with meningoencephalocele: a case report. Ann Rehabil Med. 2014;38(3):401.
32. Häberle J, Hülskamp G, Harms E, Krasemann T. Cervical encephalocele in a newborn—Chiari III malformation. Childs Nerv Syst. 2001;17(6):373–5.
33. McVige J, Leonardo J. Imaging of Chiari Type I malformation and syringohydromyelia. Neurol Clin. 2014;32(1):95–126.
34. Aboulezz A, Sartor K, Geyer C, Gado M. Position of cerebellar tonsils in the normal population and in patients with Chiari malformation. J Comput Assist Tomogr. 1985;9(6):1033–6.
35. Barkovich A, Wippold F, Sherman J, Citrin C. Significance of cerebellar tonsillar position on MR. AJNR. 1987;7:795–9.
36. Elster A, Chen M. Chiari I malformations: clinical and radiologic reappraisal. Radiology. 1992;183(2):347–53.
37. Variend S, Emery J. Cervical dislocation of the cerebellum in children with meningomyelocele. Teratology. 1976;13(3):281–9.
38. Volpe P, De Robertis R, Fanelli T, Boito S, Volpe G, Votino C, Persico N, Chaoui R. Low torcular herophili position and large brainstem–tentorium angle in fetuses with open spinal dysraphism at 11–13 weeks' gestation. Ultrasound Obstet Gynecol. 2022;59(1):49–54.
39. Hadley DM. The Chiari malformations. J Neurol Neurosurg Psychiatry. 2002;72:ii38–40.
40. Mancarella C, Delfini R, Landi A. Chiari malformations. Acta Neurochirurgica Supplement. 2019;125:89–95.
41. Peach B. Arnold-Chiari malformation: anatomic features of 20 cases. Arch Neurol. 1965;12(6):613–21.
42. Wolpert SM, Anderson M, Scott RM, Kwan ES, Runge VM. Chiari II malformation: MR imaging evaluation. Am J Neuroradiol. 1987;8(5):783–92.
43. Armonda RA, Citrin CM, Foley KT, Ellenbogen RG. Quantitative cine-mode magnetic resonance imaging of Chiari I malformations: an analysis of cerebrospinal fluid dynamics. Neurosurgery. 1994;35(2):214–24.
44. Iqbal S, Robert AP, Mathew D. Computed tomographic study of posterior cranial fossa, foramen magnum, and its surgical implications in Chiari malformations. Asian J Neurosurg. 2017;12(3):428.
45. Fujisawa H, Kitawaki J, Iwasa K, Honjo H. New ultrasonographic criteria for the prenatal diagnosis of Chiari type 2 malformation. Acta Obstet Gynecol Scand. 2006;85(12):1426–9.
46. Roser F, Ebner FH, Sixt C, Hagen JM, Tatagiba MS. Defining the line between hydromyelia and syringomyelia. A differentiation is possible based on electrophysiological and magnetic resonance imaging studies. Acta Neurochir. 2010;152(2):213–9.
47. Mori K, Uchida Y, Nishimura T, Eghwrudjakpor P. Brainstem auditory evoked potentials in Chiari-II malformation. Childs Nerv Syst. 1988;4(3):154–7.

48. Anderson RC, Dowling KC, Feldstein NA, Emerson RG. Chiari I malformation: potential role for intraoperative electrophysiologic monitoring. J Clin Neurophysiol. 2003;20(1):65–72.
49. Hersh D, Groves M, Boop F. Management of Chiari malformations: opinions from different centers—a review. Childs Nerv Syst. 2019;35(10):1869–73.
50. Novegno F, Caldarelli M, Massa A, Chieffo D, Massimi L, Pettorini B, et al. The natural history of the Chiari Type I anomaly. J Neurosurg Pediatr. 2008;2(3):179–87.
51. Ciaramitaro P, Massimi L, Bertuccio A, Solari A, Farinotti M, Peretta P, et al. Diagnosis and treatment of Chiari malformation and syringomyelia in adults: international consensus document. Neurol Sci. 2021;43(2):1327–42.
52. Schijman E, Steinbok P. International survey on the management of Chiari I malformation and syringomyelia. Childs Nerv Syst. 2004;20(5):341–8.
53. Nishikawa M, Sakamoto H, Hakuba A, Nakanishi N, Inoue Y. Pathogenesis of Chiari malformation: a morphometric study of the posterior cranial fossa. J Neurosurg. 1997;86(1):40–7.
54. Hayhurst C, Osman-Farah J, Das K, Mallucci C. Initial management of hydrocephalus associated with Chiari malformation Type I–syringomyelia complex via endoscopic third ventriculostomy: an outcome analysis. J Neurosurg. 2008;108(6):1211–4.
55. Youmans J, Winn H. Youmans & Winn neurological surgery. 7th ed. Philadelphia: Elsevier; 2017. p. 1537–9
56. Durham S, Fjeld-Olenec K. Comparison of posterior fossa decompression with and without duraplasty for the surgical treatment of Chiari malformation Type I in pediatric patients: a meta-analysis. J Neurosurg Pediatr. 2008;2(1):42–9.
57. Akbari S, Limbrick D, Kim D, Narayan P, Leonard J, Smyth M, et al. Surgical management of symptomatic Chiari II malformation in infants and children. Childs Nerv Syst. 2013;29(7):1143–54.
58. Hoffman H, Hendrick B, Humphreys R. Manifestations and management of Arnold-Chiari malformation in patients with myelomeningocele. Pediatr Neurosurg. 1975;1(4):255–9.
59. Sacco D, Scott R. Reoperation for Chiari malformations. Pediatr Neurosurg. 2003;39(4):171–8.
60. Worley G, Schuster JM, Oakes WJ. Survival at 5 years of a cohort of newborn infants with myelomeningocele. Dev Med Child Neurol. 1996;38:816–22.

Chapter 7
Porencephaly

Ali Talib Hashim, Mays Sufyan Ahmad, and Karrar Ali Idan

Test your learning and check your understanding of this book's contents: use the "Springer Nature Flashcards" app to access questions using ▶ https://sn.pub/YnQHwS
To use the app, please follow the instructions in Chapter 1.

7.1 Introduction

Porencephaly is a rare disorder causing clefts or cystic lesions lined with white matter, usually having a connection with the ventricles and/or subarachnoid space. It involves the brain's hemispheres that can be congenital or acquired [1].

The first case was described in 1859 [2]. It is believed that the main cause of it is the disturbance of the blood supply for the brain's tissue which can cause damage. This disturbance can be caused by many causes and even during child delivery like pregnancy trauma or placenta bleeding. Figure 7.1 shows an MRI of a case with porencephaly. These cysts can be located everywhere in the brain, unilateral or bilateral. Its clinical features depend on the patient and the location and also the structure involved [3].

A. T. Hashim (✉)
Golestan University for Medical Sciences, Gorgan, Iran

M. S. Ahmad · K. A. Idan
College of Medicine, University of Baghdad, Baghdad, Iraq

© The Author(s), under exclusive license to Springer Nature Switzerland AG 2024
K. F. AlAli, H. T. Hashim (eds.), *Congenital Brain Malformations*,
https://doi.org/10.1007/978-3-031-58630-9_7

Fig. 7.1 A case of porencephaly MRI. (Case courtesy of Assoc Prof Frank Gaillard, Radiopaedia.org, rID: 15928)

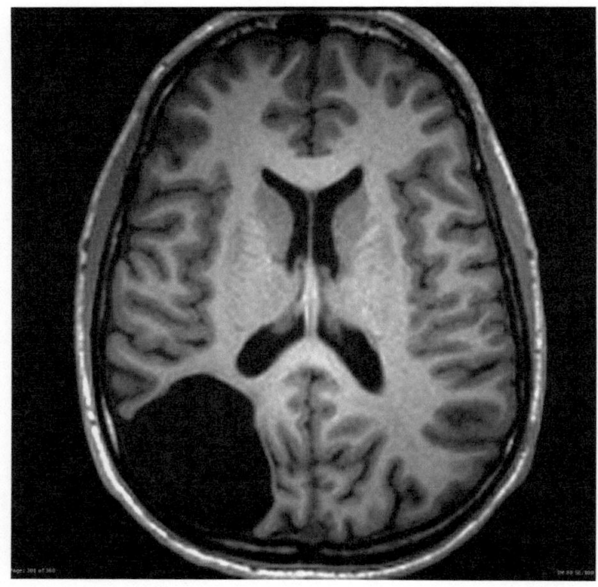

Two types of porencephaly are described:

"Type I: generally due to an antepartum intraparenchymal hemorrhage. Type II lesions are usually developmental anomalies." [4].

7.2 Epidemiology

Prevalence of porencephaly, schizencephaly, and hydranencephaly in Japan (2007–2011) was 8.3 per 100,000 births, which correlates with the USA and other European prevalence data [5].

7.3 Etiology

The disease can be congenital or acquired. Traumatic, ischemic, hemorrhagic insults in addition to infection was observed. In utero vascular injury was found to be the main contributor to porencephaly [6]. Genetic causes like a mutation in the *COL4A1 gene which is responsible for collagen*, are shown to contribute to porencephaly in humans by inducing perinatal hemorrhage. Three familial cases in unrelated Dutch families found similar results for this gene rule in hereditary porencephaly [7, 8]. A study of 61 patients with porencephaly, found a mutation in this gene in 10 of them. In addition to its cerebral vascular disease, found to cause intracranial calcification, cortical dysplasia, ocular disease and others [9].

7.4 Pathology

Porencephaly as mentioned earlier is a cleft or cyst lined by white matter, by reading schizencephaly, the same insults are found to cause both, so how can fetus develop either Porencephaly or schizencephaly, is answered by the gestational age at which the insult occurred. If the insult happened during the 4–6 months of gestation, there will be neuronal migration to produce normal or abnormal grey matter and this defines schizencephaly. If the insult occurs after 6 months of gestation, there will be no further neuronal migration and resorption will occur. If it still with no gliosis, will be called porencephaly, if gliosis occurs, then called encephalomalacia. Many confuses between those three terms although there is a difference and can't be used as synonyms [10].

Porencepaly is usually associated with other anomalies like hydrocephalus. In a study of 22 patients with porencephaly using MRI, Amygdalar and hippocampal atrophy was found in 95% of studies cases so careful looking for associated defects is essential [11].

7.5 Clinical Manifestation

The signs and symptoms depend on the location and the size of the porencephaly. Among the symptoms recorded are: mental retardation, seizure, developmental delay, Cerebral palsy, and blindness. Rare case reports mentioned Psychosis in acquired cases, otorrhea caused by a large porencephalic cyst and nystagmus [12–15].

7.6 Diagnosis

1. Ultrasound (can detect cysts prenatally).
2. MRI is the best for diagnosing different brain anomalies, including porencephaly [16].
3. CT [17].

7.7 Management

The management is conservative mainly, depending on the associated clinical manifestation (seizures, cerebral palsy and others). Surgical intervention may help in some cases. Since there is a genetic predisposition, genetic consultation is required [18].

7.8 Differential Diagnosis

1. Schizencephaly
2. Encephalomalacia
3. Neuroglial cyst
4. Hydranencephaly [17]

7.9 Prognosis

Depends on the site, size and associated anomalies.

Multiple Choice Questions
1. **Porencephaly is:**

    (a) Complicated hydrocephalus.
    (b) A cleft or cyst in the brain hemisphere lined by normal grey matter.
    (c) A cleft or cyst in the brain that is lined by abnormal grey matter.
    (d) A cleft or cyst in the brain that is lined by white matter.

Answer: d

2. **The best diagnostic way of porencephaly is:**

    (a) MRI
    (b) MRV
    (c) CT
    (d) CSF

Answer: a

3. **The prognosis of porencephaly is:**

    (a) Good
    (b) Bad
    (c) Depending on the size and severity
    (d) Depend on the management

Answer: c

4. **Porencephaly can be managed by:**

   (a) Surgery
   (b) Medical therapy
   (c) Physical and Occupational therapy
   (d) All the above

Answer: d

5. **The clinical presentation of porencephaly includes:**

   (a) Epilepsy
   (b) Respiratory failure
   (c) Abnormal limbs development
   (d) Seizures

Answer: d

6. **The medical management in porencephaly is mostly for managing:**

   (a) The seizures
   (b) The hypotonia
   (c) The paralysis
   (d) The hydrocephalus

Answer: a

7. **Among the genes involved in porencephaly pathogenesis:**

   (a) DMD
   (b) COL4A1
   (c) CACNA1A
   (d) SNCA

Answer: b

8. **Porencephaly:**

   (a) can communicate with ventricles and dura matter
   (b) cystic lesion surrounded by gliotic tissue.
   (c) Is of unilateral location only.
   (d) Includes the cranium.

Answer: a

9. **Porencephaly:**

   (a) Can come with other malformations like hydrocephalus
   (b) Can be treated prenatally
   (c) Needs no intervention
   (d) Cannot be diagnosed at birth

Answer: a

10. **Porencephaly causes:**

    (a) Are infectious in origin
    (b) Are genetic in origin
    (c) Can be caused by genetics or intrauterine infections
    (d) Drugs and radiation are the main causes.

Answer: c

References

1. Halabuda A, et al. Schizencephaly—diagnostics and clinical dilemmas. Childs Nerv Syst. 2015;31(4):551–6.
2. Heschl R. Gehirndefect und Hydrocephalus. Prag Vjschr Prakt Heilk. 1859;61:59–74.
3. Fatterpekar G, Naidich T, Som P. The teaching files: brain and spine imaging E-book. Elsevier; 2012.
4. Eller KM, Kuller JA. Fetal porencephaly: a review of etiology, diagnosis, and prognosis. Obstet Gynecol Surv. 1995;50(9):684–7.
5. Hino-Fukuyo N, Togashi N, Takahashi R, Saito J, Inui T, Endo W, Sato R, Okubo Y, Saitsu H, Haginoya K. Neuroepidemiology of porencephaly, schizencephaly, and hydranencephaly in Miyagi prefecture, Japan. Pediatr Neurol. 2016;54:39–42.e1 . ISSN0887 8994. https://www.sciencedirect.com/science/article/pii/S0887899415004270. https://doi.org/10.1016/j.pediatrneurol.2015.08.016.
6. Husain T, Langlois PH, Sever LE, Gambello MJ. Descriptive epidemiologic features shared by birth defects thought to be related to vascular disruption in Texas, 1996-2002. Birth Defects Res A Clin Mol Teratol. 2008;82(6):435–40. https://doi.org/10.1002/bdra.20449. PMID: 18383510.
7. Breedveld G, de Coo IF, Lequin MH, et al. Novel mutations in three families confirm a major role of COL4A1 in hereditary porencephaly. J Med Genet. 2006;43:490–5.
8. Gould DB, Phalan FC, Breedveld GJ, Van Mil SE, Smith RS, Schimenti JC, Aguglia U, Van Der Knaap MS, Heutink P, John SW. Mutations in Col4a1 cause perinatal cerebral hemorrhage and porencephaly. Science. 2005;308(5725):1167–71.
9. Yoneda Y, Haginoya K, Kato M, Osaka H, Yokochi K, Arai H, Kakita A, Yamamoto T, Otsuki Y, Shimizu SI, Wada T. Phenotypic spectrum of COL4A1 mutations: porencephaly to schizencephaly. Ann Neurol. 2013;73(1):48–57.
10. Griffiths PD. Schizencephaly revisited. Neuroradiology. 2018;60(9):945–60. https://doi.org/10.1007/s00234-018-2056-7. Epub 19 Jul 2018. PMID: 30027296; PMCID: PMC6096842.
11. Ho SS, Kuzniecky RI, Gilliam F, Faught E, Bebin M, Morawetz R. Congenital porencephaly: MR features and relationship to hippocampal sclerosis. AJNR Am J Neuroradiol. 1998;19(1):135–41. PMID: 9432171; PMCID: PMC8337343.ents with porencephaly-related seizures.
12. Alzahrani RA, Alghamdi AF, Alzahrani MA, Alghamdi MA, Alghamdi MF, Alzahrani AA, Alghamdi AM, Alzahrani MK, Alghamdi TS, Alghamdi RS, Alqarni FA. A giant porencephaly: a rare etiology of pediatric seizures. Cureus. 2021;13(11):e19623.
13. Puiu MG, Dionisie V, Filip AC, Manea M. Psychosis associated with acquired porencephaly—cause or incidental finding? Case report and review of literature. Medicina [Internet]. 2022;58(5):586. https://doi.org/10.3390/medicina58050586.
14. Ryzenman JM, Rothholtz VS, Wiet RJ. Porencephalic cyst: a review of the literature and management of a rare cause of cerebrospinal fluid otorrhea. Otol Neurotol. 2007;28(3):381–6. https://doi.org/10.1097/mao.0b013e31802ead9e.

15. Ishak M, Ramli R, Mohamad I. Porencephaly as a rare cause of nystagmus. Pediatria i Medycyna Rodzinna. 2020;16:227–9. https://doi.org/10.15557/PiMR.2020.0043.
16. Raafat M, Hosny SM, Sheta GA, Talaat SH, Ali EA. Role of fetal MRI to diagnose abnormal cerebral ventricular system and associated fetal brain anomalies. Egypt J Radiol Nucl Med. 2022;53(1):1–1.
17. Ho, M., Glick, Y. Porencephaly. Reference article. Radiopaedia.org.https://doi.org/10.53347/rID-7281.
18. Granata T. Porencephaly. MedLink Neurology. 2006;

Chapter 8
Septo-Optic dysplasia

Abubakar Nazir ⓘ, Usama Afzaal ⓘ, Faizan Saleem ⓘ, and Awais Nazir ⓘ

Test your learning and check your understanding of this book's contents: use the "Springer Nature Flashcards" app to access questions using ▶ https://sn.pub/YnQHwS
To use the app, please follow the instructions in Chapter 1.

8.1   Introduction

Septo-optic dysplasia is a rare genetic disease that presents with midline brain abnormalities. Once known as de Morsier syndrome, it is first described in 1941 by Reeves in 7 months old baby that presented with absent septum pellucidum and optic nerve dysfunction [1]. Its classical triad consist of optic nerve hypoplasia, pituitary hypoplasia and absence of septum pellucidum and carpus callosum. This heterogenous condition presents with variety of phenotypes together with other anomalies like grey matter heterotopias, hydrocephalus, polymicrogyria, etc. [2]. Due to variety of clinical manifestations some neurologists described it as a spectrum of disease but there is still a long ongoing to debate to decide the appropriate terminologies and nomenclature. Terminologies like SOD plus syndrome when associated with schizencephaly like cortical abnormalities and SOD spectrum when it encompasses other abnormalities like cleft lip etc. have been suggested [3]. It is most commonly confused with optic nerve hypoplasia (ONH) but it is a separate entity that doesn't fulfil the criteria of SOD and have a different etiology [2].

A. Nazir (✉) · U. Afzaal · F. Saleem · A. Nazir
King Edward Medical University, Lahore, Pakistan

K. F. AlAli, H. T. Hashim (eds.), *Congenital Brain Malformations*,
https://doi.org/10.1007/978-3-031-58630-9_8

Developed countries attribute the SOD as one of the most common causes of congenital blindness [2]. The very first presenting complain is ophthalmological involvement resulting in blindness that in most cases is bilateral but may unilateral in minority of patients. Endocrine abnormalities arise later in life that is due to hypoplasia of hypothalamic and pituitary axis [4]. But the classic triad is not present in many cases (approximately 30% have all triad symptomology) and even 40% people have intact pituitary function [5]. Various neurological manifestations have been reported that ranges from the global developmental delay, autism, sensorineural hearing loss, sleep disorders, temperature abnormalities to seizures and focal neurological deficits like hemiparesis [1]. Presumed to be equally distributed in male and female, the estimated incidence is one in 10,000 live births [6]. Occurring mostly sporadically, familial cases have also been reported indicating that genetic etiology may be present. The exact etiology is unknown but it is thought to be a result of interplay between environmental factors and various genes. Mutations in several genes have found to be associated with it [5]. Diagnosis is mainly clinical and till today there is debate going regarding the exact criteria of diagnosis. Genetic diagnosis is only made in less than 1% of the population due to its sporadic nature. Management typically involves the multidisciplinary team with routine ophthalmologic, endocrine and neurologic evaluation [1]. This chapter focuses on epidemiology, etiology, pathophysiology, clinical presentation, diagnostic, complications and management of this condition.

8.2 Embryology

Septo-optic dysplasia occurs when development of prosencephalon is affected. Nervous system development starts during third week of gestation with neurulation occurring during fourth week. The caudal part of neural tube gives rises to spinal cord and the cranial part give rises to brain. The part of neural tube giving rises to brain is divided into three primary brain vesicles after closing of anterior neuropore that are prosencephalon (forebrain), mesencephalon (midbrain), and rhombencephalon (hindbrain). In fifth week of development telencephalon (primordia of cerebral hemispheres) and diencephalon (primordia of hypothalamus, thalamus and epithalamus) arises from partial division of prosencephalon. Rhombencephalon also gives two secondary vesicles metencephalon and myelencephalon. So, there are five secondary brain vesicles [7]. Prosencephalon is highly complicated occurring during early in development of embryo during fourth to fifth week of gestational age. This is a very critical period of development and any insult during this period of development can result in the clinical manifestations. Very two important embryological developments take place in this period. First retinal ganglionic cells and optic vesicles matures and secondly fornix, corpus callosum and anterior commissure forms from the lamina terminalis when it started to thicken. Hypoplasia is generally defined as the failure of the progenitor cells to proliferate and produce the require-ment amounts of cells and subsequent maturation. Primordial tissue is generally present and in extreme cases aplasia can also occur. Any event that can affect these two developments can result in lack in ability to produce ganglionic cells of retina that leads to hypoplasia of optic nerve and failure of commissural or septal forma-tion. It can even lead to hypoplasia of structures of prosencephalon [4].

8.3 Etiology

The precise etiology of the septo-optic dysplasia is still not in the knowledge of the mankind. Numerous factors have been proposed that can contribute to the causa-tion. These factors are widely classified into the environmental aspect and genetic aspect. These two aspects interactions are responsible for variety of phenotypes that contribute to heterogeneity of disease. The disease is said to be sporadic overall but some cases tend to be run in families as well. However, the reported incidence of these cases is less than 1% and as a result genetic diagnosis can be made in less than 1% of the cases [2, 4].

Environmental factors that play role in the pathogenesis are listed as follows

- Maternal diabetes
- Young maternal age (mean age of conception or delivery is less than 22)
- Primiparity
- Ethnicity [7]
- Vascular disruption
- Alcohol
- Substance abuse
- Drugs (e.g. Valproic Acid) [5]
- Smoking
- Viral infections

All these factors have been found to have a link toward the pathogenesis of the dis-ease. They mostly contribute to the sporadic nature of the disease [2].

Genetic Factors account for the several genes that play role in the development of the embryological structure whose formation when insulted result in the develop-ment of disease. These genes have several mutations that can be inherited as auto-somal dominant or recessive. Mutations interact in several ways to contribute to the severity of disease and results in wide number of clinical manifestations. HESX1, SOX2, SOX3 and OTX2 are the genes that contribute to the pathogenesis when mutations occur in them [2, 4] (Table 8.1).

Table 8.1 Showing the factors that are involved in etiology

Environment Factors	Genes Involved
• Maternal diabetes • Young maternal age (mean age of conception or delivery is less than 22) • Primiparity • Alcohol • Substance abuse • Drugs • Smoking • Viral infections • Vascular Disruption • Ethnicity	• HESX1 • SOX2 • SOX3 • OTX2

8.4 Pathophysiology

As discussed in etiology section that this disease is multifactorial and these factors whether environmental or genetic both are important while discussing the pathogenesis of the disease. Environment and genetic factors are described separately under their respective sections as follow:

8.4.1 Environmental Factors

Vascular disruption can explain the pathogenesis according to Lubinsky's hypothesis. SOD involve structures that are generally predisposed to the vascular disruption. These structures have generally different place of origin so compromising blood supply might contribute to the hypoplasia of involved entities. The artery that is generally involved is proximal trunk of anterior cerebral artery. By focusing on some anatomy of this artery we came to know that it arises from internal carotid artery and give rise to anterior communicating artery (as a part of circle of Willis) to supply brain. Part of artery lying between its origin and origin of anterior communicating artery is lying in close association of optic nerve, chiasma, septum pellucidum and inferior pituitary. Its inferior branches supply optic tract superior part and chiasma while its superior branches supply septum pellucidum and anterior pituitary. Its disruption usually results in development of SOD [5, 8, 9]. This can be applied to broader aspect when also taking into account other arteries in circle of Willis rather anterior cerebral artery. Anterior perforated substance, mammillary bodies, optic tract, optic nerve and chiasma locating in sellar and suprasellar regions are supplied by anterior choroidal artery and perforating arteries. So, disruption of these can also result in SOD [5].

Many studies till today have identifies young maternal age is the possible risk factor towards the pathogenesis of SOD because it is much prevalent in infants born to mothers between 20 and 24 years of age [9].

Besides ethnicity have also been recognized as a risk factor being disease more prevalent in Afro-Caribbean and mixed-race groups and very much low number of cases in South Asian groups when compared with Birmingham and Midland city data [7].

Finally, alcohol, substance abuse, viral infections and some drugs exposures have also been associated in development of DOD.

8.4.2 Genetic Factors

During embryogenesis certain genes play an important role in the genesis of the structures. These are mostly transcriptional factors that act on DNA and modify the expression of other genes. By altering the functions of these genes through mutations severe events can ensue. Recently, few genes have been identified that are responsible for the development of structures that are involved in SOD. Mutations can occur in them and can contribute to the development of SOD. Many mutations can occur in a single gene that can contribute to variety of affects. Also, they can interact with environmental factors. Less than 1% of familial cases that are reported attribute their disease to the genetic dysfunction. They can occur as a result of autosomal dominant or recessive pattern. Autosomal recessive pattern has full penetrance while that of autosomal dominant has variable penetrance. These mutations can occur sporadically and as a result have a great role in sporadic nature of disease [10–13]. Following is the explanation of the genes that are detected in SOD:

HESX1 a transcriptional repressor and a paired-like homeobox gene is detected in murine pituitary development as an earliest marker. Its expression is restricted in the thickened ectoderm that will give rise to Rathke's pouch (primordia of anterior pituitary) and ventral part of diencephalon. It is expressed till 12th week of embryonic life and its expression finally disappeared by 13th week. SOD like manifestation occurs when a homozygous mutation ensues in mice. In spite of variable expression due to different mutations they are fully penetrant. Microcephaly, short forebrain, optic vesicle absence, craniofacial abnormalities, olfactory placodes absence, Rathke's pouch abnormalities and hypothalamic anomalies occur in mice [14]. Consider similar manifestations between mice and patients of SOD, homozygous mutations have been detected in siblings of consanguineous couples and thus a link is established between *Hesx1* and SOD [11, 14]. Homozygosity of mutation have been associated with severe phenotypes like aplasia of pituitary and corpus callosum. By screening a number of patients with SOD 8 heterozygous and 5 homozygous mutations have been found. They have variable phenotypes. Below there is table that list these mutations, their inheritance pattern, associated endocrine phenotype and imaging findings [4].

Next are the members of SOX family of transcription factors that are present on the sex determining region of SRY. They were first discovered on the basis of homology to the conserved binding motif of High motility group (HMG) class. About 20 distinct SOX genes have been discovered in mammals. They are grouped into different families based on the variation in homology present in HMG area. SOX2 and SOX3 are the genes that are associated with the SOD. They along with SOX1 are the members of SOXB1 subfamily [15, 16].

SOX2 is expressed in the CNS, esophagus, trachea, gut endoderm, branchial arches and sensory placodes. When both alleles are lost the results are very much lethal but heterozygous results in male infertility and reduced size in mice. When expression below 40% it results in anophthalmia. Mutations in *SOX2* results in hypoplasia of pituitary, corpus callosum defects, bilateral ophthalmia, sensorineural hearing loss, developmental delay, genital abnormalities, esophageal atresia and learning difficulties. Below table shows the SOX2 mutations and their associated ophthalmologic manifestations and pituitary phenotype [4].

SOX3 present on X chromosome is expressed throughout the nervous system and is also present in developmental early stages. It has a strong role in neurogenesis. High expressions are present in diencephalon ventral part [17–19]. In mice mutations leads to midline CNS defects, reduction in fertility and size, craniofacial defects and growth insufficiency. It also leads to hypopituitarism. It is associated with abnormal Rathke's pouch development due to higher expression in infundibulum which is a part of diencephalon [17, 19]. Duplications involving region of X-chromosome have been identified in humans. The resultant X-linked phenotype in male present with hypopituitarism along with developmental delay or mental retardation. Females can remain unaffected due to their preference of lyonization duplicated X chromosome. In rare cases females can affected that might be due to disruption of *SOX3* by duplication leading to hemizygosity in female patients. These present with hypopituitarism lead short stature, facial abnormalities, language and speech issues and hearing loss. Discovering the expansion of one of the polyalanine tracts in the gene of *SOX3* shows that it might be associated in X-linked hypopituitarism. This is due to loss of function mutation leading to hypothalamic infundibular hypoplasia. Thus, infundibular hypoplasia is strongly associated with duplication of gene and loss of function mutations due to polyalanine expansion in *SOX3* leading to pituitary hypoplasia. Therefore, normal expression of *SOX3* is very much important for appropriate development of diencephalon, infundibulum and pituitary gland [4].

8.5   Diagnosis

Diagnosis of SOD is a clinical. It is made when ≥2 of the following classic characteristics of triad is present in a patient:

- Midline brain abnormalities (Having agenesis of septum pellucidum and/or corpus callosum)
- Optic nerve hypoplasia
- Hypothalamic-Pituitary axis abnormalities

SOD can manifest soon after birth along with other congenital anomalies. It can also present later in life when growth failure occurs in child together with abnormalities of visual system like nystagmus, squint etc. Many cases have good prognosis when diagnosis is made early in the disease. This because patients are usually are suffering from hypopituitarism and when it is appropriate managed early it can lead to adrenal crisis and death. Differential diagnosis of SOD should be kept in mind when a neonate present with jaundice, cryptorchidism, micropenis, hypoglycemia with or without midline anomalies like cleft lip or palate. In such patient's ophthalmologic consultation must be taken and endocrine tests must be done to determine the baseline endocrine functions of the body. Diagnosis is made with neuroimaging such as MRI and pituitary diagnostic test. As hormonal deficiencies can be lethal so endocrine deficiencies must be managed earlier in conjunction with referral to neurodevelopmental teams for assessment of abnormalities in vision. These infants are typically referred to specialist centers for special care. Table outlines of the important points that shouldn't be missed in history, neuroimaging, endocrine tests and ophthalmologic examination [1].

8.5.1 History

Septo-optic dysplasia is a genetic disease which usually is sporadic in nature, but sometimes is found to have autosomal inheritance, most commonly recessive but sometimes dominant pattern is also observed, thus, running in families as well [1, 24, 25]. So, the first question after biodata should be about the reported cases of this disease in family.

This disease is associated with mother's age, more commonly occurring in children of younger and primigravid mothers. Maternal age should be noted. Gestational diabetes has also been found to be a risk factor for this disease. This should be included in history. Preterm birth is another associated factor [25]. This should also be asked while taking history (Table 8.2).

One of the important findings in this disease is hearing abnormality. Auditory status should be asked from the patient or attendants.

Developmental pattern should be asked. There is developmental delay in septo-optic dysplasia. Questions about growth of the patient should be asked from the parents or attendants of the patient. Loss of sense of smell is a finding in this disease. Response of the patient towards different smells and aromas should be inquired. Or if there is total lack of sense of smell, this should be asked as well. Autistic behavior is associated with disease. There should be questions to confirm it as well. It should be asked from the parents if the child shows repetitive behavior. Flapping of hands should be inquired. It should be asked if the patient has tendency to play with similar set of toys in a similar pattern. All these questions can help make diagnosis of autism in the patient. Seizures and arrhythmicity in sleep are more findings which can give clue about this disease. So, there should be questions related to pattern of sleep and if any seizures are ever observed.

Table 8.2 Important points in evaluation of septo-optic dysplasia

History	Neuroimaging

• Relation of parents before marriage i.e., Consanguinity
• Smelling status
• Hearing status
• Other birth defects like esophageal atresia or micropenis
• Seizures that might be due to structural abnormalities of brain or hypoglycemia
• Repetitive behaviors like in autism spectrum disorder
• Any abnormality in sleep i.e., arrhythmicity [20]
• Appetite abnormalities
• Temperature regulation
• Developmental milestones
• Symptomology of hormonal deficiencies like polyuria, polydipsia, fatigue etc.
	MRI is the preferred imaging because it gives detailed neuroanatomical imaging. In SOD special attention must be given to following:
	• Septum pellucidum
	• Corpus callosum
	• Optic nerve and chiasma anomalies
	• Other defects such as fornix aplasia, cerebellar hypoplasia or schizencephaly
	• Appearance of hypothalamic-pituitary axis. Is it normal or not? It must be checked specifically for
	  – Infundibular thickness
	  – Location and presence of posterior pituitary
	  – Size of anterior pituitary
	Typical MRI images shows Septum pellucidum agenesis, corpus callosum abnormalities, one sided or both sided optic nerve or chiasma hypoplasia and anomalies associated with hypothalamic-pituitary axis [21].

Pituitary Testing	Ophthalmologic Examination

• Observe pubertal changes-precocious puberty can occur due to hypothalamic dysfunction or it may result in secondary hypogonadism due to FSH and LH deficiency.
• Cortisol level
  – Children >1 year of age have early morning 8 AM cortisol test
  – Children ≤1 can undergo random cortisol test
  – Abnormal results are proceeded further by ACTH stimulation test and blood glucose levels
• Thyroid function test
• Fluid intake-if polydipsia is present than serum and urine osmolalities are calculated and diabetes insipidus is confirmed with water deprivation test.
• Growth hormone
  – Growth is monitored and if growth velocity is inadequate provocation testing is done and GH response is measured in age > 1 year.
  – History of hypoglycemia and glucose levels are measured on hydrocortisone supplementation because adrenal insufficiency is also present with hypoglycemia. If hypoglycemia is present than measure insulin growth factor-1 level and give GH hormone replacement.
	• Measure severity of visual impairment
	• See if signs of coloboma, ONH, microphthalmia, anophthalmia or other abnormalities is present or not?
	• Evaluate squint and nystagmus and if present either it is present in one or both eyes
	• Assess the presence of clinical signs of ONH such as small and pale optic disc, double ring sign and DD/DM ratios (horizontal disc diameter divided by distance between macula to temporal margin of disc; ≤0.35 is generally associated with ONH) [22].
	• Optic coherence tomography (OCT) shows thinning of several retinal layers at fovea particularly in retinal nerve fiber layer and ganglionic cell layer [23].

There is an increase in appetite in this disease. This should be asked as well, by including questions related to pattern of eating and quantity of food consumed in a day. Moreover, there should be inquiry of pattern of defecation, as constipation is a finding in this disease. There are hormonal abnormalities in this disease. One of the findings in this disease is increased sweating. Therefore, Questions about sweating should also be asked. It is found that septo-optic dysplasia is often associated with hair loss. So, hair loss should be inquired [1]. Diabetes insipidus is often associated with septo-optic dysplasia. It should be investigated that how many water is consumed by the patient in a day. Moreover, frequency of urination and urine color should be asked.

All these questions in history can help make diagnosis of this disease.

8.5.2 Examination

In order to confirm the diagnosis, multiple relevant examinations should be performed. Some of these examinations are described next.

This disease alters auditory functions. Hearing is badly affected. Usually, the hearing loss is of sensorineural type. But in some cases, mixed type of hearing loss has also been reported. Conductive type of hearing loss being equally common as mixed type, in this disease. In 63% cases sensorineural type of hearing loss was reported, in 14% cases mixed type of hearing loss was found and again in 14% cases conductive type of hearing loss was reported [26].

In order to test this, tuning fork tests should be performed. Rinne and Weber test are the most important tests to be performed. There are some other tests as well that can be performed to assess the hearing abilities of the patient suffering from septo-optic dysplasia. These tests include finger friction test, watch test and speech or voice tests. Some other tuning fork tests can also be performed. These include absolute bone conduction test, Schwabach's test and Gelle's test. Thus, all above tests can confirm the abnormalities in hearing and can determine the type of hearing loss. These tests can also give an estimate of degree of hearing loss.

Another finding in this disease is loss of sense of smell. Loss of sense of smell also can be at different levels. Multiple tests are available to assess the olfactory pathway. Physical examination can be done to check the nose. Anterior rhinoscopy can be performed to check the obstruction of olfactory cleft, but it is only 50% efficient. Nasal endoscopy can help determine the anatomical issues with olfactory bulb. Tumors can also be detected. Thus, helping to determine if the cause of loss of sense of smell is at the level of sensory organ.

Some psychological tests can also be performed, these include olfactory threshold tests and odor identification tests [27]. Hence, the above-mentioned methods of examination can be used to determine if the patient has loss of sense of smell.

Autism is another finding in this disease. In order to confirm if autistic behavior is present, the clinician has to rely on history mainly. However, some tests are available, the Autism Diagnostic Interview-Revised (ADI-R) and the Autism Diagnostic

Observation Schedule (ADOS) are considered to be gold standard tests for diagnosing autistic behavior [28]. Thus, history along with these examination tests can help determine if autistic behavior is present.

It has been found that in septo-optic dysplasia there are problems with visual system as well. Multiple examination tests are available to determine if there is any problem with vision. Ophthalmoscopy and retinoscopy can be used to assess in the inside of eye. Visual acuity is important, as it's always decreased in all types of visual problems. Strabismus and nystagmus are commonly found in individuals suffering from septo-optic dysplasia. Cover-uncover test can help determine Strabismus [29].

8.5.3 *Investigations*

After noting findings from history, clinical examinations can help in making diagnosis of septo-optic dysplasia. But to confirm the diagnosis, multiple lab investigations can be performed. All these lab investigations aim at confirming the presence of abnormalities associated with septo-optic dysplasia. Most important of the artifacts are found in brain, glands and levels of different hormones in the blood. For this purpose, MRI of brain and laboratory measurements of levels of different hormones can be done, so that diagnosis of septo-optic dysplasia can be confirmed.

MRI should be performed. There is a change in hypothalamo-pituitary axis. Moreover, sizes of anterior and posterior pituitary glands should be checked. Presence of septum pellucidum should be confirmed. Appearance of corpus callosum should be checked. In septo-optic dysplasia, typical findings in MRI are agenesis of septum pellucidum, hypoplasia (either unilateral or bilateral) of optic nerves, hypoplasia of cerebellum, aplasia of fornix and change in hypothalamo-pituitary axis.

Next, hormonal abnormalities should be assessed. Thyroid function is affected in septo-optic dysplasia. To check thyroid function, TSH levels should be checked. Cortisol levels are not normal in septo-optic dysplasia. Therefore, assessment of levels of cortisol in blood should be performed. If levels of cortisol are found to be abnormal, synacthen test should be performed. Glucose profile should also check in the presence of abnormal cortisol function.

In patients of septo-optic dysplasia, there is abnormal growth hormone function. Low levels of growth hormone with its associated effects is a common finding in patients of septo-optic dysplasia. Poor growth can hint towards this. Measurement of growth hormone levels should be done.

Pubertal status should be checked. It is found that septo-optic dysplasia is associated with precocious puberty in some cases. It is caused by abnormal function of hypothalamus. As a result of lack of Follicle Stimulating Hormone (FSH) and Leutinizing Hormone (LH), there is hypogonadotrophic hypogonadism. This leads to precocious puberty.

Diabetes insipidus is another finding in patients of septo-optic-dysplasia. To confirm the presence of diabetes insipidus, daily fluid intake by patient should be inquired. If it is found that the fluid intake is excessive, then urine osmolality and fasting plasma osmolality, both should be checked simultaneously. Moreover, water deprivation test can also be performed. All these tests can confirm the diagnosis of diabetes insipidus [1].

8.6 Treatment

Septo-optic dysplasia is a genetic disease with a wide spectrum of symptoms involving multiple systems of the body. Therefore, treatment of this disease involves multidisciplinary management. Regular follow-ups are required (at least six monthly). Management of septo-optic-dysplasia aims at identifying the existing problems associated with this disease and striving for their treatment. Abnormalities are commonly found in multiple hormonal levels, vision, growth, development of brain and associated disorders like diabetes insipidus and autism. Therefore, in management of septo-optic-dysplasia, ailments are identified and efforts are made to correct them [1, 30].

Hormonal abnormalities are commonly associated with septo-optic dysplasia. Hormonal replacement therapy is performed to rectify the issues arising due to abnormal levels of certain hormones. Most frequently affected hormones are thyroid hormone, growth hormone, LH, FSH and other pituitary hormones. The main aim of hormone replacement therapy is to bring the levels of affected hormones into normal range so that normal body functions can be maintained. Levothyroxine [31], GnRH analogs, and Growth hormone analogs are given so that normal body functions maintained by these hormones can be achieved [30]. These resolves problems caused by hormonal dysfunction like hypoglycemia, stunted growth, profuse sweating, hair loss, abnormal sexual development and diabetes insipidus.

Vision is commonly affected in patients with septo-optic dysplasia. Therefore, treatment by an ophthalmologist is also required. Aim of vision therapy is to restore normal visual function. Common visual problems encountered in septo-optic dysplasia include strabismus, nystagmus, amblyopia, poor visual acuity, abnormal pupil function and blindness. Surgery can be performed to correct strabismus [30]. For amblyopia visual therapy can be done, after correcting root cause of amblyopia. Visual acuity can be corrected by use of contact lenses or glasses. By adopting above mentioned clinical methods, problems involving vision can be corrected.

Psychiatric symptoms are also associated with septo-optic dysplasia. Autistic behavior is observed in patients suffering from septo-optic dysplasia. Psychiatric treatment along with counseling is very important. Behavioral approaches are most significant in treating the symptoms of autism [30]. Obesity is another finding in this disease. Dietary modifications is necessary to control obesity. Therefore, the patient should be provided with a proper dietary plan and it should be reviewed in follow ups. Patient should be advised to make a record of his weight. Weakness in body muscles can be corrected by physical therapy. Specific exercises should be advised. Septo-optic dysplasia has a higher chance of occurrence in consanguineous families. Therefore, counselling should be done. Parents should be advised that there is 25% chance of septo-optic-dysplasia occurring in their next child [30].

Thus, septo-optic dysplasia has a broad spectrum of symptoms and involves multiple organs of the body. Therefore, multidisciplinary approach is to be adopted and a team of specialists of different clinical fields have to work together and coordinate for the management of septo-optic-dysplasia.

Multiple Choice Questions

1. **Which of the following statements is correct?**

   (a) Septo-optic dysplasia is associated with mother's age
   (b) Gestational diabetes has also been found to be a risk factor for septo-optic dysplasia
   (c) Children of primigravid mothers are not at risk
   (d) Pre-term birth is not found to be associated with septo-optic dysplasia
   (e) Septo-optic dysplasia is an acquired disease

2. **Which one of the followings is associated with septo-optic dysplasia?**

   (a) obsessive compulsive disorder
   (b) Depression
   (c) Autism
   (d) Congestive Heart Failure
   (e) Marfan's Syndrome

3. **Diabetes found in septo-optic dysplasia is caused by:**

   (a) Less efficiency of kidneys
   (b) Over efficiency of kidneys
   (c) Lack of anti-diuretic hormone
   (d) Atrophy of bladder
   (e) Excessive drinking of water

4. **Which one of the following types is true?**

   (a) There is no hearing loss
   (b) Sensorineural type of hearing loss occurs
   (c) Conductive type of hearing loss occurs
   (d) Both conductive and sensorineural hearing loss occurs
   (e) None is correct

5. **Visual problems are associated with septo-optic dysplasia. Which one of the followings does not occur in septo-optic dysplasia?**

   (a) Strabismus
   (b) Nystagmus
   (c) Reduced visual acuity
   (d) Cataract
   (e) Amblyopia

6. **Septo-optic dysplasia is a genetic disorder affecting brain. Which of the following in a typical finding in MRI of such a patient?**

   (a) Edema in brain
   (b) Hemorrhage in cranial vessels
   (c) Change in hypothalamo-pituitary axis
   (d) Tumors in brain
   (e) Hypertrophy of pituitary gland

7. **One of the followings statements is not correct for septo-optic dysplasia. Point out:**

   (a) Thyroid hormone secretion is raised
   (b) There is excessive growth leading to gigantism
   (c) Over secretion of anti-diuretic hormone leads to stone formation in kidneys
   (d) There is lack of secretion of hormones released by hypothalamus
   (e) There are no hormonal abnormalities

8. **What is the status of blood sugar level in septo-optic dysplasia?**

   (a) Hyperglycemia is a typical finding
   (b) Hypoglycemia is a typical finding
   (c) There is no abnormality in blood glucose level
   (d) HbA1c level is raised
   (e) Fasting blood glucose level is raised

9. **Septo-optic dysplasia affects multiple organs of the body. Which of the following organs is not affected:**

   (a) Brain
   (b) Kidneys
   (c) Eyes
   (d) Ear
   (e) Nose

10. **Septo-optic dysplasia is a genetic disorder. It is true that:**

   (a) It has autosomal recessive pattern of inheritance
   (b) It has autosomal dominant pattern of inheritance
   (c) It is sporadic in nature
   (d) It is usually sporadic in nature, but sometimes has autosomal (both recessive and dominant inheritance)
   (e) None of the above is correct

Answers:
   1. a
   2. c
   3. c
   4. d

5. d
6. c
7. d
8. b
9. b
10. d

References

1. Webb EA, Dattani MT. Septo-optic dysplasia. Eur J Hum Genet. 2010;18(4):393–7. https://doi.org/10.1038/ejhg.2009.125. Epub 2009 Jul 22. PMID: 19623216; PMCID: PMC2987262.
2. Ganau M, Huet S, Syrmos N, Meloni M, Jayamohan J. Neuro-ophthalmological manifestations of septo-optic dysplasia: current perspectives. Eye Brain. 2019;11:37–47. https://doi.org/10.2147/EB.S186307. PMID: 31695544; PMCID: PMC6805786.
3. Miller SP, Shevell MI, Patenaude Y, Poulin C, O'Gorman AM. Septo-optic dysplasia plus: a spectrum of malformations of cortical development. Neurology. 2000;54(8):1701–3. https://doi.org/10.1212/wnl.54.8.1701. PMID: 10762523.
4. Kelberman D, Dattani MT. Septo-optic dysplasia—novel insights into the aetiology. Horm Res. 2008;69(5):257–65. https://doi.org/10.1159/000114856. Epub 2008 Feb 6. PMID: 18259104.
5. Chiaramonte I, Cappello G, Uccello A, Guarrera V, D'Amore A, Cavallaro T, Chiaramonte R, Ettorre GC. Vascular cerebral anomalies associated with septo-optic dysplasia. a case report. Neuroradiol J. 2013;26(1):66–70. https://doi.org/10.1177/197140091302600111. Epub 2013 Mar 8. PMID: 23859170; PMCID: PMC5278866.
6. Patel L, McNally RJ, Harrison E, Lloyd IC, Clayton PE. Geographical distribution of optic nerve hypoplasia and septo-optic dysplasia in Northwest England. J Pediatr. 2006;148(1):85–8. https://doi.org/10.1016/j.jpeds.2005.07.031. PMID: 16423603.
7. Atapattu N, Ainsworth J, Willshaw H, Parulekar M, MacPherson L, Miller C, Davies P, Kirk JM. Septo-optic dysplasia: antenatal risk factors and clinical features in a regional study. Horm Res Paediatr. 2012;78(2):81–7. https://doi.org/10.1159/000341148. Epub 2012 Aug 14. PMID: 22907285.
8. Lubinsky MS. Hypothesis: septo-optic dysplasia is a vascular disruption sequence. Am J Med Genet. 1997;69(3):235–6. PMID: 9096749.
9. Garne E, Rissmann A, Addor MC, Barisic I, Bergman J, Braz P, Cavero-Carbonell C, Draper ES, Gatt M, Haeusler M, Klungsoyr K, Kurinczuk JJ, Lelong N, Luyt K, Lynch C, O'Mahony MT, Mokoroa O, Nelen V, Neville AJ, Pierini A, Randrianaivo H, Rankin J, Rouget F, Schaub B, Tucker D, Verellen-Dumoulin C, Wellesley D, Wiesel A, Zymak-Zakutnia N, Lanzoni M, Morris JK. Epidemiology of septo-optic dysplasia with focus on prevalence and maternal age—a EUROCAT study. Eur J Med Genet. 2018;61(9):483–8. https://doi.org/10.1016/j.ejmg.2018.05.010. Epub 2018 May 10. PMID: 29753093.
10. Benner JD, Preslan MW, Gratz E, Joslyn J, Schwartz M, Kelman S. Septo-optic dysplasia in two siblings. Am J Ophthalmol. 1990;109(6):632–7. https://doi.org/10.1016/s0002-9394(14)72430-4. PMID: 2346191.
11. Wales JK, Quarrell OW. Evidence for possible Mendelian inheritance of septo-optic dysplasia. Acta Paediatr. 1996;85(3):391–2. https://doi.org/10.1111/j.1651-2227.1996.tb14044.x. PMID: 8696006.
12. Tajima T, Hattorri T, Nakajima T, Okuhara K, Sato K, Abe S, Nakae J, Fujieda K. Sporadic heterozygous frameshift mutation of HESX1 causing pituitary and optic nerve hypoplasia and combined pituitary hormone deficiency in a Japanese patient. J Clin Endocrinol Metab. 2003;88(1):45–50. https://doi.org/10.1210/jc.2002-020818. PMID: 12519827.

13. Thomas PQ, Dattani MT, Brickman JM, McNay D, Warne G, Zacharin M, Cameron F, Hurst J, Woods K, Dunger D, Stanhope R, Forrest S, Robinson IC, Beddington RS. Heterozygous HESX1 mutations associated with isolated congenital pituitary hypoplasia and septo-optic dysplasia. Hum Mol Genet. 2001;10(1):39–45. https://doi.org/10.1093/hmg/10.1.39. PMID: 11136712.

14. Dattani MT, Martinez-Barbera JP, Thomas PQ, Brickman JM, Gupta R, Mårtensson IL, Toresson H, Fox M, Wales JK, Hindmarsh PC, Krauss S, Beddington RS, Robinson IC. Mutations in the homeobox gene HESX1/Hesx1 associated with septo-optic dysplasia in human and mouse. Nat Genet. 1998;19(2):125–33. https://doi.org/10.1038/477. PMID: 9620767.

15. Stevanović M, Lovell-Badge R, Collignon J, Goodfellow PN. SOX3 is an X-linked gene related to SRY. Hum Mol Genet. 1993;2(12):2013–8. https://doi.org/10.1093/hmg/2.12.2013. PMID: 8111369

16. Pevny LH, Lovell-Badge R. Sox genes find their feet. Curr Opin Genet Dev. 1997;7(3):338–44. https://doi.org/10.1016/s0959-437x(97)80147-5. PMID: 9229109.

17. Rizzoti K, Brunelli S, Carmignac D, Thomas PQ, Robinson IC, Lovell-Badge R. SOX3 is required during the formation of the hypothalamo-pituitary axis. Nat Genet. 2004;36(3):247–55. https://doi.org/10.1038/ng1309. Epub 2004 Feb 15. PMID: 14981518.

18. Pevny L, Placzek M. SOX genes and neural progenitor identity. Curr Opin Neurobiol. 2005;15(1):7–13. https://doi.org/10.1016/j.conb.2005.01.016. PMID: 15721738.

19. Bylund M, Andersson E, Novitch BG, Muhr J. Vertebrate neurogenesis is counteracted by Sox1-3 activity. Nat Neurosci. 2003;6(11):1162–8. https://doi.org/10.1038/nn1131. Epub 2003 Sep 28. PMID: 14517545.

20. Rivkees SA. Arrhythmicity in a child with septo-optic dysplasia and establishment of sleep-wake cyclicity with melatonin. J Pediatr. 2001;139(3):463–5. https://doi.org/10.1067/mpd.2001.117074. PMID: 11562632.

21. Mehta A, Hindmarsh PC, Mehta H, Turton JP, Russell-Eggitt I, Taylor D, Chong WK, Dattani MT. Congenital hypopituitarism: clinical, molecular and neuroradiological correlates. Clin Endocrinol. 2009;71(3):376–82. https://doi.org/10.1111/j.1365-2265.2009.03572.x. Epub 2009 Mar 6. PMID: 19320653.

22. Borchert M, Garcia-Filion P. The syndrome of optic nerve hypoplasia. Curr Neurol Neurosci Rep. 2008;8(5):395–403. https://doi.org/10.1007/s11910-008-0061-7. PMID: 18713575.

23. Pilat A, Sibley D, McLean RJ, Proudlock FA, Gottlob I. High-resolution imaging of the optic nerve and retina in optic nerve hypoplasia. Ophthalmology. 2015;122(7):1330–9. https://doi.org/10.1016/j.ophtha.2015.03.020. Epub 2015 May 1. PMID: 25939636; PMCID: PMC4518044.

24. Septo-optic dysplasia. In: Diagnostic imaging: obstetrics. Elsevier; 2016. p. 126–9.

25. Signorini SG, Decio A, Fedeli C, Luparia A, Antonini M, Bertone C, et al. Septo-optic dysplasia in childhood: the neurological, cognitive and neuro-ophthalmological perspective: septo-optic dysplasia in childhood. Dev Med Child Neurol. 2012;54(11):1018–24. https://doi.org/10.1111/j.1469-8749.2012.04404.x.

26. Herrmann BW, Hathaway CR, Fadell M. Hearing loss in pediatric septo-optic dysplasia. Ann Otol Rhinol Laryngol. 2019;128(6):485–9. https://pubmed.ncbi.nlm.nih.gov/30781969/. Cited 6 Nov 2022.

27. Wrobel BB, Leopold DA. Clinical assessment of patients with smell and taste disorders. Otolaryngol Clin N Am. 2004;37(6):1127–42. https://doi.org/10.1016/j.otc.2004.06.010. Cited 6 Nov 2022.

28. Rudacille D. How many tests does it take to diagnose autism? Spectrum|Autism Research News. 2011. Available from: https://www.spectrumnews.org/news/how-many-tests-does-it-take-to-diagnose-autism. Cited 6 Nov 2022.6

29. Hull S, Tailor V, Balduzzi S, Rahi J, Schmucker C, Virgili G, et al. Tests for detecting strabismus in children aged 1 to 6 years in the community. Cochrane Libr [Internet]. 2017;2017(11):CD011221. https://doi.org/10.1002/14651858.cd011221.pub2. Cited 7 Nov 2022.

30. Septo-Optic Dysplasia (SOD). Cleveland Clinic. Available from: https://my.clevelandclinic.org/health/diseases/22793-septo-optic-dysplasia-sod. cited 7 Nov 2022.
31. Stott DJ, Gussekloo J, Kearney PM, Rodondi N, Westendorp RGJ, Mooijaart S, et al. Study protocol; thyroid hormone replacement for untreated older adults with subclinical hypothyroidism—a randomised placebo controlled trial (TRUST). BMC Endocr Disord. 2017;17(1):6. https://doi.org/10.1186/s12902-017-0156-8.

Chapter 9
Pituitary Maldevelopment

F. A. Ameer and Ibrahim Saeed Gataa

9.1 Embryology

The pituitary gland is mainly composed of three lobes, the anterior lobe, posterior lobe, and intermittent lobe each lobe have a specific function and divide from a different embryological origin, the anterior lobe is derived from ectopic, the posterior lobe in the same extension of neuro tissue of the hypothalamus (for that reason called neurohypophysis) on the other hand intermediate part of pituitary came from homogenous tissue contain mainly melanocyte cell that produces α-methanotrophic (αMSH) (Fig. 9.1).

The anterior pituitary gland produces mainly five hormones (adrenocorticotrophin (ACTH), gonadotrophs, somatotrophs, lactotrophs, thyrotrophin), and also support cells (folliculostellate). The neural part or posterior lobe contains mainly the projection of hypothalamus cells that produce mainly two hormones (Vasopressin

F. A. Ameer (✉)
College of Medicine, University of Al-Qadisiyah, Al Diwaniyah, Iraq

I. S. Gataa
Oral and Maxillofacial Surgery, University of Warith Al-Anbiyaa, Karbala, Iraq
e-mail: ibraheem@uowa.edu.iq

© The Author(s), under exclusive license to Springer Nature Switzerland AG 2024
K. F. AlAli, H. T. Hashim (eds.), *Congenital Brain Malformations*,
https://doi.org/10.1007/978-3-031-58630-9_9

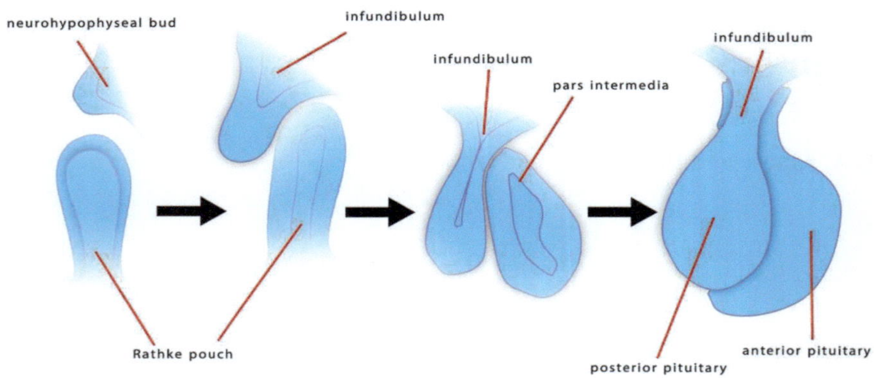

Fig. 9.1 Show normal development of the pituitary gland from week5–18, starting as Rathke pouch protrusion interacted with neurohypophyseal bud early in development, contacting the two layers to make new develop structure the pars intermedia and infundibulum on late development stage to for the three structures of adult pituitary gland anterior (endocrine) and posterior and infundibulum

and Oxytocin) and support cells. The intermediate part regresses embryologically on the 15th week, absent in adult humans.

9.1.1 Rathke Pouch

The Rathke pouch form the frontal part of the ectoderm, this part form the glandular or endocrine pituitary gland in the future. Fate-mapping study showing the central part of the oral ectoderm that invaginates to become the pituitary anlage [1]. Except for the pouch level, this invagination will form from continuous sustainable contact between two tissue neuroepithelium and the oral ectoderm. Due to genetic modification, this contact, which is crucial for the development of the pouch and pituitary development, is disturbed, resulting in an interruption of the pituitary development process [1, 2].

The data shows the importance of the development of this tissue with exchange signal and transcription factor between the diencephalon and pituitary development, so diencephalon development failure leads to secondary pituitary failure. According to data, the SOX3 mutation has been interconnected to pituitary insufficiency, anterior endoderm homeobox gene Rpx/Hesxl overexpression during gastrulation, and late Rathke pouch formation [3–5].

9.1.2 *Signals Controlling Pituitary Development*

Several, intricate expression patterns, as well as numerous signaling pathways, are involved in the organogenesis and development of the pituitary gland. BMP is well demonstrated in this complex process. Noggin antagonizes BMP4 blockade signaling and arrests the pituitary in the pouch stage, so Ectodermal pituitary anlage induction by BMP4 is commonly recognized [6, 7].

Shut down the Noggin gene critical to the important role of the BMP gene in the induction pathway, another expression that may regulate BMP signaling is Lhx3, Pitx factor [8]. Sonic Hedgehog (Shh) is one of the most important genes in expression during pituitary development although the Shh−/−mutant in mouse not heavily informative about the precise function of the Shh gene during the development of this structure main bulk. Furthermore, HIP overexpression which antagonizes the Shh gene shut down the development of the Rathke pouch [9] (Fig. 9.2).

Despite the presence of numerous Wnt molecules and receptor expressions near the pituitary structure, it is still challenging to create a comprehensive roadmap and understand the Wnt pathway's involvement in pituitary development. Prop1 expression has been attributed to cases of unidentified pituitary hormone deficiency, and Notch signaling is crucial for Prop1 expression throughout embryonic development. Notch2 signaling has no impact on early pituitary development [10, 11].

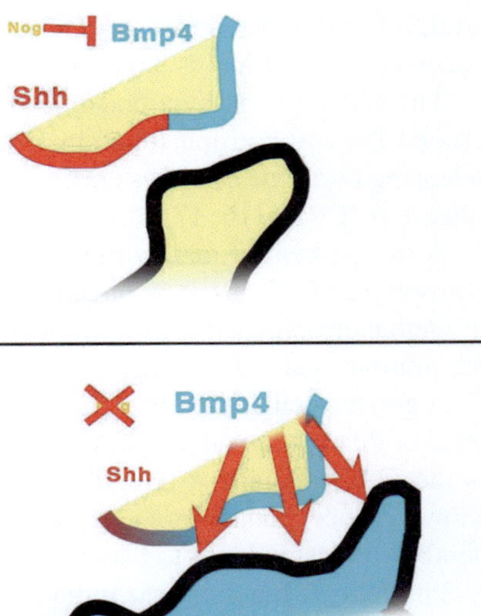

Fig. 9.2 Show the Innumerable anomalous invaginations of the oral ectoderm, Noggin's role in regulating Bmp4 during the development of the Rathke pouch, the effect of Bmp4 on the ventral diencephalon in blue, the lower domain in red, and a Noggin mutation embryo where the suppression effect is missed and the Bmp4 effect is increased

9.1.3   Cells Differentiation

Mature adult pituitary gland appears to be known by highly differentiated cell type, initial sight In the epithelial portion of the Rathke pouch, where corticotrophs differentiate from a common stem pool and thyrotrops develop from two lineages, early development is also influenced by a transcription factor that marks terminal differentiation, which is typically expressed hours before the hormone gene. Most assessments of this transcription factor mutation, in study demonstrating three lineages, to acquire appropriate insight into the link between distinct lineages. A transcription factor is required for somatotrophs, lactotrophs, and thyrotrophs. Pit-1 in Missense Mutation promotes Differentiation (Snell dwarf mouse) [12]. Pit-1-dependent compared clearly delineated melanotroph and gonadotroph lineages support the binary paradigm of pituitary cell differentiation [13].

Stem/Progenitor cell that is different from any terminal cell doesn't have any marker due to the rapid proliferation of these cells, These cells can participate in significant growth and development of the gland, We can identify at first time Putative pituitary stem through a cell sphere assay by using other tissue cell marker [14].

The first cell that reaches terminal differentiation is corticotroph, in fact, Pitx1/2 or Lhx3/4 mutant pituitary only cell to appear [8] Tpit gene Inactivation of the mouse showed corticotroph differentiation essential required for Tpit gene accordantly block the termination of corticotrophs cell lineage [13]. Tpit is a relatively straightforward performance indicator of corticotroph adenoma cells, in particular, because glucocorticoids have had no impact on its expression [15].

The activation by hypothalamic signals and the feedback by glucocorticoids are crucial for corticotroph function. The main mechanism by which corticotrophin-releasing hormone activates corticotroph function, POMC transcription, and ACTH release is (CRH) [16, 17].

A few percent of melanotrophs express POMC, but Tpit is necessary as a corticotroph for POMC expression. On the other hand, distinct regulators of the function of methanotrophic, which is predominantly secreted from the intermediate region of the pituitary gland [13, 18].

A gonadotroph function expression of the different transcription factors, the high level of Pitx1 in gonadotrophin compare to another lineage [19], another contributor is the GATA-2 gene to gonadotroph differentiation because shut down GATA-2 shows reduce gonadotroph expression, [20] Another window for FSH independently expression upon LH seen affected by Foxl2 gene (Fig. 9.3).

Pit1 loss-of-function was initially discovered when the Jackson and Snell dwarf mice were examined and found to possess Pit1 gene mutations. The Pit1 transcription factor is a Pou homeodomain that is necessary for labeling three lineages of somatotrophs, lactotrophs, and thyrotrophs for terminal differentiation. Since the

Fig. 9.3 Shows the effect of the Smad1/4 complex induced by Bmp (Smad complex translocates to the nucleus), leading to disrupts transcription activity of the Pitx and Tpit

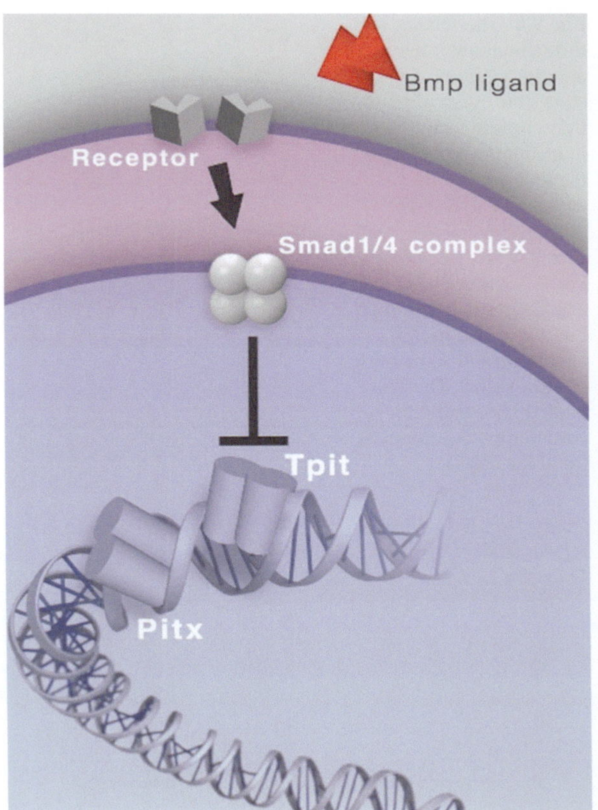

three Pit1-expressing lineages are lacking in these Pit1 mutant mice, this factor is essential for their final differentiation [21].

CPHD is caused becausea ofmutation in the Pit1 gene and PROP1 [12, 22]. The bHLH required Growth hormone and GHRH receptor expression as factor NeuroD4 (Math3) that is dependent on its expression on Pit1 [23].

Estrogen is a strong activator of lactotroph function this action is sustained mainly by the suppression of hypothalamic dopamine this function express by Prl, ERF estrogen repressor factor makes Prl a promotor and suppressor of dopamine [24].

Thyortrophs cells lineage is related to somatotroph and lactotrophs and also depends on GATA-2 on expressions such as factor shared with gonadotrophs Field [25]. Mutations in the genes Pit1, Prop1, SF1, Tpit, and Pax7 is one of the leading cause of pituitary hormone deficiencies (Fig. 9.4).

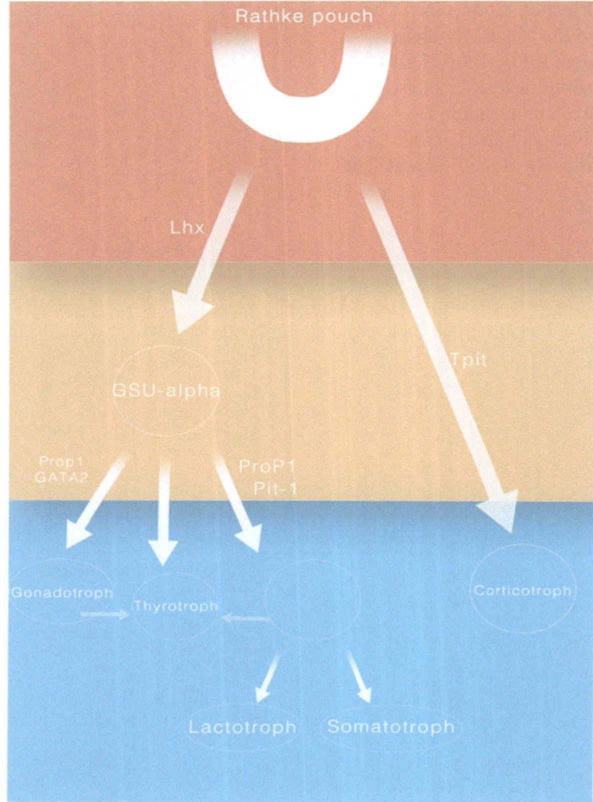

Fig. 9.4 The scheme on differentiation of the anterior pituitary gland shows the effect of transcription factor and homeodomain marker on the lineage of cell development, Rathke pouch stem cell affected by Lhx and Tpit (red color), Prop1 and GATA2 marker expressed in gonadotroph Pit1 expressed in lactotroph and somatotroph (yellow color). The Tpit marker is essential for corticotroph development (red-blue color)

9.2 Anatomy and Physiology

9.2.1 Anatomy

The pituitary gland is most a unique and interesting part of our body as anatomic speech, this small structure is located in a very special, protected in our skull. The blood supply very unique and different in how the vascular bed and portal get communicated or how the neuron part gets linked to the vascular part of the gland, and by far how this gland gets communicated literally with every glandular part in our body is just like a small hand that protruded from our brain to get control into everything glandular in the human body in a such complex way mostly consisting of three parts: (1) Pars distalis (2) Pars tuberalis (3) pars intermedia. Pars intermedia thought to produce POMC peptide regress and disappear in the adult pituitary gland, lifting two other components, tuberalis anatomically Speaking linking the pars distalis below to the hypothalamus above [26].

Adenohypophysis

The hypothalamus secretes inhibitory factors which in turn work as a signal to hormone release from the distal part which is mainly endocrine in nature through a capillary network linking these parts to each other [27]. (Fig. 9.5).

The distalis part is composed of five hormones secreted tissue that is named on the function of hormones also the hypothalamus secreted hormone may be the inhibitory or stimulatory name on the effect of this hormone, e.g.: Growth hormone-releasing factor from the hypothalamus that affects the somatotroph cell that in return secret Growth hormone which is responsible for many functions related to growth in human [26].

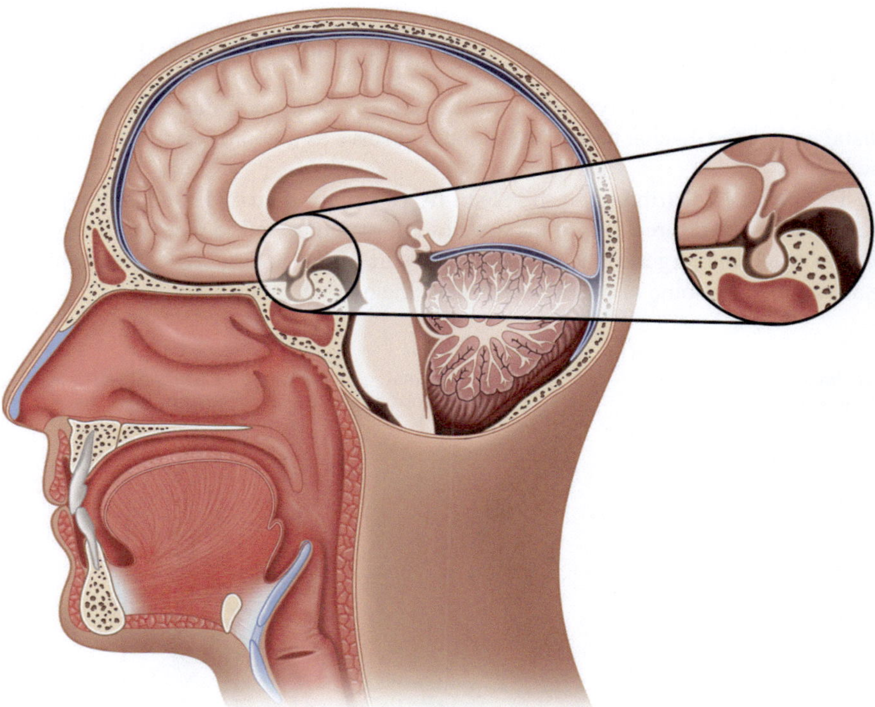

Fig. 9.5 The pituitary gland anatomy

Neurohypophysis

The neuron part of the pituitary gland work as a connection between the hypothalamus and the anterior part of the gland, in fact, it is a continuation of the hypothalamus itself [26, 27].

As we discussed in the embryology part is derived mainly from the neuroectoderm of the diencephalon.

As the name applied (the posterior pituitary) is located mainly behind the anterior part (adenohypophysis), That downward to form what is called the pituitary stalk which is mainly a large bundle of nerves, [27].

Vascularization

The main supply to the pituitary gland is by superior and inferior hypophysial arteries (Fig. 9.6).

The portal vein, supply vein! Join the network with the pituitary artery in the distal end of the distalis part of the gland and serve as a connection to the vascular bed [26].

The blood is distributed in the gland by two main roads: (1) adenohypophysis hormone secreted directly into the arteries and vascular bed to the circulatory system to reach the target tissue in a different part of the body (2) Neurohypophysis part supplied by some of this blood reaches the hypothalamus [28, 29].

Fig. 9.6 Cavernous sinus (Frontal section)

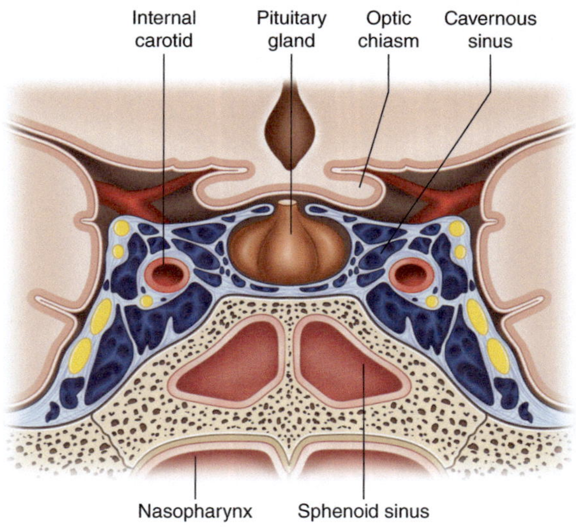

Fontal section: Cavernous sinus

Innervation

In fact, there is no direct nerve supply to the endocrine part of the gland, the main neuron part is a posterior gland, which serves as a communication or connection neuron bundle between the hypothalamus and anterior (endocrine part).

9.2.2   Physiology

CRH stands for corticotrophin-releasing hormone; GHRH stands for growth hormone-releasing hormone; and GnRH stands for gonadotrophin-releasing hormone. TSH stands for thyroxin-stimulating hormone. ACTH stands for adrenocorticotropic hormone. GH stands for growth hormone. LH stands for luteinizing hormone. FSH stands for follicle-stimulating hormone (Table 9.1).

First off, the brain signal acts differently throughout the course of a day, changing from a peak curve into a pulsatile and target pulse. The signal is sent to the hypothalamus, which in turn may stimulate or inhibit the pituitary gland, which in turn releases hormones known as trophs. Every gland in our body receives feedback from the pituitary trophs, which release hormones, so each gland either sends a signal to tissue to secrete more hormone or not, the level of each hormone in our body has the feedback on its gland secretion eg: Thyrotrophs releasing hormone secreted from the hypothalamus has an effect on the pituitary gland to secret the TSH which has a direct effect on a receptor found in the thyroid gland to release more T3/T4, this hormone has the negative feedback on TSH itself so when the T3/T4 increase in blood TSH decrease in response (Fig. 9.7).

Table 9.1 The hormonal effects and stimulations of the body

		Hypothalamus	Pituitary	Target
Stimulatory	TRH	Paraventricular	Thyrotroph, Lactotroph & **TSH**	Thyroid & T4, T3
	CRH	Paraventricular	Corticotroph & **ACTH**	Adrenal cortex & Cortisol androgens
	GHRH	Arcuate ventromedial	Somatotroph & **GH**	Liver & IGF-1
Inhibitory	GnRH	Mediobasal, infundibular, periventricular regions	Gonadotroph & **LH, FSH**	Gonads & Estrogen, testosterone progesterone
	Somatostatin	Periventricular paraventricular arcuate ventromedial	Somatotroph, thyrotroph, corticotroph & **GH, TSH, ACTH**	
	Dopamine	Arcuate periventricular	Lactotroph, thyrotroph, melanotroph & **GH, TSH, ACTH**	

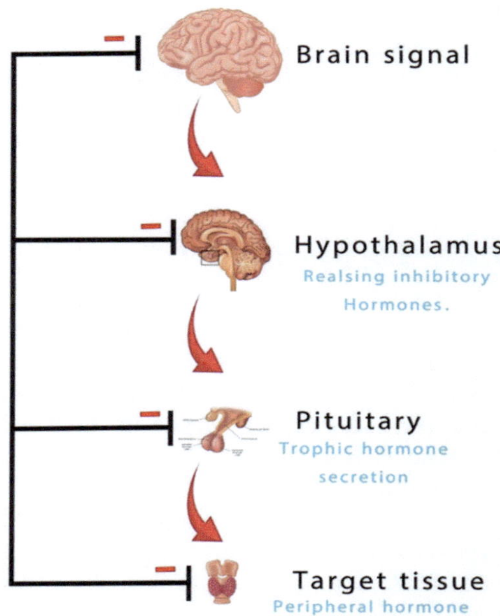

Fig. 9.7 Augmented the brain-hypothalamus-pituitary-target axis's physiological feedback

9.3 Pituitary Developmental Factor Mutation

9.3.1 *Prop1*

The Prop1 transcription-specific factor to pituitary development as discussed above, anterior pituitary restricted development depends mainly on this gene expression [10, 11]. New studies and evidence suggest Prop1 act an essential role in developing and stimulating the stem cells and pituitary structure organogenesis also necessary for cell migration and differentiation. Which is the most frequent cause of hypopituitarism and combined pituitary hormone insufficiency in humans are mutations in PROP1 [30, 31].

The variation and spectrum effect on the transcription factor defect show in patients with Prop1 mutation, even if the patient has an identical phenotype [32–34].

The wide open probability of Prop1 mutation, interesting cases showing before hypoplasia affect the hyperplasia changes, [35] dynamic effects of mutation from showing hypogonadism patient to develop another endocrine issue like adrenal insufficiency [32, 36, 37].

9.3.2 *Pit1*

Mutation in the Pou1f1 family which is a group of transcription factors in humans responsible for the development, in general, leads to a restricted anterior (endocrine) part of the pituitary [38, 39].

As we discussed previously Pit1 is essential and specific for the development of Somatotroph, Lactotrophs, and Thyrotrophs [12, 21, 22]. There is 28 different mutations have been discovered and described, for autosomal dominant was 5 and 23 autosomal recessives, so by far the recessive expression most common 78, also by far the most common mutation is R271W which leads to impaired dimerization through dominant inhibitor to transcription factor [40]. Many other point mutation has been described as affecting Pit1 leading to CPHD, some show shut or eliminate the transactivation of gene [41].

9.3.3 Shh–Gli2

Sonic hedgehog gene as previously mentioned one of the major genes in our system that play a critical role in urgent many tissues to differentiate and proliferated, in the pituitary gland organogenesis system act as a control expression of the Rathke pouch, ventral diencephalon [9].

As simple as that, in mice, if the Gli2 deficit leads to undifferentiated many structures but still pituitary development (for that and many reasons not considered as two mentioned above specific to the pituitary gland) but the three lineages will affect Corticotroph, somatotroph, lactotrophs [42].

In order to talk about Gli2 mutation, the first thing to mention there is no combined effect or disease as seen in specific type transcription factors, in addition, there is an unrelated endocrine association like polydactyly. Via one or more anterior pituitary lineage hormone deficiencies without the stated posterior section that may or may not be afflicted or hypoplastic in this problem, GH hormone deficiency alone may be identified without holoprocephalon or other defects [43].

9.3.4 Hesx1

Hesx1 mutations may lead to solitary growth hormone insufficiency or mixed pituitary hormone deficiency, either with or without septo-optic dysplasia. Qing Fang's study show patients who presented variable level and problem regarding pituitary development start from ACTH, TST, and GH deficiencies and end varying type of hypoplasia and aplasia in a different part of the pituitary gland, interestingly Hesx1 was shown to suppress the Prop1 transcription factor activation [44].

Variety in Hesx1 mutation has been investigated well regarding congenital hypopituitarism. Paul Q. Thomas scan 288 patients this patient was having broad-spectrum disease on the level of Hesx1 mutation and hypopituitarism, showing the association variety that came with mutation: 85 patients with isolated pituitary hypoplasia, 105 with septo-optic dysplasia, 38 with holoprosencephaly [45].

9.3.5 Lhx 3/4

The anterior and intermediate pituitary glands, as well as other regions like the spinal cord and the hindbrain, are affected by the expression of Lhx 3, which also acts as a transcription factor for a portion of the anterior and intermediate pituitary gland. In addition, well to mention associated expression and common projector stem cells through Lhx3 show expression of alfa–glycoprotein subunit which is, in turn, suggestive of the precursor of three lineages Corticotroph, Thyrotroph and somatotrophs, furthermore, expression of GH hormone and Prolactin [46, 47].

Lhx3 is one of the rare causes of CPHD [48], Lhx4 has the same impact as Lhx3 on disease and expression, a wide variety of diseases associated with a mutation from panpituitarism into IGHD with or without pituitary hypoplasia or with or without carpus callosum hypoplasia [49].

9.3.6 Other Transcription Factor Deficiency

Due to the role this gene plays in the expression and development of the rostral brain, Otx2 gene expression mutation has been linked to a variety of disorders, and pituitary shortages are linked to anomalies and issues [50].

Sox2 is one having an effect on pituitary development starting from early development on stem cell/progenitor cell level, this patient reported eye abnormalities [51] [52].

The FGF8 and FGFR1 genes have been historically reported in a patient with solitary hypogonadotropic hypogonadism [53].

Multiple Choice Questions
1. **A middle-aged patient from Iraq presented as a short, seemingly hypogonadal man with a height of less than 130 cm. Laboratory tests confirmed hypogonadotropic hypogonadism with low LH and FSH stimulation levels and testosterone below the detection threshold. Additional dynamic assessment of pituitary function revealed insufficient levels of somatotrope, thyrotrope, and lactotrophs. The anterior pituitary lobe was severely hypoplastic on MRI, although the posterior pituitary and the pituitary stalk appeared normal. The most common Transcription factor mutation leads to this condition?**

   (A) Prop1
   (B) Shh
   (C) Lhx3
   (D) Gli2

2. **A girl born consanguineously to parents of average height displayed slowed growth (height 90 cm) at their first presentation at age 5. Analysis in the lab revealed a GH deficit. The results of TSH and fT4 tests showed secondary hypothyroidism, although the levels of PRL serum were within the healthy range. The anterior pituitary lobe was hypoplastic on MRI, but the pituitary stalk and neurohypophysis were normal, as per MLPA analysis. PCR results will most likely suggest?**

   (A) Complete, homozygous loss of PROP1
   (B) Partial, heterozygous loss of Shh
   (C) Complete, homozygous loss of Gli2
   (D) Complete, heterozygous loss of Lhx3

3. **One girl and three boys from a consanguineous Iraqi marriage were among the four affected children. He did not exhibit any indicators of the beginning of puberty at age 17. While ACTH secretion was normal, laboratory tests revealed deficiencies in GH, TSH, gonadotropins, and PRL. Four unaffected brothers, a healthy sister, the parents, and all but one of their siblings had hemizygous PROP1 deletions, according to MLPA analysis. The affected people also had a complete loss of PROP1. Which of the following is suggesting the diagnosis if Prop1 mutation?**

   (A) Craniofacial abnormalities
   (B) slightly enlarged adenohypophysis
   (C) Posterior pituitary hypoplasia
   (D) Polydactyly
   (E) SOD

4. **A 43-year-old patient from Southern Iraq presented as a short, 120.4 cm tall female who was apparently hypogonadal. Additional dynamic assessment of pituitary function revealed insufficiency of somatotrope, thyrotrope, and lactotroph., On cranial nerve examination the patient suffered from hearing loss further follow-up and test show sensorineural type, Which of the following gene mutation did you expect the main cause of this presentation?**

   (A) HESX1
   (B) Prop1
   (C) SOX2
   (D) GLI2

5. **A male patient in his twenties who complained of nausea, vomiting, headaches, and dizziness underwent additional laboratory testing, which revealed a lack of GH, TSH, gonadotropins, and PRL, although ACTH secretion was normal. A hypoplastic Corpus callosum was discovered using magnetic resonance imaging (MRI), which type of mutation?**

   (A) Gli2
   (B) Shh

(C) Lhx 3/4
(D) Prop1
(E) Hox3

6. **Asian baby girl, 8 days old. After a routine pregnancy, she was born by a cesarean section at 39 weeks and 4 days of gestation due to fetal distress. Her parents have no blood ties. She had phototherapy and infusion therapy as well as being treated for hypoglycemia and jaundice. At 6 days old, we discovered that her TSH level was less than 0.01 IU/ml and her FT4 level was 0.4 pg/ml. What do you expect on MRI?**

   (A) Normal pituitary structure
   (B) Decrease size of the hypothalamus
   (C) Shrink pituitary gland
   (D) Non visible anterior pituitary gland
   (E) Non visible posterior pituitary gland

7. **A second-degree consanguineous family of four siblings, two of whom have combined pituitary hormone insufficiency. TSH, FSH/LH, and prolactin deficit were observed in two brothers, 32 and 35 years old. MLPA analysis confirms the diagnosis with Prop1 mutation. Which other hormone suggests the diagnosis?**

   (A) GH decrease
   (B) Cortisol increase
   (C) Aldosterone increase
   (D) Cortisol decease

8. **Which of the following gene act as a repressor to the Bmp4 transcription factor during the development of the Rathke pouch embryo?**

   (A) Shh
   (B) Wnt
   (C) Smad1/4
   (D) Sox2
   (E) Noggin

9. **A laboratory study of pituitary hormones in a 13-year-old boy with severe growth retardation revealed total or almost complete loss of somatotrope, lactotroph, and thyroidotrope, but normal corticotrope and gonadotrope activity. The anterior pituitary gland was found to be hypoplastic on magnetic resonance imaging (MRI). Which transcription factor mutation suggests this finding?**

   (A) Lhx3
   (B) Shh
   (C) Pouf1
   (D) Gli2

10. Which type of gene mutation is associated with Polydactyly?

(A) SOX2
(B) OTX2
(C) GLI2
(D) Prop1

Answers and Explanation

1. Ans A: By far the most cause is Prop1 mutation
2. Ans A: exhibited severe hypoplasia of the anterior pituitary lobe, whereas the pituitary stalk and posterior pituitary looked to be normal. This observation is consistent with the Prop1 mutation.
3. Ans B: hyperplasia then hypoplasia is one of the interesting finds in patients with Prop1 mutation, other choice suggests the transcription mutation.
4. Ans C: this presentation is typical for SOX mutation patients who suffer from deafness and other CPHD symptoms.
5. Ans C: hypoplastic corpus callosum with symptoms suggest CPHD most likely cause is Lhx mutation
6. Ans D: this patient shows signs and symptoms of congenital GH deficiency combined with other anterior pituitary endocrine defects, this suggests transcription factor mutation by fat the most common is Prop1.
7. Ans D: Prop1 associated reported in some cases associated with cortisol deficiency.
8. Ans E: effect of Noggin during Rathke pouch development regulating Bmp4, in Noggin mutation embryo the suppression effect is missed leading to an increase in the effect of the Bmp4.
9. Ans C: Pituitary hormone study in the lab revealed normal corticotrope and gonadotrope function, but total or virtually total loss of somatotrope, lactotroph, and thyrotrope.
10. Ans C: Polydactyly associated with Gli2 (Table 9.2)

Table 9.2 The genes and their associated findings

Gene	Association finding
Prop1	Other endocrine problems & hypoplasia to hyperplasia
GLI2	Polydactyly
HESX1	Optic nerve hypoplasia
LHX3	Cervical spine/vertebral anomalies
LHX4	Hypoplastic corpus callosum
OTX2	Micro- or anophthalmia
SOX2	Sensorineural hearing loss
SOX3	Craniofacial abnormalities

References

1. Daikoku S, Chikamori M, Adachi T, Maki AY. Effect of the basal diencephalon on the development of Rathke's pouch in rats: a study in combined organ cultures. Dev Biol. 1982;90:198–202. Received 26 May 1981; accepted in revised form 8 Oct 1981.
2. Kawamura K, Kikuyama S. Induction from posterior hypothalamus is essential for the development of the pituitary proopiomelacortin (POMC) cells of the toad (*Bufo japonicus*). Cell Tissue Res. 1995;279:233–9. Received 2 Feb 1994/Accepted 24 June 1994.
3. Rizzoti K, Brunelli S, Carmignac D, Thomas PQ, Robinson IC, Lovell-Badge R. SOX3 is required during the formation of the hypothalamo-pituitary axis. Nat Genet. 2004;36:247–55.
4. Zhao Y, Mailloux CM, Hermesz E, Palkovits M, Westphala H. A role of the LIM-homeobox gene Lhx2 in the regulation of pituitary development. Dev Biol. 2009;337:313–23.
5. Hermesz E, Williams-Simons L, Mahon KA. A novel inducible element, activated by contact with Rathke's pouch, is present in the regulatory region of the Rpx/Hesx1 homeobox gene. Dev Biol. 2003;260:68–78.
6. Treier M, Gleiberman AS, O'Connell SM, Szeto DP, McMahon JA, McMahon AP, Rosenfeld MG. Multistep signaling requirements for pituitary organogenesis in vivo. Genes Dev. 1998;12:1691–704.
7. Davis SW, Camper SA. Noggin regulates Bmp4 activity during pituitary induction. Dev Biol. 2007;305:145–60.
8. Nudi M, Ouimette J-F, Drouin J. Bone morphogenic protein (Smad)-mediated repression of proopiomelanocortin transcription by interference with Pitx/Tpit activity. Mol Endocrinol. 2005;19:1329–42.
9. Botermann DS, Brandes N, Frommhold A, Heß I, Wolff A, Zibat A, Hahn H, Buslei R, Uhmann A. Hedgehog signaling in endocrine and folliculo-stellate cells of the adult pituitary. J Endocrinol. 2021;248:303–16.
10. Nantie LB, Himes AD, Getz DR, Raetzman LT. Notch signaling in postnatal pituitary expansion: proliferation, progenitors, and cell specification. Mol Endocrinol. 2014;28:731–44.
11. Hamdi-Rozé H, Ware M, Guyodo H, Rizzo A, Ratié L, Rupin M, Carré W, Kim A, Odent S, Dubourg C, David V, de Tayrac M, Dupé V. Disrupted hypothalamo-pituitary axis in association with reduced SHH underlies the pathogenesis of NOTCH-deficiency. J Clin Endocrinol Metab. 2020;105:dgaa249.
12. Cohen LE, Radovick S. Molecular basis of combined pituitary hormone deficiencies. Endocr Rev. 2002;23(4):431–42.
13. Pulichino AM, Vallette-Kasic S, Tsai JP, Couture C, Gauthier Y, Drouin J. Tpit determines alternate fates during pituitary cell differentiation. Genes Dev. 2003;17:738–47.
14. Chen J, Hersmus N, Van Duppen V, Caesens P, Denef C, Vankelecom H. The adult pituitary contains a cell population displaying stem/progenitor cell and early embryonic characteristics. Endocrinol. 2005;146:3985–98.
15. Vallette-Kasic S, Figarella-Branger D, Grino M, et al. J Clin Endocrinol Metab. 2003;
16. Smith GW, Aubry JM, Dellu F, et al. Corticotropin releasing factor receptor 1-deficient mice display decreased anxiety, impaired stress response, and aberrant neuroendocrine development. Neuron, 20. 1998:1093–102.
17. Bale TL, Picetti R, Contarino A, Koob GF, Vale WW, Lee KF. J Neuro Sci. 2002;22(1)
18. Bilodeau S, Roussel-Gervais A, Drouin J. Mol Cell Biol. 2009;29(7)
19. Lanctôt C, Gauthier Y, Drouin J. Pituitary homeobox 1 (Ptx1) is differentially expressed during pituitary development. Endocrinol. 1999;140(3):1416–22.
20. Acampora D, Mazan S, Tuorto F, Avantaggiato V, Tremblay JJ, Lazzaro D, di Carlo A, Mariano A, Macchia PE, Corte G, Macchia V, Drouin J, Brûlet P, Simeone A. Transient dwarfism and hypogonadism in mice lacking Otx1 reveal prepubescent stage-specific control of pituitary levels of GH, FSH and LH. Development. 1998;125(7):1229–39.
21. Andersen B, Rosenfeld MG. Endocrine revision. 2001;22(1)

22. Wei W, Cogan JD, Pfäffle RW, Dasen JS, Frisch H, O'Connell SM, Flynn SE, Brown MR, Mullis PE, Parks JS, Phillips III JA, Rosenfeld MG. Mutations in PROP1 cause familial combined pituitary hormone deficiency. Nat Genet. 1998;18:147–9.
23. Zhu X, Zhang J, Tollkuhn J, Ohsawa R, Bresnick EH, Guillemot F, Kageyama R, Rosenfeld MG. Sustained notch signaling in progenitors is required for sequential emergence of distinct cell lineages during organogenesis. Genes Dev. 2006;20:2739–53.
24. Liu JC, Baker RE, Sun C, Sundmark VC, Elsholtz HP. Activation of Go-coupled dopamine D2 receptors inhibits ERK1/ERK2 in pituitary cells. A key step in the transcriptional suppression of the prolactin gene. J Biol Chem. 2002;277(39):35819–25.
25. Dasen JS, O'Connell SM, Flynn SE, Treier M, Gleiberman AS, Szeto DP, Hooshmand F, Aggarwal AK, Rosenfeld MG. Reciprocal interactions of Pit1 and GATA2 mediate signaling gradient–induced determination of pituitary cell types. Cell. 1999;97:092–8674.
26. Asa KK, Sylvia L. Functional endocrine pathology. Arch Pathol Lab Med. 2000;
27. Moore K, Persaud T. Before we are born: essentials of embryology and birth defects. 5th ed. Philadelphia: Elsevier; 1998. p. 9780721673776.
28. Dietrich RB, Lis LE, Greensite FS, Pitt D, et al., editors. Normal MR appearance of the pituitary gland in the first 2 years of life. AJNR; 1995. p. 1413–9. PMC8338052.
29. Bergland RM, Page RB. Pituitary-brain vascular relations: a new paradigm. Science. 1979;4388:18–24.
30. Millan MIP, Brinkmeier ML, Mortensen AH, Camper SA. PROP1 triggers epithelial-mesenchymal transition-like process in pituitary stem cells. Elife. 2016;5:e14470.
31. Böttner A, Keller E, Kratzsch J, Stobbe H, Weigel JFW, Keller A, Hirsch W, Kiess W, Blum WF, Pfäffle RW. PROP1 mutations cause progressive deterioration of anterior pituitary function including adrenal insufficiency: a longitudinal analysis. J Clin Endocrinol Metab. 2004;89(10):5256–65.
32. Flück C, Deladoey J, Rutishauser K, Eblé A, Marti U, Wu W, Mullis PE. Phenotypic variability in familial combined pituitary hormone deficiency caused by a PROP1 gene mutation resulting in the substitution of Arg-->Cys at codon 120 (R120C). J Clin Endocrinol Metab. 1998;83:3727–34.
33. Vieira TC, da Silva MR, Abucham J. Endocrine. 2006;30:365–9.
34. Lebl J, Vosáhlo J, Pfaeffle RW, Stobbe H, Cerná J, Novotná D, Zapletalová J, Kalvachová B, Hána V, Weiss V, Blum WF. Auxological and endocrine phenotype in a population-based cohort of patients with PROP1 gene defects. Eur J Endocrinol. 2005;153:389–96.
35. Himes AD, Raetzman LT. Premature differentiation and aberrant movement of pituitary cells lacking both Hes1 and Prop1. Dev Biol. 2009;325:151–61.
36. Böttner A, Keller E, Kratzsch J, Stobbe H, Weigel JFW, Keller A, Hirsch W, Kiess W, Blum WF, Pfäffle RW. PROP1 mutations cause progressive deterioration of anterior pituitary function including adrenal insufficiency: a longitudinal analysis. J Clin Endocrinol Metab. 2004;89:5256–65.
37. Deladoëy J, Flück C, Büyükgebiz A, Kuhlmann BV, Eblé A. "Hot spot" in the PROP1 gene responsible for combined pituitary hormone deficiency. J Clin Endocrinol Metab. 1999;84:1645–50.
38. Bodner M, Castriilo J-L, Theill LE, Deerinck T, Ellisman M, Karin M. The pituitary-specific transcription factor GHF-1 is a homeobox-containing protein. Cell. 1988;55:391–535.
39. Simmons DM, Voss JW, Ingraham HA, Holloway JM, Broide RS, Rosenfeld MG, Swanson LW. Pituitary cell phenotypes involve cell-specific Pit-1 mRNA translation and synergistic interactions with other classes of transcription factors. Genes Dev. 1990;4:695–711.
40. Jacobson EM, Li P, Leon-del-Rio A, Rosenfeld MG, Aggarwal AK. Structure of Pit-1 POU domain bound to DNA as a dimer: unexpected arrangement and flexibility. Genes Dev. 1997;11:198–212.
41. Romero CJ, Nesi-Franca S, Radovick S. The molecular basis of hypopituitarism. Trends Endocrinol Metab. 2009;20:506–16.

42. Park HL, Bai C, Platt KA, Matise MP, Beeghly A, Hui CC, Nakashima M, Joyner AL. Mouse Gli1 mutants are viable but have defects in SHH signaling in combination with a Gli2 mutation. Development. 2000;127:1593–605.
43. Arnhold IJP, França MM, Carvalho LR, Mendonca BB, Jorge AAL. Role of GLI2 in hypopituitarism phenotype. J Mol Endocrinol. 2015;54:R141–50.
44. Fang Q, Benedetti AFF, Ma Q, Gregory L, Li JZ, Dattani M, Sadeghi-Nejad A, Arnhold IJP, Mendonca BB, Camper SA, Carvalho LR. HESX1 mutations in patients with congenital hypopituitarism: variable phenotypes with the same genotype. Clin Endocrinol. 2016;85:408–14.
45. Thomas PQ, Dattani MT, Brickman JM, McNay D, Warne G, Zacharin M, Cameron F, Hurst J, Woods K, Dunger D, Stanhope R, Forrest S, Robinson IC, Beddington RS. Heterozygous HESX1 mutations associated with isolated congenital pituitary hypoplasia and septo-optic dysplasia. Hum Mol Genet. 2001;10:39–45.
46. Zhadanov AB, Bertuzzi S, Taira M, Dawid IB, Westphal H. Expression pattern of the murine LIM class homeobox gene Lhx3 in subsets of neural and neuroendocrine tissues. Dev Dyn. 1995;202:354–64.
47. Sheng HZ, Zhadanov AB, Mosinger B Jr, Fujii T, Bertuzzi S, Grinberg A, Lee EJ, Huang SP, Mahon KA, Westphal H. Specification of pituitary cell lineages by the LIM homeobox gene Lhx3. Sci. 1996;272:1004–7.
48. Pfaeffle RW, Savage JJ, Hunter CS, Palme C, Ahlmann M, Kumar P, Bellone J, Schoenau E, Korsch E, Brämswig JH, Stobbe HM, Blum WF, Rhodes SJ. Four novel mutations of the LHX3 gene cause combined pituitary hormone deficiencies with or without limited neck rotation. J Clin Endocrinol Metab. 2007;92:1909–19.
49. O'Neill C, Gangat M, Radovick S. Growth hormone deficiency. Endocrine. 2022;3:736–44.
50. Lamonerie T, Tremblay JJ, Lanctôt C, Therrien M, Gauthier Y, Drouin J. Ptxl, a bicoid-related homeo box transcription factor involved in transcription of the pro-opimelanocortin gene. Genes Dev. 1996;10:1284–95.
51. Castinetti F, Reynaud R, Saveanu A, Jullien N, Quentien MH, Rochette C, Barlier A, Enjalbert A, Brue T. MECHANISMS IN ENDOCRINOLOGY: an update in the genetic aetiologies of combined pituitary hormone deficiency. Eur J Endocrinol. 2016;174:R239–47.
52. Kelberman D, Rizzoti K, Avilion A, Bitner-Glindzicz M, Cianfarani S, Julie Collins W, Chong K, Kirk JMW, Achermann JC, Ross R, Carmignac D, Lovell-Badge R, Robinson ICAF, Dattani MT. Mutations within Sox2/SOX2 are associated with abnormalities in the hypothalamo-pituitary-gonadal axis in mice and humans. Clin Invest. 2006;116:2442–55.
53. Raivio T, Avbelj M, McCabe MJ, Romero CJ, Dwyer AA, Tommiska J, Sykiotis GP, Gregory LC, Diaczok D, Tziaferi V, Elting MW, Padidela R, Plummer L, Martin C, Bihua. Genetic overlap in Kallmann syndrome, combined pituitary hormone deficiency, and septo-optic dysplasia. J Clin Endocrinol Metab. 2012;97:E694–9.

Chapter 10
Posterior Fossa Malformation

Hadi Mroueh, Nooralhuda Sameer Alash, and Hashim Talib Hashim

Test your learning and check your understanding of this book's contents: use the "Springer Nature Flashcards" app to access questions using ▶ https://sn.pub/YnQHwS
To use the app, please follow the instructions in Chapter 1.

10.1   Introduction

To understand the posterior fossa malformation, it is crucial to grasp some of the key embryological stages that result in the formation of the cerebellum. The neural tube serves as the foundation for all of the brain's components. The major brain vesicles which are the forebrain, the midbrain, and the hindbrain are created by the neural tube fusion in the cranial region and the rostral neuropore closure by the fourth gestational week. The hindbrain is the primary vesicle, while the secondary vesicles are metencephalon and myelencephalon. Metencephalon develops from the rostral rhombencephalon, gives rise to cerebellum and pons. Cerebellum functions as center of coordination and posture, as well as the proliferation of the neuroecto-derm cells give rise to cerebellar nuclei, purkinje cells and golgi cells at the

H. Mroueh (✉)
Carol davila University of Medicine and Pharmacy, Bucharest, Romania

N. S. Alash
College of Medicine, University of Baghdad, Baghdad, Iraq

H. T. Hashim
Department of Research, University of Warith Al-Anbiyaa, College of Medicine, Karbala, Iraq

K. F. AlAli, H. T. Hashim (eds.), *Congenital Brain Malformations*, https://doi.org/10.1007/978-3-031-58630-9_10

ventricular zone, to basket, granule, stellate cells at the external germinal layer, to astrocytes, oligodendrocytes and bergmann cells at the external and internal germinal layers. On the other hand the pons serve a road for nerve fibers between cerebrum, cerebellum and the spinal cord [1].

The fourth ventricle, a pyramid-shaped chamber located ventral to the cerebellum and dorsal to the brainstem. The choroid plexus is pushed inferiorly by the cerebellum's growth and rearward extension. The fourth ventricle's posterior membranous area then grows like the finger of a glove developing a noticeable caudal protrusion, which has been named as Blake's pouch. The Blake's pouch is formed of ventricular ependyma with some mesenchymal tissues and it is a closed cavity that has no communication with the subarachnoid space of the cisterna magna surrounding it [2]. The foramen of Magendie is formed as a result of the condensation of the network between the Blake's pouch and the vermis and as the permeabilization of the pouch occurs the foramen is finally formed. At around six weeks of gestation, the cisterna magna, which connects to the fourth ventricle by the foramen of Magendie, is thought to form.

The cerebellum's morphology reflects how it developed embryologically. Phylogenetically, the archicerebellum (flocculonodular lobe) is the earliest component. It is interconnected with the vestibular system.

The anterior lobe of the paleocerebellum and the vermis are phylogenetically more recent. It is connected to limb density data.

Phylogenetically, the neocerebellum is the newest component. Selective control of limb movements is linked to this region of the cerebellum [3].

10.2   Malformations of the Posterior Fossa

The vermis and paravermis hemispheres emerge from the cerebellum, which begins to develop at the end of the fourth week. The cerebellar hemispheres begin to form in the fifth week and keep developing until the second year of life. The majority of cerebellar abnormalities, such as cerebellar and pontine hypoplasia (primordial tissue that is histologically normal but incompletely developed), and dysplasia, are thought to be caused by proliferation abnormalities [4].

10.2.1   Diseases with Cerebellar Agenesis, Aplasia or Hypoplasia

Complete absence of the cerebellum is termed cerebellar agenesis and it is rare. A deformity phenotype caused by mutations in the PTF1A gene on chromosome 10, has been described in recent genetic studies. These genetic studies also explain the permanent neonatal diabetes mellitus in these patients since the studied gene is linked to the development of the pancreas.

Imaging studies show small remnants of cerebellar tissues and hence subtotal agenesis would be a more suitable term. The posterior fossa may be normal in size or may be expanded, with increment in the total cerebral spinal fluid and pontine hypoplasia. hydranencephaly and anencephaly are the cerebral abnormalities to be expected in total agenesis [4].

Unilateral agenesis cases have been documented, and they typically lead to secondary contralateral hypoplasia of the inferior olivary nuclei and the pontine with pons asymmetry, hypoplasia of the contralateral substantia nigra and red nucleus and hypoplastic ipsilateral middle and superior cerebellar peduncles and superior colliculus. MRI is used to show these findings particularly for identifying accurately the remnants of the cerebellum.

There is variability in the clinical presentation and compensation by the cerebral cortex may cause the diagnosis to be delayed and the patients would most likely be asymptomatic. However, the more complex cognitive functions will be affected, problems would arise in speech and language as well as affective, executive and spatial cognitive impairment due to the cerebellar contribution to these functions. There will also be in some patients impairment with movement coordination, as well as truncal ataxia if the cerebellar vermis is involved in patients with unilateral cerebellar hypoplasia [5].

10.2.2   *Rhombencephalosynapsis*

The fusion or merger of the cerebellar hemispheres with the total or partial loss of the vermis, dentate nuclei, and cerebellar peduncles is known as rhombencephalosynapsis. Signs of cerebellar dysfunction, such as nystagmus, ataxia, delayed motor development and head stereotypies are the signs to be expected in affected individuals. Rhombencephalosynapsis is infrequent, the majority of the patients are found to be nonsyndromic. However, it may also occur in VACTERL syndrome (Vertebral anomalies, Anal atresia, Cardiac defects, Tracheoesophageal fistula and/or Esophageal atresia, Renal anomalies, and Limb defects).

As well as Gomez-Lopez-Hernandez syndrome (parietal alopecia, craniofacial dysmorphic signs and trigeminal anesthesia) [5].

The significant neuroimaging findings are:

- Partial or complete absence of the vermis.
- The fourth ventricle is keyhole shaped.
- the dentate nuclei and the superior cerebellar peduncle fusion.
- cerebellar folia extending horizontally across the midline with fused hemispheres of the cerebellum.
- Absent vermian primary fissure on midsagittal plane

10.2.3 Vermian-Cerebellar Hypoplasia

Vermian-cerebellar hypoplasia describes various degrees of inadequate vermis and cerebellar development. It is crucial to distinguish between cerebellar hypoplasia and cerebellar atrophy because the latter usually refers to volume loss brought on by a developing injury rather than a true developmental anomaly [6].

Cerebellar hypoplasia has been attributed to genetic and metabolic factors such as trisomies 9, 13, and 18, glycosylation disorders, migration disorders, and congenital muscular dystrophies. Cerebellar hypoplasia can also occur when teratogenic substances like cocaine and anticonvulsants, as well as infectious agents like the cytomegalovirus, interfere with the cerebellum's normal development.

Vermian–cerebellar hypoplasia imaging features include:

A normal-sized posterior fossa which contains the vermis and cerebellum with various degrees of hypoplasia.

Characteristic is a big fourth ventricle that connects to the posterior cerebellar region via a passively expanded vallecula [7].

A large cisterna magna and hydrocephalus are common associated abnormalities.

These patients exhibit hypotonia, abnormal eye movements, and ataxia clinically. However, the degree of additional findings including delayed developmental milestones and intellectual disabilities varies.

10.2.4 Lhermitte–Duclos Disease

Dysplastic cerebellar gangliocytoma, commonly known as Lhermitte-Duclos disease, is a rare lesion of the cerebellum that is characterized by distortion of the normal laminar pattern. There is no known genetic or pathogenic etiology. It is sometimes linked to Cowden syndrome and is regarded as a benign hamartomatous tumor. Patients might present clinically in a variety of ways, ranging from being completely asymptomatic to having symptoms including headache, blurred vision, and papilledema that are linked to elevated intracranial pressure. The presence of obstructive hydrocephalus is common [8].

MRI is the preferred test for diagnosing Lhermitte-Duclos illness. The traditional signs are a non-enhancing striated mass with an associated mass effect over the fourth ventricle in the posterior fossa, which causes hydrocephalus and the patient's symptoms.

10.2.5 Walker–Warburg Syndrome

Walker–Warburg syndrome is an autosomal recessive disorder that affects multiple systems in the body. It is rare and it is characterized by ocular and cerebral anomalies and congenital muscular dystrophy.

The disease results from defects in the O-glycosylation of alpha-dystroglycan which is crucial for cerebellar neuronal migration and is extensively expressed in pial membranes. Muscle dystrophy, cataracts, microphthalmia, detachment of the retina, and hypoplastic and/or atrophied optic nerve are some of its distinguishing features [9].

Seizures and missed developmental milestones are symptoms of this illness in patients. By their third year of life, most patients die.

10.2.6 Joubert Syndrome

The term "Joubert syndrome" refers to a collection of rare diseases, often known as "ciliopathies," that are caused by defects in the primary non motile cilium, a cellular organelle. Cilia are involved in the cerebellum and brainstem's axonal migration and neuronal cell proliferation in the central nervous system (CNS). Hypotonia, irregular respiratory patterns, varying intellectual impairment, ataxia, and ocular motor apraxia are typical neurologic signs.

10.2.7 Cystic Posterior Fossa Anomalies

The majority of these aberrations are thought to have a common genesis in defects with mesenchymal neuroepithelial signaling.

Dandy–Walker malformation: It results from the anterior membrane portion of the plica choroidal failing to integrate. The nonintegrated anterior membranous area expands posteriorly within the posterior fossa as a result of cerebral spinal fluid pulsations, creating a sizable posterior cyst that represents the fourth ventricle. Non-communicating hydrocephalus will result due to the accumulation of the cerebro-spinal fluid in the ventricles as a result of blockage of its flow from the fourth ventricle into the subarachnoid space. This will lead to high intracranial pressure and macrocephaly. Spina bifida is a common occurrence due to its association with Dandy-Walker syndrome. Dandy-Walker syndrome signs and symptoms frequently appear at or shortly after birth. Vomiting, irritability and seizures can be expected. Infants may gradually develop delays in their ability to walk and crawl. Ataxia, nystagmus, muscular paralysis or spasticity, as well as abnormal breathing patterns, can all result from cerebellar dysfunction. Dandy–Walker syndrome is frequently detected during pregnancy using ultrasonography, and the diagnosis can be verified after birth with an MRI. A ventriculoperitoneal shunt is frequently implanted as part of treatment. Additionally, physiotherapy is frequently helpful for patients to improve their motor skills [10].

Arachnoid cyst: Arachnoid cysts are benign leptomeningeal cysts that form when the arachnoid membrane splits or duplicates, and the extra membrane is then filled with cerebrospinal fluid. Arachnoid cysts are typically accidental, asymptomatic abnormalities that have no communication with the ventricular system or the arachnoid space surrounding it. Up to two thirds of them can be located in the middle cranial fossa, though their locations vary. They are uncommon in the posterior fossa, and they may resemble other cystic abnormalities of the posterior fossa. The sellar area, as well as the prepontine and interpeduncular cisterns, are other locations where arachnoid cysts have been observed. The age of the patient, the size of the cyst, and how much pressure the cyst puts on the nearby structures all affect how the posterior fossa arachnoid cysts present clinically. Adults may experience acute symptoms when an arachnoid cyst expands due to hemorrhage [11], increasing its pressure. This expansion and pressure can also occur due to osmotic shifts, fluid discharge from the cyst wall cells, a ball-valve mechanism, and other factors. Cyst enlargement in children may result in hydrocephalus and mass effect, which enlarges the head and causes symptoms of cerebellar compression. Arachnoid cysts appear as big cystic formations with smooth, well-defined edges on imaging, the cysts may be linked to hydrocephalus and cause a bulk effect and displacement of the nearby cerebellum without invading. The neighboring bone may become scalloped as a result of pulsation. Unless there are issues like hemorrhage or infection, computed tomography (CT) density values and magnetic resonance (MR) signal intensity are equivalent to cerebrospinal fluid.

Blake's pouch cyst: The Blake's pouch cyst is an embryological anomaly of the posterior membranous region that results in the failure of Blake's pouch to regress as a result of the foramen of Magendie's foramen not being fenestrated. The supratentorial and fourth ventricles can grow diffusely because of flow blockage at the bigger foramen of Magendie since the foramina of Luschka form at a later stage and by then it cannot correct this enlargement. This cystic lesion, which is an outgrowth of the fourth ventricle and blocks free communication with the subarachnoid space, has a mass effect on the nearby structures. The location of the choroid plexus within the fourth ventricle, curving around the vermis to lay within the Blake's pouch cyst along its superior wall, is an important finding that helps to distinguish this abnormality from comparable entities. In addition, the fourth ventricle involvement in diffuse hydrocephalus is important since it differentiates it from posterior fossa arachnoid cysts, the latter's obstruction is due to compression at the level of the fourth ventricle. Clinical manifestation can vary. There have been reports of severe cases of intracranial hypertension, which are typically caused by issues with the cyst itself, such hemorrhage or infection. However, some people may not exhibit any symptoms or may only have minor neurologic impairment and in these patients the pouch is usually found incidentally. The best imaging technique for detecting it is MRI [12].

Mega Cisterna magna Although the megacisterna magna technically isn't a cyst, it is an essential differential diagnosis because its imaging look is similar to that of the cystic posterior fossa anomalies mentioned above. Megacisterna magna is a frequent anomaly defined by aberrant enlargement of the cisterna magna with a cerebellar vermis and hemispheres that appear normal. It is thought to happen as a result of Blake's pouch's late permeabilization, which enables the pouch to extend and widen the posterior fossa before its fenestration. As a result, the fourth ventricle has a normal size and the cisterna magna can freely communicate with the nearby subarachnoid areas. Most individuals are asymptomatic, and there is typically no hydrocephalus. A normal vermis with nine lobules distinguishes the disorder from Dandy-Walker malformation and vermian-cerebellar hypoplasia, two conditions that share some imaging characteristics with it. Megacisterna magna can be distinguished from a chronic Blake's pouch by the absence of hydrocephalus. The abnormality can be distinguished from an arachnoid cyst by its lack of mass influence on the nearby cerebellum and cerebellar falx.

10.2.8 Chiari Malformations

The cerebellum of the brain can protrude into the spinal canal in a disease known as a Chiari malformation, which prevents the cerebrospinal fluid from flowing normally. Typically, it results from the posterior fossa of the skull's underdevelopment during fetal development. The deformed posterior fossa, where the cerebellum is still growing and developing, eventually pushes it down into the foramen magnum. The two main types of Chiari malformation which are type I and type II are distinguished based on the structures which herniate. When only the cerebellar tonsils herniate into the foramen magnum, this is known as a type I Chiari malformation. The fourth ventricle may become compressed as a result, which prevents the cerebrospinal fluid from flowing normally from the ventricles into the subarachnoid space. Which consequently lead to increased intracranial pressure and hydrocephalus [13].

Cerebrospinal fluid may accumulate in the spinal canal over time, though the precise mechanism is still not understood. This pooling can lead to a syrinx. This is a condition known as syringomyelia. The spinothalamic tract and other surrounding nerve fibers are destroyed as the syrinx grows and starts to spread outward from the spinal cord's core. Type I Chiari malformations are typically asymptomatic or discovered by accident, hence they are typically only identified during adolescence or maturity. A type II Chiari malformation, also known as an Arnold-Chiari malformation, is significantly more severe and, as a result, is more easily recognized in children. Cerebellar tonsils herniate in type II Chiari malformations, just like in type I, but there is also herniation of the cerebellar vermis. Furthermore, a myelomeningocele, a type of spina bifida, is a common association. According to some research, type II Chiari malformations may actually be caused by myelomeningoceles, with the degree of herniation being a complication. It has been demonstrated that type II Chiari malformations can frequently be stopped or reversed through fetal surgery to treat myelomeningoceles. Occipital headaches are a common symptom of type II Chiari malformations, and they can get worse with valsalva actions like yawning, sneezing, and coughing. If there's cerebellar dysfunction it can cause vertigo, nystagmus or ataxia. The cough and gag reflexes can be hampered by excessive pressure on the medulla oblongata, which can also lead to breathing problems and sleep apnea. Finally, the symptoms of hydrocephalus itself include headache and vomiting. And if there is syringomyelia, due to the destruction of the spinothalamic tract at the level of the cervical spine, typically C4-C6, there will be a loss of pain and temperature sensation in the shoulders and arms in a "cape-like" distribution. On brain MRI cerebellar structures that are visible more than 5 millimeters below the foramen magnum are usually a sign that a Chiari malformation is present. The posterior fossa decompression procedure can be used to treat neurological symptoms in a person with a Chiari malformation. In the presence of hydrocephalus, a ventriculoperitoneal shunt, for example, can be used to treat it and lower intracranial pressure [14].

References

1. Shekdar, K. (2011). Posterior fossa malformations. In Seminars in ultrasound, CT and MRI (Vol. 32, 3, pp. 228–241). WB Saunders.
2. Forzano F, et al. Posterior fossa malformation in fetuses: a report of 56 further cases and a review of the literature. Prenat Diagn. 2007;27(6):495–501.
3. Altman NR, Naidich TP, Braffman BH. Posterior fossa malformations. Am J Neuroradiol. 1992;13(2):691.
4. Severino M, Huisman TAGM. Posterior fossa malformations. Neuroimaging Clinics. 2019;29(3):367–83.
5. Garel C. Posterior fossa malformations: main features and limits in prenatal diagnosis. Pediatr Radiol. 2010;40:1038–45.
6. D'Antonio F, et al. Systematic review and meta-analysis of isolated posterior fossa malformations on prenatal imaging (part 2): neurodevelopmental outcome. Ultrasound Obstet Gynecol. 2016;48(1):28–37.
7. Widjaja E, Blaser S, Raybaud C. Diffusion tensor imaging of midline posterior fossa malformations. Pediatr Radiol. 2006;36:510–7.
8. Aldinger KA, et al. Cerebellar and posterior fossa malformations in patients with autism-associated chromosome 22q13 terminal deletion. Am J Med Genet A. 2013;161(1):131–6.
9. McCormick WF, Hardman JM, Boulter TR. Vascular malformations ("angiomas") of the brain, with special reference to those occurring in the posterior fossa. J Neurosurg. 1968;28(3):241–51.
10. Niesen, Charles E. Malformations of the posterior fossa: current perspectives. Seminars in pediatric neurology. Vol. 9 4. WB Saunders, 2002.
11. Batjer H, Samson D. Arteriovenous malformations of the posterior fossa: clinical presentation, diagnostic evaluation, and surgical treatment. J Neurosurg. 1986;64(6):849–56.
12. Frieden IJ, Reese V, Cohen D. PHACE syndrome: the association of posterior fossa brain malformations, hemangiomas, arterial anomalies, coarctation of the aorta and cardiac defects, and eye abnormalities. Arch Dermatol. 1996;132(3):307–11.
13. Munshi I, et al. Effects of posterior fossa decompression with and without duraplasty on Chiari malformation-associated hydromyelia. Neurosurgery. 2000;46(6):1384–9.
14. Sgouros S, Kountouri M, Natarajan K. Posterior fossa volume in children with Chiari malformation Type I. J Neurosurg Pediatr. 2006;105(2):101–6.

Chapter 11
Microcephaly

Ali Qais Hasan and Moath Mohammed Madlool

Test your learning and check your understanding of this book's contents: use the "Springer Nature Flashcards" app to access questions using ▶ https://sn.pub/YnQHwS
To use the app, please follow the instructions in Chapter 1.

11.1 Introduction

Microcephaly can be defined in simple words as a head size smaller than average for age and sex. Either due to abnormalities in brain development hindering the brain from reaching its full size or sudden stoppage of brain growth for many reasons, one of which is exposure to insults during pregnancy.

As for the detailed definition of microcephaly, there is an ongoing debate among experts to define it; most experts state that microcephaly is *An (OFC) equal to or more than two standard deviations (SD) below the mean occipitofrontal head circumference for age and sex (OFC ≤ −2SD)* [1]. While other experts define it as OFC equal to or more than three standard deviations (SD) below the mean for age and sex (OFC ≤ −3SD) [2]. Statistics have shown that about 2% of the population would be deemed microcephalic if we utilized the former cutoff point (OFC ≤ −2SD) for measurement; however, many of those people fall on the lower end of the demographic distribution and are neurologically healthy. In contrast, the percentage of individuals considered to have microcephaly drastically drops to as low as 0.1% if

A. Q. Hasan (✉) · M. M. Madlool
College of Medicine, University of Baghdad, Baghdad, Iraq

© The Author(s), under exclusive license to Springer Nature Switzerland AG 2024
K. F. AlAli, H. T. Hashim (eds.), *Congenital Brain Malformations*,
https://doi.org/10.1007/978-3-031-58630-9_11

(OFC ≤ -3) was used as a standardized cutoff point for measurement, and thus the majority of these individuals suffer from severe mental disabilities. These statistics made it clear that using any of those two definitions at the expense of the other as a standard would deem it incorrect. As a result, this debate gave birth to a dilemma yet to be solved [3] to minimize further confusion and misunderstanding, we will adopt a modified definition for microcephaly and classify it as "mild" microcephaly and "severe" microcephaly (also termed "true" microcephaly). This way, it is simpler to describe the (−3SD) as nothing more than a cutoff point in determining when to consider microcephaly severe rather than being a definition for microcephaly [Fig. 11.1] [4]. On the other hand, the severity of microcephaly is not determined only by measuring the occipitofrontal circumference but also depending on the presence of neuroanatomical anomalies, including cerebral atrophy, latency in myelination, and

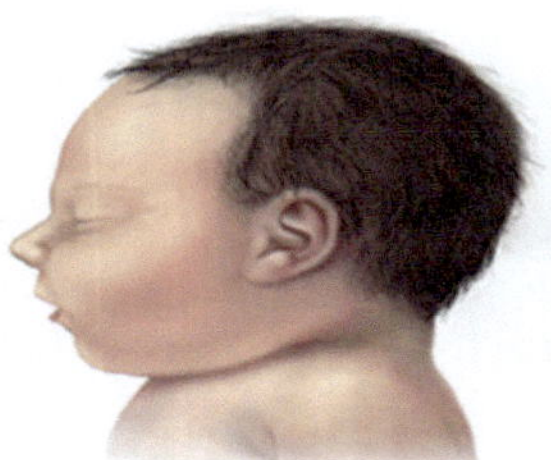

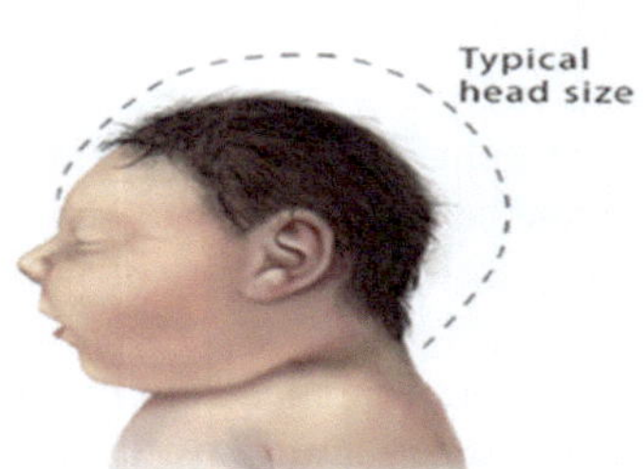

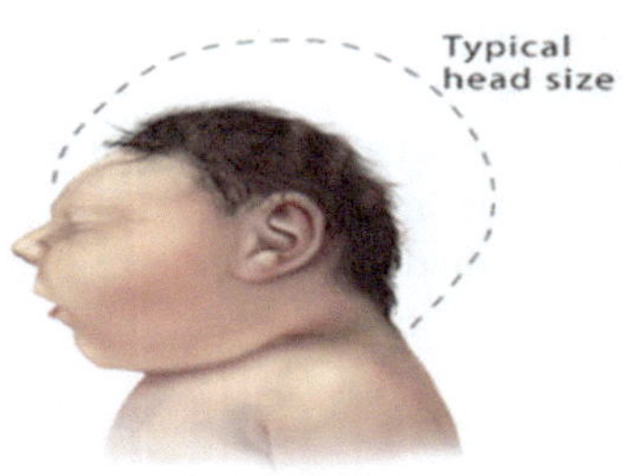

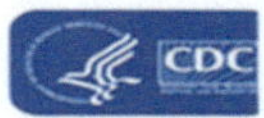

Fig. 11.1 Normocephalic baby in comparison with microcephalic babies at different severity levels (Image attributes to the Centers for Disease Control and Prevention, National Center on Birth Defects and Developmental Disabilities). https://www.cdc.gov/ncbddd/birthdefects/microcephaly.html

white matter hypoplasia. These abnormalities were more predictive of poor cognitive and developmental performance [5].

Both genetic and environmental factors play a role in causing microcephaly. If microcephaly is associated with other congenital defects, it is classified as syndromic microcephaly; if not, then it is isolated microcephaly. Whether the cause was genetic or environmental, isolated, or syndromic, microcephaly can either present at birth and is termed "Primary" microcephaly, or later in life due to sudden stoppage of average brain growth, such condition is termed "secondary" microcephaly [6]. Hence We will be focusing more on primary microcephaly rather than secondary microcephaly.

Microcephaly affects both developmental milestones and intellectual abilities, whether it is isolated or syndromic. This is attributed to the abnormal and incomplete development of the cerebral cortex; whose grey matter is responsible for developmental performance. Hence, individuals with a small cortex suffer from numerous problems, including delayed motor and language abilities and faulty development of visual capabilities; furthermore, it can lead to epilepsy, hearing loss, cerebral palsy, and mental retardation in correlation with the severity of microcephaly [7]. On the other hand, a strong association between the severity of microcephaly and low IQ. A study that was conducted on 212 microcephalic children showed that "the median IQ decreased with decreasing head circumference; in children with OFC between 2 and 2.1 SD, the mean IQ was 62 versus a mean IQ of 35 when OFC was (> −3SD) below the mean" [3]. Epidemiologically speaking, it is difficult to precisely point at a range of numbers within which the prevalence of microcephaly in the population falls. This is attributed to discrepancies in the overall incidence rates, poor precision, and completeness of reports [8].

A thorough history and good physical exam are the initial steps in diagnosing microcephaly, followed by needed investigations depending on history and examination, such as virology tests, neuroimaging and even gene sequencing in certain cases.

With no known definitive remedy, microcephaly is considered a lifelong affliction. Therefore, management is mainly supportive for the child to improve the developmental performance while focusing on preventing possible complications [9].

11.2 Etiology and Pathogenesis

Typically, the natural developmental milestone of the cerebral cortex reaches most of its final stage in the middle of the gestational age. Although the cellular proliferation of glial cells continues after birth, adding more to the eventual volume of the brain [10]. This process and multiple other developmental processes control the final size of the brain; those processes themselves are affected by multiple factors, some are genetic factors, and some are environmental factors. If any of these factors (genetic or environmental) negatively affect the balance between progenitor cell proliferation and cell death which is considered an essential developmental process within which the brain can reach its eventual growth capacity, this can cause microcephaly [11]. Therefore, microcephaly can be classified according to the etiology into genetic and environmental microcephaly.

11.2.1   Genetic Etiologies of Primary Microcephaly

A variety of genetic etiologies play a role in the causation of primary microcephaly. These genetic disorders can either render the baby to show nothing more than a small head size at birth, with no other apparent defects or malformations (isolated microcephaly); on the other hand, the effect of the genetic disorders can be more profound and may manifest as a syndrome (syndromic microcephaly). The former subgroup which is also termed "Microcephaly primary hereditary" has heterogeneous pathogenesis with about 28 MCPH-associated gene loci according to the database published by the Online Mendelian Inheritance in Man (OMIM) (accessed as of 2022) [12, 13].

These different genes convey a variety of essential cellular processes. *"CENPJ, STIL, CEP135, CEP152 and SASS6 (MCPH6, MCPH7, MCPH8, MCPH9 and MCPH14 respectively) are the genes responsible for centriole biogenesis"*, whereas *"WDR62, CDK5RAP2, KNL1, ASPM, CENPE, CIT, KIF14 and MAP 11 (MCPH2, MCPH3, MCPH4, MCPH5, MCPH13, MCPH17, MCPH20 and MCPH25 respectively) are the genes responsible for microtubule dynamics such as (PCM scaffold, microtubule nucleation, centriolar engagement, cytokinesis, spindle orientation, et cetera.)"*. Furthermore, some MCPH-associated genes are responsible for DNA dynamics (chromosome condensation, cell cycle checkpoint regulation, DNA damage response, transcription regulation, chromatin remodeling, nuclear envelope disassembly, et cetera.) and signaling (BBB lipid transport, WNT signaling, cellular trafficking, et cetera.) those genes are the *"MCPH1, MCPH10, MCPH11, MCPH16, MCPH21, MCPH22, MCPH23, MCPH24, MCPH12, MCPH15, MCPH18 and MCPH19 that are named (MCPH1, ZNF335, PHC1, ANKLE2, NCAPD2, NCAPD3, NCAPH, NUP37, CDK6, MFSD2A, WDFY3 and COPB2 respectively)"*[14].

Autosomal recessive Mendelian inheritance is the most common mode of inheritance for these genes; however, some genes have an autosomal dominant (WDFY3) or an X-linked mode of inheritance. Although it is rare for the genetic factors to be seen in the form of mosaicism or ring chromosomes, it is still worth mentioning that such modes can be found in some cases of microcephaly primary hereditary (MCPH) [3].

Despite the different cellular processes conveyed by the different genes (MCPH1-28) and the various modes of inheritance, mutations in one or more of these genes tend to cause microcephaly in their own way. Most commonly, the mutations are in the form of premature stop codons (trinucleotide in a molecule of DNA or mRNA that codes for a specific amino acid responsible for signaling a halt to intracellular protein syntheses), interrupting the progression of the cell cycle, which in turn, leads to abnormalities in the centromere ending with premature cellular apoptosis and on a larger scale can lead to smaller brain size [15].

A single gene mutation leads mostly to isolated microcephaly of an autosomal recessive mode of inheritance, whereas multiple gene mutations yield other obvious congenital defects along with small head size (syndromic microcephaly). Among the known over 800 syndromes associated with microcephaly, diagnosis of a respectable number of these syndromes is reached mainly by assessing the head size, as microcephaly is their key sign. In contrast, other syndromes show microcephaly as an associated yet less diagnostic finding [9]. Among the former group of syndromes are the Wolff-Hirshhorn syndrome, cri-du-chat syndrome, Williams syndrome, DiGeorge syndrome and Miller-Dieker syndrome (4p deletion, 5p deletion, 7q11 deletion, 22q11 and 17p11 microdeletion respectively) other monogenic syndromes include Renpenning syndrome (X-linked), Rett syndrome (X-linked), Cohen syndrome (AR), Rubinstein-Taybi syndrome and others [4].

It is worth mentioning that numerous neurometabolic disorders are also capable of causing microcephaly. However, these inborn errors of metabolism are more likely to cause syndromic microcephaly rather than isolated microcephaly. Among these disorders are serine deficiency (Neu-Laxova syndrome) which occurs due to genetic mutation in the PHGDH gene, and Asparagine synthetase deficiency (ASNS gene mutation) which leads to flat brain gyri and loss of cerebral cortical thickness. Moreover, many other metabolic disorders such as phenylketonuria type 2, Amish lethal microcephaly, Smith-Lemli-Opitz syndrome and the list goes on [16].

11.2.2 *Environmental Etiologies of Primary Microcephaly*

Environmental causes of microcephaly include a variety of factors that a baby can be exposed to during the period of pregnancy, such as hypoxic-ischemic encephalopathy, intrauterine growth restriction (IUGR), poorly controlled maternal diabetes, inborn errors of metabolism like maternal phenylketonuria syndrome and Adenylosuccinate Lyase deficiency. Exposure to teratogenic factors during pregnancy is also a renowned causative agent, including radiation, alcohol (Fetal alcohol syndrome), heroin, cocaine and anti-epileptic drugs (carbamazepine, phenytoin, et cetera.). Furthermore, multiple intrauterine infections, among which are the TORCH infections (toxoplasmosis, others, rubella, cytomegalovirus, and herpes virus) and Zika virus infection. Before the Zika virus outbreak in Brazil 2015–2016, TORCH infections were the most common pre-natal infections associated with microcephaly, with cytomegalovirus (CMV) having the highest rates of microcephaly (20% of CMV cases under the condition that the infection is symptomatic). Currently, the Zika virus is the most common for many reasons, one of them being the decrease in the incidence of some TORCH infections, including rubella, due to vaccination against it. Other causes are attributed to the appearance of a larger number of Zika virus cases and the strong relationship between pre-natal infection and microcephaly, as stated by the CDC in April 2016. The mechanism within which Zika virus causes microcephaly was closely observed by conducting multiple in vitro studies; those studies showed that the mechanism is similar to the mechanism found in autosomal recessive primary microcephaly, explained in the section above. Even though most of the environmental factors are acquired (with some exceptions), i.e., there is no foundation for the genetic defects in the genomic sequence prior to exposure to the factors (i.e., not De novo mutations), they still share similar mechanisms with microcephaly caused primarily by genetic predisposition [3, 7, 9].

Moreover, approximately 59% of 680 microcephalic children who underwent a cohort retrospective etiological analysis in 2014 in Berlin-Germany showed a well-known etiology, among which 50% were genetic etiologies, 45% were attributed to injuries during birth, and only 3% was the share of injuries later in life [17].

Understanding the different etiologies of microcephaly and their mechanism holds great importance in enabling physicians to distinguish between genetic and environmental microcephalies, despite being quite challenging due to the above-mentioned reasons. This, in turn, permits for future prevention of such conditions, providing plans for early interventions that might aid in the minimization of their various effects on the fetal developmental and intellectual abilities and further prepare the parents for the possible outcomes of their baby's condition [9].

11.3   Diagnosis

11.3.1   History and Clinical Presentation

Babies with microcephaly can be presented clinically with different symptoms and features depending on the cause and severity of microcephaly; however, almost all cases of microcephaly share a common list of symptoms and clinical features, and babies have somewhat similar facial features.

Detailed medical history is the initial move in evaluating a microcephalic baby. This step includes assessing the various risk factors the individual might have been exposed to, whether during pregnancy, at delivery or even postnatally. Regarding the pregnancy period, exposure to the numerous causative agents of microcephaly, among which are the pre-natal TORCH infections and Zika virus infections, must be thoroughly asked for, including the timing of infection (i.e., trimester), severity and if the condition was managed accordingly. Other significant exposures that need to be assessed are maternal smoking, alcohol intake, and drug misuse such as cocaine, heroin, carbamazepine phenytoin and other anti-epileptic drugs. Microcephaly is the most seen manifestation in pre-natal radiation exposure; hence it should be assessed. Maternal conditions (e.g., uncontrolled maternal diabetes, phenylketonuria, malnutrition, maternal hypothyroidism and systemic illness) also must be evaluated. Perinatal period complications (asphyxia) and infections are considered as a part of the detailed history [3, 9, 18].

To differentiate whether microcephaly is primary or secondary to reach a suggestive idea of the possible etiology, precise questions about postnatally acquired causes of microcephaly must be directed to the mother, including questions about past-medical conditions such as chronic renal failure, meningitis, anemia, malnutrition, and exposure to heavy metals such as copper. As explained in [Sect. 11.2.1] above, genetic etiologies play a significant role in causing microcephaly; hence, asking about family history (other family members with a similar condition or any syndromes that reflect genetic predisposition for microcephaly) along with consanguinity is a mandatory step to minimize the list of possible causes which in turn may change the pathway of treatment.

11.3.2 Physical Examination

The fundamental point of examining a microcephalic baby is to measure the occipitofrontal head circumference to assess the size of the head, which reflects the size of the brain. The standardized method of measurement is described by the American Academy of Neurology (AAN) as *"Accurate head circumference (HC) measurement is obtained with a flexible non-stretchable measuring tape pulled tightly across the most prominent part on the back (occiput) and front (supraorbital ridges) of the head."* [18].

Moreover, abnormal head shape, prematurely fused skull sutures, early or late fontanelle closure, the presence of dysmorphic facial features, and other congenital defects must all be looked for as they reflect the syndromic type of microcephaly, therefore redirecting the management plan towards another path. Syndromes like cri-du-chat, trisomy 21 and Rubinstein-Taybi are closely linked with late closure of the anterior fontanelle, whereas early closure indicates craniosynostosis. Among the dysmorphic features commonly seen in syndromes that cause microcephaly are hypertelorism and nasal bridge depression, commonly seen in 1q42-q44 deletion syndrome. Greek helmet appearance, cleft lip, and large ears in Wolff-Hirshhorn syndrome patients and numerous other features that develop due to syndromes like cri-du-chat, Williams DiGeorge syndromes, et cetera. Furthermore, many syndromes are associated with congenital heart defects and abnormalities in muscular tone, power, and reflexes, while some metabolic disorders are associated with hepatosplenomegaly; thereby, a complete systemic examination of cardio-vascular, gastro-intestinal and nervous systems is advised as well. Along with exams conducted by an ophthalmologist, audiologist, and dermatologist to assess the presence of visual or hearing defects, determine the degree of impairment caused by microcephaly, and further link skin manifestations with the corresponding etiology such as hypertrichosis in Cornelia De Lange syndrome patients [4, 19].

The physician must also evaluate the child's growth by measuring and recording his/her weight, height and head circumference with each visit to further compare it with the older results because microcephaly may or may not be associated with growth delay and short stature. Additionally, measuring the OFC of family members is necessary to exclude familial causes of microcephaly. Developmental and intellectual performance are among the key factors to be examined, as they reflect the severity of microcephaly. Suppose the child has nothing more than a small head which is proportional to his/her height and weight at the time, with no pronounced effect on growth and development as of now, with the absence of neurological signs and symptoms, no congenital defects or other facial dysmorphic features and no family history of similar condition or other neurological conditions. It is advisable in this case to only closely follow this child up and monitor the development without additional investigations. On the other hand, if the ratio between head size and child's weight and height was off, or in case the other criteria mentioned above are present, then it is crucial to conduct further more in-depth investigative measures such as magnetic resonance imaging (MRI) and even gene sequencing if needed [4, 9].

11.3.3 Neuroimaging

As explained in the paragraph above, diagnosing microcephaly does not mandatorily require neuroimaging in every single case. The choice of resorting to neuroimaging relies heavily on the careful history and physical exam conducted by medical personnel. In certain situations, neuroimaging is needed, one of them being an individual with an occipitofrontal head circumference more than six standard deviations below the mean for age and sex (OFC < −6SD). Other situations include having significant neurological signs such as motor dysfunction or the child is suffering from epileptic seizures early in life, moreover, in situations where the diagnosis has already been reached, imaging can be used to determine the prognosis of the condition. While in cases where the OFC is 3SD below the mean, yet it has not reached more than the 6SD cutoff point, and there are no additional clinical features, then it is illogical to use neuroimaging [19, 20]. It is also important to mention that in cases of microcephaly of a known genetic etiology, MRIs will only show minimal neuroanatomical changes or anomalies (mainly migration disorders alone) and occasionally the presence of MRI findings is hardly noticeable and can be neglected. Thus, it will be of no benefit to expose the baby to such procedures as they will not change the management plan, nor will they add to the prognostic expectations of the patient [21].

The imaging modalities primarily used for diagnosing microcephaly are magnetic resonance imaging (MRI), computed tomography (CT) and ultrasound. Each modality has its advantages and disadvantages over the other, with magnetic resonance imaging having the highest sensitivity due to being more informative regarding soft tissue; thereby, it outperforms CT scans in diagnosing neuroanatomical anomalies. Pre-natal neuroimaging involves the utilization of two modalities which are ultrasound and MRI. Ultrasound is the one primarily used in diagnosis due to its cost-effectiveness and lesser time consumption. Whereas abdominal CT scan is

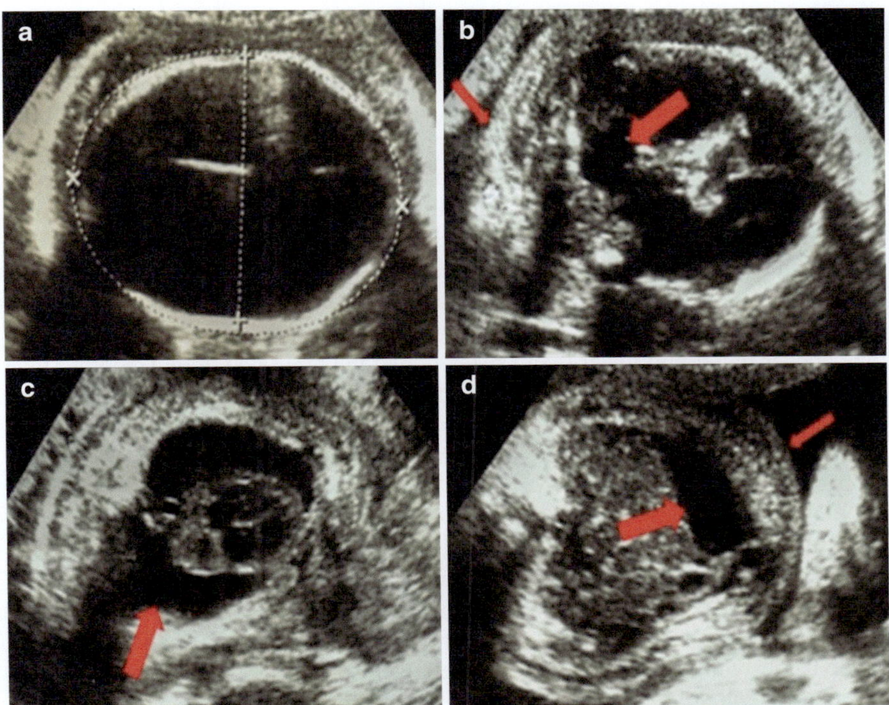

Fig. 11.2 Axial sonography of a fetus at 30 weeks of gestation showing: (**a**) Severely microcephalic head; (**b**) Decimated cerebellar vermis; (**c**) Pleural effusion; (**d**) Ascites. [Image file from Sarno M, Sacramento G, Khouri R, do Rosário M, Costa F, Archanjo G, Santos L, Nery N, Vasilakis N, Ko A, de Almeida A (2016). "Zika Virus Infection and Stillbirths: A Case of Hydrops Fetalis, Hydranencephaly and Fetal Demise". PLOS Neglected Tropical Diseases. DOI:https://doi.org/10.1371/journal.pntd.0004517. PMID 26914330. PMC: 4767410]

contraindicated in pregnancy as it exposes the fetus to radiation that might cause further harm. The current evolvement of sonography techniques enabled it to diagnose microcephaly and other malformations accompanying it, which can help direct the physicians towards a specific etiology [Fig. 11.2], with the emphasis on the link between the timing of performance of ultrasound (gestational age) and the accuracy of the results. The earlier the ultrasound is taken, the less accurate its results are. Nevertheless, antenatal sonography works great in excluding microcephaly. However, the diagnostic yield of antenatal ultrasound in cases suspected with microcephaly has not yet been established. This can be attributed to the presence of many obstacles that hinder the accuracy of sonography; one of these obstacles is the fact that there is no standardized table for average values or fixed cutoff points for the variables that sonography measures (biparietal diameter, occipitofrontal diameter, total area of fetal head, et cetera.), below which we can state that this is considered microcephaly even though some experts state that *"Microcephaly is a head circumference of more than three standard deviations below the mean for gestational age"* as a cutoff point for diagnosing microcephaly via fetal sonography. However, the head circumference can vary depending on numerous variables; thus, there is a debate on using these standards for diagnosis. Another obstacle is ultrasound's inaccuracy and overall low sensitivity in distinguishing microcephaly from normal head size in fetuses with unproportionate head to abdomen size, such as in intrauterine growth restriction (IUGR) [22–24]. Antenatal fetal MRI, however, has higher sensitivity than US. It is capable of additionally assessing fetal brain size rather than relying mainly on skull diameter, along with the ability to detect various anomalies in the brain, which in turn reflects the presence of a possible etiological factor; for instance, the cerebral cortex and cerebellum appear small, the stem of the brain loses its normal thickness, while ventricles get larger; moreover, fetal brain's gyri may appear flatter and fewer than expected, and the brain may look smoother than normal (lissencephaly-pachygyria spectrum), all these features can all be seen antenatally by MRI [22, 25].

Postnatally, US becomes of less importance except when the size of the baby's anterior fontanelle is favorable to perform brain sonography; otherwise, we can rely on MRI with the addition of CT scan. Post-natal MRI shows the same findings mentioned above [Fig. 11.3], whereas CT is less informative, thus used less than MRI. Computed tomography is primarily helpful for checking skull sutures in more detail to exclude premature fusion of the sutures and additionally in cases where we suspect the presence of micro-calcifications inside the brain, especially in microcephalic babies with pre-natal TORCH infections [19].

Neuroimaging of microcephalic babies is known to deliver non-specific findings that physicians cannot rely entirely on to reach the diagnosis. However, with a good history and physical exam, neuroimaging can help direct physicians towards a specific diagnosis or even give a clue on the subsequent logical investigative study to be

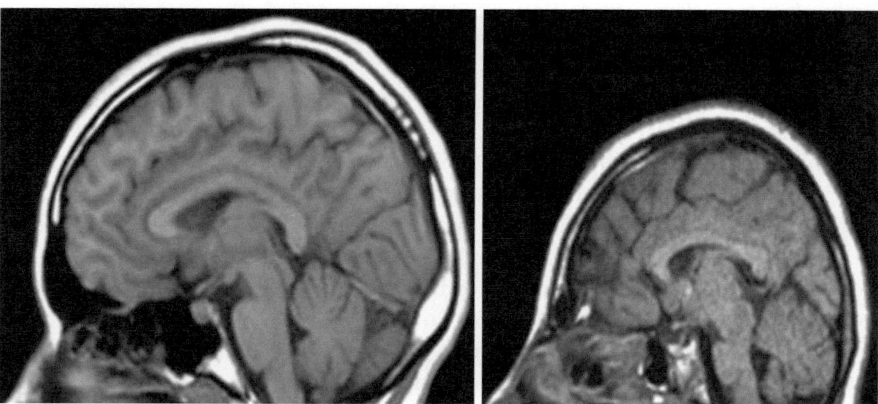

Fig. 11.3 MRI of a normal baby side by side with an MRI of a baby with microcephaly caused by a genetic mutation, it is obvious how the microcephalic brain looks smoother and has fewer gyri, is smaller in size and lacks brainstem thickness. [Image by an unknown author—(2004) Evolutionary History of a Gene Controlling Brain Size. PLoS Biol 2 (5): e134. https://doi.org/10.1371/journal.pbio.0020134]

done. Thus, neuroimaging was found to have excellent diagnostic yield overall, ranging from approximately 40% in cases of mild microcephaly to nearly 80% in patients with an OFC < −3SD up to nearly 80%. Therefore, neuroimaging of microcephalic individuals has lately been advised [9, 26, 27].

11.3.4 Biochemical Tests and Virology

During pregnancy, biochemical and virology tests are considered the next step in diagnosis after a suspicion of metabolic or infectious etiology for microcephaly is made using US and/or MRI in addition to history and exam, and the diagnosis is not yet confirmed.

As explained above in the etiology paragraph, various metabolic disorders and pre-natal infections can cause microcephaly. Thus, it is beneficial to conduct these tests to confirm the diagnosis. Biochemistry is utilized in selected situations, commonly in cases suspected with maternal phenylketonuria, Amish lethal microcephaly, phosphoglycerate dehydrogenase deficiency, et cetera. Furthermore, since inborn errors of metabolism are more commonly associated with post-natal microcephaly; thereby, it is logical to perform biochemical tests on the baby after delivery as it is shown to have better diagnostic yield [26]. These tests vary depending on the suspected disorder; for example, in GLUT1 deficiency, measuring CSF glucose can have a diagnostic yield. Furthermore, urine purine levels can detect disorders with purine metabolism, which also can cause microcephaly [19].

DNA polymerase-chain-reaction (PCR) aided by serological studies can additionally give a better picture of the infectious causative agent of microcephaly. Maternal TORCH and Zika virus infections may be asymptomatic in some cases. Thus, laboratory testing is not performed, and the infection can be missed and not treated accordingly, leading to fetal microcephaly. When microcephaly is detected, and the medical history and physical examination suspect an infectious etiology, then it is advised to conduct virology tests. The method of testing for antenatal infections depends on two significant procedures; the first is identifying the antigen in the serum, amniotic fluid or other possible body fluids harboring the organism. The second method relies on testing for antibodies in the serum (IgG and IgM). The results of these tests are variable and depend primarily on the time they are performed; for instance, it is not possible to detect the presence of herpes simplex virus antigen nor IgM antibodies if there are no visible legions in the oral cavity and external genitalia at the time of performing PCR or serology tests. Furthermore, some viruses such as Zika virus and rubella cease to exist in serum after ten weeks and two weeks, respectively; thereby, it will be of no benefit to perform PCR after that. IgG and IgM vary depending on the organism some will have increased titers of IgG and IgM within a shorter period, and in some viruses, it takes longer for the titers to raise, and the titers decrease variably depending on the virus. Moreover, in the same virus, both IgG and IgM titers differ in the timing at which they increase and decrease, with IgM being quicker but having a shorter staying period, whereas

IgG stays for more extended periods. ELISA is the gold standard test in distinguishing acute from chronic infections. It is also worth mentioning that despite having exceptionally high sensitivity, PCR still cannot have accurate results all the time, and it was found that PCR gives the best results when performed between 20 to 21 weeks of gestation [7, 8, 26].

11.3.5   Genetic Studies

Genetic sequencing can be more challenging to use in detecting genetic etiologies of microcephaly due to the wide variety of genes and the different mutations that can be responsible for microcephaly. However, it has lately become more available for use, and it was found in a study to have high diagnostic yields of 15.3% up to 52%. Genetic studies are recommended as a last resort when other investigative methods fail to detect the etiology of microcephaly [9, 28].

The most sensitive method is to sequence the entire genome in a study called whole-exome sequencing (WES), which focuses only on the regions of the DNA that is responsible for coding proteins, unlike whole-genome sequencing (WGS), which sequences the genome regardless of its regions; however, this method comes with its disadvantages as it is known to be time-consuming and costly. A quicker and cheaper method to detect genetic anomalies would be selected gene sequencing, which relies on the information provided about genes associated with microcephaly, as many of these genes are being discovered with time and linked with the corresponding phenotypical form of microcephaly. This way, it is possible to rely on history, examination and other tests to guide the physician on which genes to be sequenced selectively rather than squandering resources to sequence the whole genome. Many possible mutations like deletion mutations, duplication mutations and others can be detected with sequencing. Another genetic study that can be used is comparative genomic hybridization (CGH) micro-array, which functions by analyzing copy number variations on a molecular basis and can confirm the diagnosis in 15–20% of the cases. This method helps in accelerating genetic study with less time consumption; however, it has low sensitivity and can have false negative results or, in some cases, detect minor genetic anomalies while the individual does have a significant genetic anomaly when tested with whole gene sequencing. This issue, along with other issues, is faced by the physicians when it comes to genetic studies as a whole and not just CGH. Among these problems is the possibility of detecting harmless genetic anomalies that are not the cause of microcephaly; this can lead to mistreatment of the patient and panic among other family members. It is recommended for the physicians to approach the patient initially with simpler genetic studies (comparative genomic hybridization micro-array) to have an initial thought about the possible cause while saving time and resources. If no definitive cause is found, the physician can jump to the next step and order selected gene sequencing. When all these studies fail to confirm the diagnosis, the last resort would be whole-exome sequencing (WES) and/or whole-genome sequencing (WGS) [17, 19, 26].

11.4 Management and Prevention

Managing microcephaly relies solely on its etiology; hence, it is crucial to determine the etiology after reaching the diagnosis as soon as possible. Environmental etiologies are somewhat more modifiable, and their effect can be minimized to some degree if the diagnosis was reached early enough (during pregnancy). For instance, the severity of microcephaly and the degree of damage in fetal brain tissue caused by heroin, cocaine or alcohol (fetal alcohol syndrome) being misused by the mother could be reduced by simply preventing their use and providing aid and rehabilitation for the mother [7, 19]. Following a strict low protein diet for mothers with phenylketonuria and controlling maternal diabetes can improve microcephaly's outcomes.

TORCH and Zika virus infections are also among the modifiable etiologies, as some are preventable with vaccines, like rubella, while others are treated accordingly to minimize their effect on the fetal brain. Although even in such individuals, it is still quite challenging to manage microcephaly if the damage was already done, despite modification of risk factors. The baby could still suffer from severe microcephaly associated with neuroanatomical anomalies and delayed developmental and intellectual performance.

On the other hand, microcephaly with a genetic etiological basis is mostly unpreventable nor treatable due to the non-modifiable nature of the cause.

The treatment choices for varies due to microcephaly having a severity ranging from mild, all the way to severe microcephaly. Besides their tiny head, infants with mild microcephaly usually have no other health issues and require nothing more than growth and development monitoring [29].

On the other hand, for severely microcephalic babies, the management plan can take two pathways; the first path is followed if the diagnosis was made early in pregnancy, and this path relies on assessing the condition of the fetus, severity of microcephaly and the prognosis by conducting extensive investigations by a qualified multi-disciplinary team. According to the findings, the team can decide whether to counsel the parents about terminating the pregnancy [7]. However, this is not a definitive solution for the problem as it is more like running away from the real problem. Furthermore, parents can reject this solution or even simply, this solution would not be possible to implement if the diagnosis was reached late, as in cases diagnosed at birth or in cases of secondary microcephaly where the symptoms develop later in life. Here comes the second pathway of management, which includes providing aid for the child, and supporting him/her through life, especially the first years of life. Regarding delivery, the physicians need to discuss the mode of delivery with the parents after taking a thorough history and conducting studies to exclude any contraindications for vaginal delivery as it is the preferred mode of delivery in such cases [30]. These supportive measures aim to ensure that the child reaches the developmental milestones for his/her age. With a specific focus on preventing, early recognizing, and treating the various microcephaly complications that may evolve as time passes, among which are epilepsy which complicates roughly about 40% of cases of microcephaly, other complications include visual and hearing loss and mental retardation. All of that is provided via the help of a multi-disciplinary team that should be assigned to a child as soon as being diagnosed. This team must include community and general pediatricians to prevent and treat complications, follow up the development of the child and refer to other specialists or sub-specialists when needed. Due to the reason that children with microcephaly could suffer from visual and hearing problems, both an ophthalmologist and a hearing aid expert should also be on the team, providing their knowledge to spot the presence of any visual or hearing deficit by performing electronic hearing tests and visual tests such as visual acuity and others. To support the child's vision with glasses or surgically when in need and check if the child needs a hearing aid. Moreover, it is mandatory to include psychologists in the team to nourish the child with stable psychological status and acceptance of his condition. The ability to follow the developmental milestone for language is supported by speech and language experts who are also among the multi-disciplinary team along with teachers to sculpt the child's personality further and intellectual abilities to as near to normal as possible. Besides children, parents need much support because raising a child with a disability is challenging as it is mentally draining and requires close monitoring of their child's condition. Hence, parents should receive mental support and go through educational plans to explain how this condition affects their child and the common complications to keep an eye out for, such as learning about the distinct types of seizures, how to spot them, and when to visit the specialist [19].

11.5 Complications

Many complications and problems may be present in children with microcephaly, which are usually life-long, so early diagnosis and interventions might attenuate these sequences and improve the life quality of the affected child [8].

Even though the heads of microcephalic babies are usually smaller than average for age and sex, some of those babies still gain developmental milestones. On the other hand, the most common complications encompass:

- Seizures
- Delay in Walking, standing, sitting, speech and other developmental milestones
- Mental disability
- Dysphagia
- Ophthalmologic and audiological disorders
- Epilepsy
- Cerebral palsy
- Impaired Coordination and balance
- Hyperactivity
- Facial deformities and short stature (dwarfism) may be found

A wide variety of factors can determine the complications mentioned above and affect their presence, but the most significant factors are the etiology of microcephaly and its seriousness [29].

There are priorities for the appropriate timing to intervene; for example, hearing problems should be screened and managed as early as possible to improve language evolution, whereas other problems, such as psychological complications, the treatment can be delayed until childhood [8].

11.6 Prognosis

Since microcephaly is a lifelong condition, the prognosis is usually terrible. In general, the development of the affected baby (whether disabled baby or not) is determined by many factors, mainly by the underlying cause and severity of the condition; for example, mild forms of microcephaly are usually not associated with other complications in contrast to severe forms leading to normal development. On the other hand, infectious, genetic and metabolic causes of microcephaly are usually associated with a bad prognosis and can end up with mental retardation and sometimes cerebral palsy [7, 17].

Multiple Choice Questions
1. **Which one of the following environmental factors is the least likely to cause primary microcephaly?**

    (a) Rubella infection
    (b) Intra uterine growth restriction (IUGR)
    (c) Recurrent UTI
    (d) Uncontrolled maternal DM
    (e) Alcohol addiction

2. **One of the following medications has the potential to causes primary microcephaly if it was taken during pregnancy:**

    (a) Alpha methyldopa.
    (b) Doxycycline.
    (c) Metoclopramide.
    (d) Acetaminophen.
    (e) Carbamazepine.

3. **Microcephaly is defined as head circumference of…...:**

    (a) $\geq$ 1SD below the mean for age and sex.
    (b) $\geq$ 3SD below the mean for age and sex.
    (c) $\leq$ 6SD below the mean for age and sex.
    (d) $\geq$ 2SD below the mean for age and sex.
    (e) $\leq$ 2SD below the mean for age and sex.

4. **In genetically induced microcephaly, the most common mode of inheritance is?**

   (a) Autosomal dominant mendelian inheritance.
   (b) Autosomal recessive mendelian inheritance.
   (c) X-linked dominant inheritance.
   (d) X-linked recessive inheritance.
   (e) Mitochondrial inheritance.

5. **A 25yo woman who is currently pregnant and in her 32nd week of gestation comes to you for a regular antenatal care visit, she mentions that she missed her last visit (26th week's visit) due to being on a vacation in Brazil for the last 2 months; during sonography, you noticed that the fetal head size parameters are abnormally small for his gestational age and no other significant findings. You suspected that the baby is microcephalic. What is the next initial step to be taken?**

   (a) Reassure the mother, send her home, and tell her to visit after 2 weeks to repeat the US.
   (b) Immediate referral to take Magnetic Resonance Imaging (MRI) of the fetal brain.
   (c) Send for Enzyme-linked Immunosorbent Assay (ELISA).
   (d) Send for Reverse Transcription Polymerase Chain Reaction (RT-PCR).
   (e) Schedule an appointment for a Whole-exome Sequencing (WES) to exclude genetic defects.

6. **All the following genes can cause microcephaly by affecting centriole biogenesis in neuronal cell DNA except:**

   (a) CENPJ
   (b) STIL
   (c) CEP135
   (d) CEP152
   (e) CDK5RAP2

7. **A 32yo pregnant woman was referred to you from a primary health-care center located in a rural area with a suspicion of microcephalic fetus. During history taking, she mentioned that 3 weeks ago a rash showed up on her face and then spread all over her body till it disappeared after 3 days, she also was febrile and had a headache and a sore throat 2 days before the appearance of the rash. Other than that, nothing was significant. A recent MRI report that was brought by the mother states that there are multiple micro-calcifications in the fetal brain. What is your provisional diagnosis for the etiology of microcephaly in this case?**

   (a) Genetic mutation in the (CENPJ) gene affecting fetal brain development.
   (b) Rubella infection.
   (c) Maternal Exposure to radiation.

(d) Zika virus infection.
(e) Cytomegalovirus (CMV) infection.

8. **Regarding the case above (MCQ number 7) what is the next initial step to confirm your diagnosis?**

(a) Send for Ultrasound.
(b) Repeat the MRI scan.
(c) Send for (RT-PCR) assay to look for rubella antigen.
(d) Send for (ELISA) to confirm the presence of rubella-specific antibodies in maternal blood.
(e) Counsel the mother and take consent to terminate the pregnancy.

9. **A 2-month-old male infant is brought to you by his mother who is afraid that his head might be smaller than normal. After a thorough history was taken, there was no history of antenatal incidents, no rashes no infections, the mother did not get exposed to radiation, does not smoke or drink alcohol and she had good antenatal care; furthermore, her drug history was negative. Regarding the delivery of the baby, she mentions that the baby was delivered vaginally with no complications weighing (2600 g). Upon physical examination of the infant, you found that his OFC lies 2 standard deviations below the mean for his age and sex; however, it is proportionate with the baby's weight and length. And there were no facial dysmorphic features Moreover, the baby does not show any signs of neurological impairment and his head, and his developmental milestones are reached for his age. MRI showed no significant findings.**

    You complete the examination by measuring the mother's head circumference and find out that it is slightly smaller than normal for her age and sex, she justifies that by telling you that it is normal as her husband and other children have small heads as well, yet they are healthy. What will your next step be?

(a) Reassure the mother that it is normal and send her home.
(b) Schedule the baby for Comparative Genomic Hybridization (CGH).
(c) Prepare a multi-disciplinary team to ensure that the baby gets normal development and prevent complications of microcephaly.
(d) Conduct an EEG study on the baby.
(e) Send for (RT-PCR) and (ELISA) to exclude congenital TORCH infections.
(f) Reassure the mother that it is normal and schedule a monthly visit plan for her baby to follow up his growth and development.

10. **In the same case above (MCQ number 9) what would be the next step if family history showed that the baby's older brother suffers from Down syndrome and has mental retardation, and the examination of the infant showed of trisomy 21 facies?**

(a) brain ultrasound as the anterior fontanelle is favorable.
(b) Karyotyping.

    (c) CT scan.
    (d) Comparative Genomic Hybridization (CGH).
    (e) Whole-genome Sequencing.
    (f) Whole-exome Sequencing.

Answers and Explanation

1. ***The answer is (c)*** it is less likely for urinary tract infections to cause microcephaly.

2. ***The answer is (e)*** Carbamazepine use during is proven to be linked with high incidence of congenital defects such as neural tube defects and microcephaly, along with other anti-epileptic drugs. Whereas other drugs (a, b, c and d) are approved to be safe during pregnancy.

3. ***The answer is (d)*** although there is a debate on defining microcephaly, OFC $\geq$ 2SD is the right definition while OFC $\geq$ 3SD means that microcephaly is severe.

4. ***The answer is (b)*** [explained in the above paragraph Sect. 11.2.1].

5. ***The answer is (d)*** this is a case of microcephaly caused by Zika virus infection because the mother was in a Zika virus endemic region. Hence, the next initial move to confirm the diagnosis is to send for (RT-PCR) looking for Zika virus antigen in maternal blood since Zika virus can be detected for the first 10 weeks after getting infected.

6. ***The answer is (e)*** [explained in the above paragraph Sect. 11.2.1].

7. ***The answer is (b)*** this is a typical presentation of rubella infection

8. ***The answer is (d)*** the symptoms showed 3 weeks ago thereby, rubella antigens will not be detected by (RT-PCR) because the antigens cease to exist after 2 weeks of the emergence of the rash. Whereas Immunoglobulins (IgM and IgG) against rubella, can be detected for longer period. So the best step is to send for (ELISA).

9. ***The answer is (f)*** this is a case of familial microcephaly and since the baby has no neurological deficit or developmental delay, and his head size is proportionate with the rest of his body, then it is best to just follow up his development.

10. ***The answer is (b)*** there is a strong connection between microcephaly and down syndrome. Because this case shows a suspicion to be caused by genetic mutation (most likely trisomy 21) then to confirm the diagnosis we should send for karyotyping.

References

1. Opitz JM, Holt MC. Microcephaly: general considerations and aids to nosology. J Craniofac Genet Dev Biol. 1990;10(2):175–204.
2. Dolk H. The predictive value of microcephaly during the first year of life for mental retardation at seven years. Dev Med Child Neurol. 1991;33(11):974–83.
3. Abuelo D. Microcephaly syndromes. Semin Pediatr Neurol. 2007;14(3):118–27.
4. Passemard S, Kaindl A, Verloes A. Microcephaly. Handb Clin Neurol. 2013;111:129–41.

5. Custer D, Vezina G, Vaught D, Brasseux C, Samango-Sprouse C, Cohen M, et al. Neurodevelopmental and neuroimaging correlates in nonsyndromal microcephalic children. J Dev Behav Pediatr. 2000;21(1):12–8.
6. Woods CG. Human microcephaly. Curr Opin Neurobiol. 2004;14(1):112–7.
7. Nawathe A, Doherty J, Pandya P. Fetal microcephaly. BMJ. 2018;361:k2232.
8. Devakumar D, Bamford A, Ferreira MU, Broad J, Rosch RE, Groce N, Breuer J, Cardoso MA, Copp AJ, Alexandre P, Rodrigues LC, Abubakar I. Infectious causes of microcephaly: epidemiology, pathogenesis, diagnosis, and management. Lancet Infect Dis. 2018;18(1):e1–e13.
9. Hanzlik E, Gigante J. Microcephaly. Children (Basel). 2017;4(6):47.
10. Spalding KL, Bhardwaj RD, Buchholz BA, Druid H, Frisén J. Retrospective birth dating of cells in humans. Cell. 2005;122(1):133–43.
11. Barkovich AJ, Kuzniecky RI, Jackson GD, Guerrini R, Dobyns WB. A developmental and genetic classification for malformations of cortical development. Neurology. 2005;65(12):1873–87.
12. Jayaraman D, Bae BI, Walsh CA. The genetics of primary microcephaly. Annu Rev Genomics Hum Genet. 2018;19:177–200.
13. Farooq M, Lindbæk L, Krogh N, Doganli C, Keller C, Mönnich M, Gonçalves AB, Sakthivel S, Mang Y, Fatima A, Andersen VS, Hussain MS, Eiberg H, Hansen L, Kjaer KW, Gopalakrishnan J, Pedersen LB, Møllgård K, Nielsen H, Baig SM, Tommerup N, Christensen ST, Larsen LA. RRP7A links primary microcephaly to dysfunction of ribosome biogenesis, resorption of primary cilia, and neurogenesis. Nat Commun. 2020;11(1):5816.
14. Jean F, Stuart A, Tarailo-Graovac M. Dissecting the genetic and etiological causes of primary microcephaly. Front Neurol. 2020;11:570830.
15. Thornton GK, Woods CG. Primary microcephaly: do all roads lead to Rome? Trends Genet. 2009;25(11):501–10.
16. Kempińska W, Korta K, Marchaj M, Paprocka J. Microcephaly in neurometabolic diseases. Children (Basel). 2022;9(1):97.
17. von der Hagen M, Pivarcsi M, Liebe J, von Bernuth H, Didonato N, Hennermann JB, Bührer C, Wieczorek D, Kaindl AM. Diagnostic approach to microcephaly in childhood: a two-center study and review of the literature. Dev Med Child Neurol. 2014;56(8):732–41.
18. Ashwal S, Michelson D, Plawner L, Dobyns WB, Quality Standards Subcommittee of the American Academy of Neurology and the Practice Committee of the Child Neurology Society. Practice parameter: evaluation of the child with microcephaly (an evidence-based review): report of the Quality Standards Subcommittee of the American Academy of Neurology and the Practice Committee of the Child Neurology Society. Neurology. 2009;73(11):887–97.
19. Seregni F, Parker A. How to assess and support the child with microcephaly. Paediatr Child Health. 2018;28(10):468–73.
20. Woods CG, Parker A. Investigating microcephaly. Arch Dis Child. 2013;98(9):707–13.
21. Sugimoto T, Yasuhara A, Nishida N, Murakami K, Woo M, Kobayashi Y. MRI of the head in the evaluation of microcephaly. Neuropediatrics. 1993;24(01):4–7.
22. Counsell SJ, Arichi T, Arulkumaran S, Rutherford MA. Fetal and neonatal neuroimaging. Handb Clin Neurol. 2019;162:67–103.
23. Chervenak FA, Jeanty P, Cantraine F, Chitkara U, Venus I, Berkowitz RL, Hobbins JC. The diagnosis of fetal microcephaly. Am J Obstet Gynecol. 1984;149(5):512–7.
24. Kurtz AB, Wapner RJ, Rubin CS, Cole-Beuglet C, Ross RD, Goldberg BB. Ultrasound criteria for in utero diagnosis of microcephaly. J Clin Ultrasound. 1980;8(1):11–6.
25. Yaniv G, Katorza E, Tsehmaister Abitbol V, Eisenkraft A, Bercovitz R, Bader S, Hoffmann C. Discrepancy in fetal head biometry between ultrasound and MRI in suspected microcephalic fetuses. Acta Radiol. 2017;58(12):1519–27.
26. Chu A, Heald-Sargent T, Hageman J. Primer on microcephaly. Neo Reviews. 2017;18(1):e44–51.
27. Kirkham FJ. Indications for the performance of neuroimaging in children. Handb Clin Neurol. 2016;136:1275–90.

28. den Hollander NS, Wessels MW, Los FJ, Ursem NT, Niermeijer MF, Wladimiroff JW. Congenital microcephaly detected by pre-natal ultrasound: genetic aspects and clinical significance. Ultrasound Obstet Gynecol. 2000;15(4):282–7.
29. Mai C, Kucik J, Isenburg J, Feldkamp M, Marengo L, Bugenske E, et al. Selected birth defects data from population-based birth defects surveillance programs in the United States, 2006 to 2010: featuring trisomy conditions. Birth Defects Res A Clin Mol Teratol. 2013;97:709–25.
30. Jauniaux E, Alfirevic Z, Bhide A, Belfort M, Burton G, Collins S, et al. Placenta praevia and placenta accreta: diagnosis and management. BJOG. 2018;126(1):e1–e48.

Chapter 12
Megalencephaly and Hemimegalencephaly

Aalaa Saleh, Farah Shibli, Hadi Mouslem, Rayan Awada, and Abbas Fadhil Abdul Hussein

Test your learning and check your understanding of this book's contents: use the "Springer Nature Flashcards" app to access questions using ▶ https://sn.pub/YnQHwS
To use the app, please follow the instructions in Chapter 1.

12.1 Introduction

Megalencephaly refers to the excessive expansion of the brain's cerebral lobes as a result of aberrant postnatal events or developmental anomalies that affect neuronal migration and/or proliferation during the various stages of brain development. The traditional definition of MEG, initially put forth by DeMyer in 1986, is a large brain with weight and size that deviates at least 2 standard deviations from the mean for age, gender, and race. Head size has been utilized in place of brain weight because it is not measurable in real life. Despite the fact that occipitofrontal circumference (OFC) is an inaccurate reflection for brain weight, we can define MEG as an OFC of at least 3 standard deviations above the mean for age and gender after ruling out other causes of excessive head size or macrocephaly including hydrocephalus, arachnoid cysts, subdural hemorrhage, or bone overgrowth. Although it can be

A. Saleh · F. Shibli · H. Mouslem · R. Awada
Faculty of Medical Sciences, Lebanese University, Beirut, Lebanon

A. F. A. Hussein (✉)
College of Medicine, Babylon University, Babil, Iraq

© The Author(s), under exclusive license to Springer Nature Switzerland AG 2024
K. F. AlAli, H. T. Hashim (eds.), *Congenital Brain Malformations*,
https://doi.org/10.1007/978-3-031-58630-9_12

congenital, MEG is typically discovered after 1 year of age, particularly the first 4 months, when the head size has grown extremely quickly [1, 2].

In this chapter, we will highlight the etiologies of megalencephaly, then we review the clinical presentation, diagnosis, and management.

12.2 Pathogenesis

The pathogenesis of megalencephaly vary based on the underlying etiology.

12.2.1 Metabolic Megalencephaly

Three types of metabolic disorders can be accompanied by megalencephaly: organic acid defects, lysosomal storage diseases, and metabolic leukoencephalopathies [3, 4].

Megalencephaly leads to brain dysfunction through edema and accumulation of metabolic products, abnormal in type or amount, in the absence of any inherent abnormalities [5–7].

Physical examination in pediatrics reveals neurological abnormalities, such as enlarged fontanels and sutures, lethargy, hypotonia, irritability, development delay, and seizures. A more wholistic physical examination may reflect pathognomonic features of the associated metabolic disease, like hepatosplenomegaly [8].

12.2.2 Anatomic Megalencephaly

Anatomic megalencephaly is the result of a monogenic mutation affecting brain cells growth, migration, or multiplication. Mutations in the mammalian Target of Rapamyicin (mTOR), Mitogen-Activated Protein Kinase or Extracellular Signal-Regulated Kinases (MAPK/ERK), and Sonic hedgehog (SHH) pathways are frequently associated with megalencephaly [3].

Gene mutations can lead to somatic overgrowth, skeletal dysplasia, chromosomal abnormalities, neuro-cardio-facio-cutaneous manifestations, Greig cephalopolysyndactyly, and acrocallosal syndromes [9].

The expansion in the number of cells can be attributed to either an increase in their proliferative capacity or a decrease in their apoptosis [5, 6, 10]. The result of the increase in the number and/or the size of neural or glial cells would be an increase in the overall brain size.

12.3 Classifications

12.3.1 Megalencephaly

Megalencephaly had been classified into benign (idiopathic), anatomical and metabolic subtypes, where these subtypes have considerable differences in the underlying genetic etiologies, pathophysiology, clinical symptoms and medical management [8].

12.3.2 Benign Familial Megalencephaly (BFM)

It is the most common form [2]. Children with BFG have mild megalencephaly with occipito-frontal circumference (OCF) +2–3 SD above the mean without any neurological impairments [8]. Recurrences are reported in parents, siblings, and second-degree relatives [11].

12.3.3 Metabolic Megalencephaly

It is associated with other metabolic disorders characterized by the accumulation of abnormal type or quantity of metabolic product without any increase in cell number [2]. However, the subsequent cell death will eventually lead to brain atrophy [8]. The metabolic disorders that are shown to be associated with megalencephaly are organic acid defects, metabolic leukoencephalopathies, and lysosomal storage diseases [3, 4]. Even though these metabolic pathways are critical, they affect a limited type of affected cells [3]. For example, metabolic leukoencephalopathies affect preferentially astrocytes and oligodendrocytes [3].

12.3.4 Defects of Organic Acids

Type 1 Glutaric acidiuria is caused by insufficiency in glutaryl-CoA dehydrogenase required for the metabolism of lysine and tryptophan amino acids [12]. Glutaryl-CoA dehydrogenase deficiency causes the accumulation of glutaric acid and 3-hydroxyglutaric acid in the neurons and oxidative stress which contributes to neuronal impairment [12]. The neonate will have macrocephaly, hypotonia, poor feeding, and irritability [13]. Among these defects, L-2 hydroxyglutaric aciduria is the most frequent and severe form, and it is characterized by megalencephaly, neurological impairment, cerebellar signs, and epileptic seizure [14]. D-2–hydroxy-glutaric aciduria is manifested by megalencephaly, cardiomyopathy, hypotonia, and intellectual delay [15].

12.3.5 Metabolic Leukoencephalopathies

Canavan disease is an autosomal recessive disease. It is due to a mutation in the gene encoding aspartoacylase which catalyzes the hydrolysis of N-acetylaspartic acid (NAA) to acetate [16]. The buildup of N-acetylaspartic acid will cause mega-lencephaly, hypotonia, and seizures in 3–6 months old infants [17]. Alexander dis-ease's etiology is a mutation in the glial fibrillary acidic protein in astrocytes [16]. The glial fibrillary acidic protein aggregates into Rosenthal fibers causing astrocyte death and impaired myelination due to abnormal astrocyte–oligodendrocyte inter-action [18].

12.3.6 Lysosomal Storage Diseases

Tay-Sachs disease is caused by mutation in HEXA gene encoding the alpha subunit of β-hexosaminidase A. β-hexosaminidase A is responsible for the conversion of ganglioside GM3 into GM2. Accumulation of ganglioside GM2 causes hypotonia and progressive delay at age of 6 months and apparent megalencephaly at age of 1 year. Short height, progressive spasticity, seizures with visual problems, deafness, and cherry red spots are the most important clinical manifestations [19]. These clin-ical signs are similar to Sandhoff disease which is caused by an inherited mutation in HEXA and HEXB. These enzymes are essential for the degradation of GM2, its derivative GA2, and glycolipid globoside [20].

12.3.7 Anatomical Megalencephaly

It is defined as an enlarged brain due to increased number of cells, size or both with-out any metabolic abnormalities [2]. Its etiology is a single gene mutation involved in cell growth, migration, and replication like mTOR, Ras/MAPK, or SHH path-ways [3]. Megalencephaly could be a unique manifestation or it might be associated with other structural anomalies [3].

12.3.8   *Megalencephaly with Dwarfism [23]*

The corresponding etiology is a mutation in the FGF3 gene. The patient presented with a cranium that is disproportional to their height. The patient at birth has prominent forehead, flat nasal bridge, and small chest. Their cognitive function is normal but they might have cerebral complications.

12.3.9   *Megalencephaly with Gigantism [21]*

Sotos syndrome is an overgrowth syndrome in the prenatal and postnatal period caused by a mutation in the nuclear receptor set domain containing protease 1 (NSD1) gene. The clinical presentation is tall stature, megalencephaly, seizures, abnormal craniofacial features, and gait dyspraxia. Height becomes normal but the head circumference will remain large.

12.3.10   *Megalencephaly with Syndromes [22, 23]*

Megalencephaly- polymicrogyria–polydactyly–hydrocephalus (MPPH) is caused by de novo germline mutation in APT3, and PIK3R2. This syndrome is distinguished by megalencephaly with head size more than 10 SD, hydrocephalus, cerebellar tonsillar ectopia, and polymicrogyria. Megalencephaly Capillary Malformation (MCAP) is caused by mutation in genes involved in the phosphatadylinositol-3 kinase. It has same clinical features as MPPH but without postaxial polydactyly.

12.3.11   *Pretzel Syndrome [8, 24, 25]*

The etiology of Polyhydramnios, megalencephaly, and symptomatic epilepsy syndrome (PMSE), or Pretzel syndrome is homozygous deletions of exons 9 to 13 in the upstream inhibitor of the mammalian target of rapamycin complex 1. It is characterized by infantile-onset epilepsy, hypotonic muscles, craniofacial dimorphism and neurocognitive delay. Megalencephaly is due to extracerebral fluid, or hydrocephalus. mTORC1 signaling pathway activation is reported in the basal ganglia, hippocampus, frontal cortex and spinal cord.

12.4   Hemimegalencephaly

Hemimegalencephaly (HME) is a relatively rare disorder caused by cortical malformation leading to cortical asymmetry [26]. Hemimegalencephaly can occur in isolation or in association with other genetic disorders; however, the real prevalence of each type is not documented in the literature [27].

12.4.1   Isolated [28]

It occurs without any association with other cutaneous or systemic disorders. It occurs in different ethnic groups and equally in both genders. It is initial representation consists of early-onset epilepsy, psychomotor retardation and hemiparesis and hemianopia on the contralateral part of the body.

12.4.2   Syndromic [29–31]

It is hemisphere dysplasia associated with cutaneous or neurological syndromes such as Epidermal nerves syndrome, Klippel-Trenauny Syndrome, McCune Albright syndrome, Proteus syndromes, Unilateral hypomelanosis of Ito, Neurofibromatosis type 1 (NF1), Tuberous sclerosis, and CLOVES syndrome.

12.4.3   Total Hemimegalencephaly [28]

It is associated with hypertrophy of the brainstem and the cerebellum.

12.5   Clinical Presentation

Presentation of megalencephaly can range from being clinically insignificant to etiology-dependent significant features.

Clinically-significant megalencephaly may affect one or both hemispheres. In unilateral forms (hemimegaloencephaly), associated clinical features vary according to the underlying etiology. Patients can possibly present with somatic hemihypertrophy, extraneural hamartomatous lesions, intractable seizures, mental retardation, hyperreflexia, hypotonia, unilateral infantile spasms, Chiari I malformation with holocord syrnix, or even unilateral alopecia [2, 31–37].

However, megalencephaly may be present without any of the pathognomonic findings of the associated syndromes. For example, the most common type of megalencephaly, benign familial megalencephaly, may not have any associated pathologic features [9, 35].

12.5.1 Clinically Significant Megalencephaly Are Characterized by 1 or More of the Following: [38]

1. Head circumference measured either at birth or later in infancy reveal a head size >2 standard deviations above the mean in an otherwise normal individual. Successive measurements may demonstrate an accelerated growth rate.
2. Mental or psychomotor retardation, learning difficulties, or seizures.
3. Stigmata associated with neurocutaneous syndromes.
4. Somatic anomalies, including excessive stature, dwarfism, abnormal facies, or other developmental malformations.

Clinically-insignificant or benign/primary megalencephaly is characterized by the following criteria [29]:

1. Head circumference greater than 2 standard deviations above the mean.
2. No clinical evidence of increased intracranial pressure.
3. Normal developmental and neurologic examinations.
4. Absence of any constellation of neurocutaneous stigmata and craniofacial or somatic anomalies suggesting a specific syndrome.
5. One or both parents or siblings has a large occipital-frontal circumference (OFC) but is neurologically normal, or the enlarged OFC can be traced through several generations.
6. Clinical monitoring at follow-up visits establishes normal development and slowing of the rate of head growth so that the growth acceleration begins to parallel the normal curve.

Note that individuals with anatomic megalencephaly often have a large head circumference with normal intracranial pressure at birth. Although head size crosses the 98th percentile within the first few months of life, it will eventually parallel the upper percentiles on occipital-frontal circumference (OFC) growth curves. In contrast, patients with metabolic megalencephaly typically present without macrocephaly but rather developmental and neurological examination abnormalities at birth, followed subsequently with a relatively rapid head growth rate [5, 6, 9].

12.6   Diagnosis

12.6.1   Megalencephaly [39, 40]

The diagnosis of megalencephaly depends on physical examination. The physical examination should start by inspection of general appearance to search for dysmorphic characteristic which are suggestive of specific anomalies. Occipital-frontal circumference (OFC), weight, and suture are measured and plotted on a standard curve. The head of the child should be observed to check for any abnormalities in the fontanelles and auscultation of the intracranial bruits. The parents' OFC should be obtained to determine if there are any genetic influences on the child's megalencephaly.

Radiologic evaluation of megalencephaly could be done by different modalities including radiographs, ultrasound, CT scan, and MRI.

Ultrasonography identifies ventricular and subarachnoid space enlargement, with a normal neurological examination, absence of elevated intracranial pressure, and an open anterior fontanelle.

MRI and CT scan should be done for infants with neurological abnormalities, increasing intracranial pressure, and enlarging occipital-frontal circumference.

MRI is done to evaluate the size and position of the ventricles, width of the subarachnoid space, changes in the white matter, mass lesions, vascular malformations, subdural fluid collections, and porencephalic cysts. The MRI findings of MPPH and MCAP is characterized by the presence of megalencephaly, polymicrogyria, and periventricular ribbon-like heterotopia with predominance in the temporal and occipital regions.

CT scan can identify intracranial calcifications, tubers in tuberous, and asymmetry of the cerebral hemisphere in infants with sebaceous nevus syndrome.

It is essential to rule out other causes of megalencephaly such as hydrocephalus and ventriculomegaly.

Other additional tests might be required in order to rule out any associated genetic disorders [35, 36].

12.6.2   Hemimegaloencephaly

Many neuroimaging techniques are able to diagnose Hemimegalencephaly like ultrasound, CT scan, and MRI; however, MRI will give the best imaging [29].

Prenatal diagnosis is done by CNS ultrasound or MRI. It shows asymmetrical cerebral hemispheres, midline shift, displaced occipital lobe, and dilated posterior horn of the lateral ventricles [37].

Regarding postnatal diagnosis, a review done by Salamon et al. on 16 cases of hemimegaloencephaly showed that all cases have enlargement of the affected cerebral hemisphere with thickened gray matter and poor gray-to-white matter differentiation. About 11 of these cases showed ipsilateral ventricular enlargement with straightened lateral horn. In 6 cases, there was enlargement of the caudate nucleus, thalamus, basal ganglia, and the olfactory bulb. White and gray matter anterior to the corpus collosum, medial to the ventricles were enlarged in half of the cases [27].

12.7 Management and Prognosis

The prognosis of the disease is highly dependent on the etiology and the associated neurological manifestation [38], but generally, the patients have a bad prognosis [39].

For the severely mentally disabled hemimegalencephalic patients, hemispherectomy should be performed to seize the seizures and their consequences [39].

Carbamazepine showed a neuro-protective role against megalencephaly through its anti-epileptic role in lab mice [40], which suggests that Carbamazepine could be a future treatment for specific types of megalencephaly [41].

There are studies that suggest the use of mTOR inhibitors (rapamycin, ridaforolimus, everolimus, temsirolimus) not only for the treatment but also for the prevention of epilepsy and other neurological symptoms in megalencephalic patients [39].

Moreover, for patients with an increased intracranial pressure, surgical intervention is required [42]. Surgery could also be performed in case of failure of previous methods in controlling the symptoms, where resection of the focal encephalopathy without the alteration of the normal growth would be appropriate [33].

Multiple Choice Questions
1. **Which of following Is incorrect regarding MRI findings In hemimegaloencephaly?**

   (A) Give Information about the affected hemisphere such as ventricle size
   (B) Showed white matter calcification, polymicrogyria and hemicranium
   (C) Enlargement of cerebellum and brainstem
   (D) For identify the seizures associated with hemimegaloencephaly

2. **Patient diagnosis with hemimegaloencephaly associated with seizures, patient was treated by antiepileptic drugs but it isn't response for this medication, then patient was treated by surgery use hemispherectomy, after first week complications occurred. What is likely complication?**

   (A) Difficult in speech and memory
   (B) Paralysis
   (C) Facial nerve damage.
   (D) Fever

3. **Regarding causes of megalencephaly, all of following is true, except:**

   (A) Defect of organic acid
   (B) Mutation in MTOR pathway
   (C) Neurofibromatosis
   (D) Mutations in the FLNA

4. **Pediatric department show case of the syndrome rare to see, so the syndrome called MPPH, all of which is neurological disorders associated with MPPH, except:**

   (A) Shizencephaly
   (B) Hydrocephalus
   (C) Bilateral perisylvian polymicrogyria (BPP).
   (D) Megalencephaly

5. **All of following is true regarding hemimegaloencephaly except:**

   (A) Homonymous hemianopsia
   (B) Problems with breathing, heart rate, and swallowing
   (C) Lost lamination of cortex
   (D) Hamartomatous overgrowth of one cerebral

6. **Regarding diagnosis of megalencephaly, all of following is correct except:**

   (A) Uses EEG to identify seizures
   (B) Head circumference measurement that is smaller two standard deviations above the age-related mean of population
   (C) Uses MRI to gives information for size and shape of brain and confirms diagnosis
   (D) Ultrasound test is performed before birth

7. **Megalencephaly is commonly seen:**

   (A) Turner syndrome
   (B) Down syndrome
   (C) Tay Sach's disease
   (D) Intrauterine infection

8. **Which one of following causes of a large head is least likely to be associated with mental retardation:**

   (A) Subdural effusion
   (B) Hydrocephalus
   (C) Megalencephaly
   (D) Hydranencephaly

9. **Regarding megalencephaly, Identify false statement:**

   (A) Megalencephaly is autosomal recessive disease
   (B) It uses EEG to identify seizures associated with megalencephaly.

   (C) It is condition in which the brain cerebral hemispheres are absent and replaced by sacs filled with CSF

   (D) Megalencephaly occurs alone or associated with neurological disorders

10. **1 year old male child came to pediatric clinic complain with overgrowth on left side of face, left upper and lower limb. Examination showed macrocephaly, speech delay, syndactyly of third and four toes, intellectual disability and capillary malformation of middle face. MRI revealed asymmetry between right and Left side of body. There was ventriculomegaly on right side. What the most likely diagnosis?**

   (A) Megalencephaly polymicrogyria polydactyly hydrocephalus

   (B) Megalencephaly capillary malformation syndrome

   (C) Hydrocephalus

   (D) Schizencephaly

Answer and Explanations

1. *The answer is (D)* the seizures associated with hemimegaloencephaly is diagnosed by EEG.
2. *The answer is (A)* the common complication with hemispherectomy is difficult in memory and speech
3. *The answer is (D)* defect of organic acids, mutations in MTOR pathway and neurofibromatosis are all causes megalencephaly
4. *The answer is (A)* MPPH is associated with hydrocephalus, bilateral perisylvian polymicrogyria (BPP) and megalencephaly
5. *The answer is (B)* problems with breathing, heart rate, and swallowing are not associated with hemimegaloencephaly
6. *The answer is (B)* head circumference measurement that is more two standard deviations above the age-related mean of population in megalencephaly
7. *The answer Is (C)* megalencephaly is commonly seen in a Tay sach's disease
8. The answer is (C) megalencephaly is least associated with mental retardation
9. *The answer Is (C)* condition in which the brain cerebral hemispheres are absent and replaced by sacs filled with CSF is hydrocephalus instead megalencephaly
10. *The answer is (B)* Diagnosis is megalencephaly capillary malformation syndrome.

References

1. DeMeyer W. Megalencephaly in children. Clinical syndromes, genetic patterns, and differential diagnosis from other causes of megalocephaly. Neurology. 1972;22(6):634–43.
2. DeMyer W. Megalencephaly: types, clinical syndromes, and management. Pediatr Neurol. 1986;2(6):321–8.
3. Winden KD, Yuskaitis CJ, Poduri A. Megalencephaly and macrocephaly. Semin Neurol. 2015;35(3):277–87.

4. Mirzaa GM, Poduri A. Megalencephaly and hemimegalencephaly: breakthroughs in molecular etiology. Am J Med Genet C Semin Med Genet. 2014;166C(2):156–72.

5. Olney AH. Macrocephaly syndromes. Semin Pediatr Neurol. 2007 Sep;14(3):128–35.

6. Williams CA, Dagli A, Battaglia A. Genetic disorders associated with macrocephaly. Am J Med Genet A. 2008;146A(15):2023–37.

7. Renaud DL. Leukoencephalopathies associated with macrocephaly. Semin Neurol. 2012;32(1):34–41.

8. Pavone P, Praticò AD, Rizzo R, Corsello G, Ruggieri M, Parano E, et al. A clinical review on megalencephaly: a large brain as a possible sign of cerebral impairment. Med. 2017;96(26):e6814.

9. Pina GE. Fenichel's clinical pediatric neurology. 8th ed. St. Louis: Elsevier; 2019.

10. Mittal K, Kaushik JS, Kaur G, Aamir M, Sharma S. Unusual presentation of Sturge-Weber syndrome: progressive megalencephaly with bilateral cutaneous and cortical involvement. Ann Indian Acad Neurol. 2014;17(2):207–8.

11. Whitehouse AJO, Hickey M, Stanley FJ, Newnham JP, Pennell CE. Brief report: a preliminary study of fetal head circumference growth in autism spectrum disorder. J Autism Dev Disord. 2011;41(1):122–9.

12. Redcay E, Courchesne E. When is the brain enlarged in autism? A meta-analysis of all brain size reports. Biol Psychiatry. 2005;58(1):1–9.

13. Mraz KD, Dixon J, Dumont-Mathieu T, Fein D. Accelerated head and body growth in infants later diagnosed with autism spectrum disorders: a comparative study of optimal outcome children. J Child Neurol. 2009;24(7):833–45.

14. Day RE, Schutt WH. Normal children with large heads—benign familial megalencephaly. Arch Dis Child. 1979;54(7):512–7.

15. Jafari P, Braissant O, Bonafé L, Ballhausen D. The unsolved puzzle of neuropathogenesis in glutaric aciduria type I. Mol Genet Metab. 2011;104(4):425–37.

16. Hedlund GL, Longo N, Pasquali M. Glutaric acidemia type 1. Am J Med Genet C Semin Med Genet. 2006;142C(2):86–94.

17. Steenweg ME, Jakobs C, Errami A, van Dooren SJM, Adeva Bartolomé MT, Aerssens P, et al. An overview of L-2-hydroxyglutarate dehydrogenase gene (L2HGDH) variants: a genotype-phenotype study. Hum Mutat. 2010;31(4):380–90.

18. Nyhan WL, Shelton GD, Jakobs C, Holmes B, Bowe C, Curry CJ, et al. D-2-hydroxyglutaric aciduria. J Child Neurol. 1995;10(2):137–42.

19. Rodriguez D. Leukodystrophies with astrocytic dysfunction. Handb Clin Neurol. 2013;113:1619–28.

20. Traeger EC, Rapin I. The clinical course of Canavan disease. Pediatr Neurol. 1998;18(3):207–12.

21. Swaiman KF, Wright FS, editors. The practice of pediatric neurology. Saint Louis: Mosby; 1975. p. 2.

22. Krivit W, Desnick RJ, Lee J, Moller J, Wright F, Sweeley CC, et al. Generalized accumulation of neutral glycosphingolipids with GM2 ganglioside accumulation in the brain. Sandhoff's disease (variant of Tay-Sachs disease). Am J Med. 1972;52(6):763–70.

23. Bouali H, Latrech H. Achondroplasia: current options and future perspective. Pediatr Endocrinol Rev. 2015;12(4):388–95.

24. Mauceri L, Sorge G, Baieli S, Rizzo R, Pavone L, Coleman M. Aggressive behavior in patients with Sotos syndrome. Pediatr Neurol. 2000;22(1):64–7.

25. Mirzaa G, Graham JM, Keppler-Noreuil K. PIK3CA-related overgrowth spectrum. In: Adam MP, Everman DB, Mirzaa GM, Pagon RA, Wallace SE, Bean LJ, et al., editors. Gene Reviews® [Internet]. Seattle: University of Washington, Seattle; 1993. Available from: http://www.ncbi.nlm.nih.gov/books/NBK153722/. Cited 13 Nov 2022.

26. Mirzaa GM, Conway RL, Gripp KW, Lerman-Sagie T, Siegel DH, de Vries LS, et al. Megalencephaly-capillary malformation (MCAP) and megalencephaly-polydactyly-polymicrogyria-hydrocephalus (MPPH) syndromes: two closely related disorders

of brain overgrowth and abnormal brain and body morphogenesis. Am J Med Genet A. 2012;158A(2):269–91.
27. Parker WE, Orlova KA, Parker WH, Birnbaum JF, Krymskaya VP, Goncharov DA, et al. Rapamycin prevents seizures after depletion of STRADA in a rare neurodevelopmental disorder. Sci Transl Med. 2013;5(182):182ra53.
28. Puffenberger EG, Strauss KA, Ramsey KE, Craig DW, Stephan DA, Robinson DL, et al. Polyhydramnios, megalencephaly and symptomatic epilepsy caused by a homozygous 7-kilobase deletion in LYK5. Brain. 2007;130(Pt 7):1929–41.
29. Friede RL. Developmental neuropathology. Second rev. and expanded edition. Berlin/Heidelberg: Springer Berlin Heidelberg; 1989.
30. Salamon N, Andres M, Chute DJ, Nguyen ST, Chang JW, Huynh MN, et al. Contralateral hemimicrencephaly and clinical–pathological correlations in children with hemimegalencephaly. Brain. 2006;129(2):352–65.
31. Hemimegalencephaly F-SL. Part 1. Genetic, clinical, and imaging aspects. J Child Neurol. 2002;17(5):373–84. discussion 384.
32. Tjiam AT, Stefanko S, Schenk VW, de Vlieger M. Infantile spasms associated with hemi-hypsarrhythmia and hemimegalencephaly. Dev Med Child Neurol. 1978;20(6):779–98.
33. Pelayo R, Barasch E, Kang H, Marion R, Moshé SL. Progressively intractable seizures, focal alopecia, and hemimegalencephaly. Neurology. 1994;44(5):969–71.
34. Flores-Sarnat L, Sarnat HB, Dávila-Gutiérrez G, Alvarez A. Hemimegalencephaly: Part 2. Neuropathology suggests a disorder of cellular lineage. J Child Neurol. 2003;18(11):776–85.
35. Maria BL. Child neurology. 7th ed. Lippincott Williams & Wilkins; 2006.
36. Baskan O, Silav G, Demirci S, Canoz O, Turanli G, Elmaci I. Focal megalencephaly: intraoperative ultrasound imaging in epilepsy surgery. J Med Ultrason. 2015;42(1):127–31.
37. Segal D, Heary RF, Sabharwal S, Barry MT, Ming X. Severe holocord syrinx in a child with megalencephaly-capillary malformation syndrome. J Neurosurg Pediatr. 2016;18(1):79–82.
38. Megalencephaly _ MedLink Neurology.html.
39. Macrocephaly in infants and children_ Etiology and evaluation—UpToDate.html.
40. Kobayashi Y, Magara S, Okazaki K, Komatsubara T, Saitsu H, Matsumoto N, et al. Megalencephaly, polymicrogyria and ribbon-like band heterotopia: a new cortical malformation. Brain Dev. 2016;38(10):950–3.
41. Alvarez RM, García-Díaz L, Márquez J, Fajardo M, Rivas E, García-Lozano JC, et al. Hemimegalencephaly: prenatal diagnosis and outcome. Fetal Diagn Ther. 2011;30(3):234–8.
42. Megalencephaly _ National Institute of Neurological Disorders and Stroke.html.

Chapter 13
Neurocutaneous Syndromes

Ta'ef Mohammed and Zaher Odai Khudher

Test your learning and check your understanding of this book's contents: use the "Springer Nature Flashcards" app to access questions using ▶ https://sn.pub/YnQHwS
To use the app, please follow the instructions in Chapter 1.

13.1   Introduction

Neurocutaneous syndromes (also called phakomatoses) are group of congenital and inherited disorders, as the name suggest they involve the nervous system and the skin, although this definition may involves a wide variety of disorders like SLE and certain vitamins deficiencies (e.g. Pellagra), but we are focusing on congenital and inherited disorders here.

They may involve all the three germ cell layers, but mostly the ectoderm (which encompass retina, skin and nervous system) and mesoderm are involved [1].

Phakomatoses refers to two of the most common types, these are neurofibromatosis and tuberous sclerosis.

Some of these disorders may continue to progress, thus increasing the risk of tumor formation [2]. Among which are neurofibromatosis type 1 and type 2, von Hippel Lindau and tuberous sclerosis.

Over all, tumors caused by these disorders and other inherited disorders that increase the risk of tumor formation and cancer accounts for 10% of childhood malignancies [2].

Ta'ef Mohammed (✉) · Z. O. Khudher
College of Medicine, University of Baghdad, Baghdad, Iraq

© The Author(s), under exclusive license to Springer Nature Switzerland AG 2024
K. F. AlAli, H. T. Hashim (eds.), *Congenital Brain Malformations*,
https://doi.org/10.1007/978-3-031-58630-9_13

13.2 Etiology & Pathophysiology

As a group, neurocutaneous syndromes caused by genetic mutations of certain genes that has inhibition properties over several oncogenes.

Neurofibromatosis type 1 is the commonest among neurocutaneous syndromes; mutation of NF1 gene located on chromosome region 17q11.2 (responsible for production of protein called neurofibromin) is involved in the development of this disorder. Naturally, neurofibromin is responsible for inhibition of an oncogene called RAS, without this inhibition the RAS overactivation will lead to tumor formation like optic nerve glioma and plexiform neurofibroma [3, 4].

Neurofibromatosis inherited as autosomal dominant with penetrance of 100% although 50 & of cases occur as de novo mutation [5–7].

In neurofibromatosis type 2, NF2 gene encodes for Merlin protein which is located on chromosome 22q1.11.is mutated. Like neurofibromatosis type 1, neurofibromatosis type 2 is autosomal dominant with half the cases being new mutations [8].

In tuberous sclerosis, mutation occurs on TSC1 gene (encodes for Hamartin protein) located on chromosome 9q34.13 or TSC2 gene (encodes for Tuberin protein) located on chromosome 16p13.3 is the causative mechanism, like the above disorders, tuberous sclerosis is autosomal dominant with complete penetrance and 50% of the cases being de novo [9–12].

13.3 Clinical Features

The clinical features of neurocutaneous syndromes varying among these disorders, in fact some of these disorder presents with many manifestations at presentation, while others present with sole manifestation at the start.

We will be discussing the clinical features of the most common disorders among neurocutaneous syndromes.

13.3.1 Neurofibromatosis Type 1

Some the clinical manifestation of this disease presents at birth such as café-au-lait spots and become increasingly more during the first year of life, they are flat hyperpigmented lesions that are found on the trunk and limbs, at least six café-au-lait spots or more [7] is required to suspect the diagnosis [13].

Axillary and groin freckling also occur in NF1 and they usually appear in preschool and school age, they are similar to café-au-lait spots but are smaller in size [14].

Lisch nodules, which are hamartoma of the iris also occurs in pre-school and through school age, lisch nodules never effect vision but its benefit lies in detection if one of the parents is affected and also for establishing the diagnosis [15].

Cutaneous and subcutaneous neurofibroma: these are benign peripheral nerve sheath tumors, as the name suggests [16]. they may occur in the skin or beneath it along peripheral nerves, the former is soft and domed shape and can be depressed in the center and usually painless, while the latter is round, hard and sometimes painful, they occur in school-age to adolescent [17].

Plexiform neurofibroma: these lesions present at birth they arise from the nerve sheath and unlike the cutaneous neurofbroma, they grow larger causing disfigurement, they may extend deep inside the body to involve the fascia or the muscle, they may cause airway obstruction or involve the spinal cord and causing compression [18].

They occur in different parts of the body, like the orbit, causing sphenoid wing dysplasia, plexiform neuro fibroma represents an important cause for morbidity and mortality in patient with NF1, because of the airway and neural tissue compression, and on the other hand because they have the potential to transform into malignant peripheral nerve sheath tumors (MPNSTs) [19–22].

Other clinical manifestations include optic nerve glioma, these are low grade pilocytic astrocytoma [23]. Most of them are asymptomatic but visual loss has been reported [24]. Gliomas also occurs in other parts of the CNS like the brainstem [25]. Seizure, macrocephaly, cognitive deficits and learning disability have been reported.

13.3.2 Neurofibromatosis Type 2

Unlike NF1, the cutaneous manifestations like café-au-lait and neurofibroma and others are rarely presenting in NF2, rather NF2 usually present with sole manifestation and the most common one is vestibular shwanoma which can be bilateral and presents with dizziness, tinnitus and hearing loss [26–28].

Other clinical manifestation includes, shwanoma of cranial nerves other than the eighth, intracranial meningioma, spinal tumors, peripheral neuropathy.

Eye manifestations include cataract, retinal hamartomas and epi retinal membrane and these can cause visual disturbance. Skin tumors, skin plaques and subcutaneous tumors are all reported.

13.3.3 Tuberous Sclerosis

Like other neurocutaneous disorders, TS clinical features include dermatological and other organs signs and symptoms.

Dermatological

Dermatological features were suggested as clinical criteria for diagnosis by the Tuberous Sclerosis Complex Consensus Conference in 1998 [29].

Those include hypopigmented lesions known as (Ash leaf spots), the are mainly located in the trunk [30] and limbs, however it can be found in any part of the body but never in the palms or soles. It associated with poliosis if they affect hair. The appears at birth and never changed during lifetime.it is presence is due to decreased number of melanosomes in otherwise normal numbered melanocytes at the affected area [31].

This feature is characteristic and present in about 90% of affected patients and every suspected case should be examined using wood's lamp [32].

Other Dermatological Features Include

1. Facial angiofibromas.
2. Fibrous cephalic plaque (face or scalp)
3. Ungula fibromas
4. Shegreen patches (a skin colored well demarcated lesion found mainly in the back)
5. Confetti skin lesions.
6. Cafe-au-lait spots.
7. Dental enemal pits.
8. Oral cavity fibromas.

Other Organs

Many ophthalmic findings were described, it includes retinal hamartomas which if multiple considered as significant and included as major criteria in the diagnosis of TS. Those lesions are usually benign and clinically silent, but in rare cases it can cause vision deterioration if macula was affected. Retinal achromia which are simply areas of hypopigmentation on the retina was also described [33].

CNS features include seizures, which appear early in life and may occur in form of infantile spasm. Other neurological manifestation includes neurocognitive problems and autism [34].

Rhabdomyoma involves heart in 50% of children with TS [35]. Pulmonary lymphangioleiomyomatosis (LAM) is considered as a major criterion in diagnosis of TS. Kidney involvement by angiomyolipoma which is a benign tumour that could present as heamaturea or flank pain, large mass can cause renal hypertension and renal failure, however renal involvement is not common [36]. Endocrine and gastrointestinal involvement is extremely rare, mainly as hamartomas and angiomyolipoma [37].

13.3.4 Sturge-Weber Syndrome

Cutaneous findings in SWS appear at birth, allowing clinical suspicion of the diagnosis. It includes the characteristics finding (port wine nevus) which associated with 8% risk of having SWS [38].

It consists of dilated capillaries and venules. Appear as flat, pink to red, blenching lesion. Usually locate in the distribution of the ophthalmic nerve V1; it may involve V2 V3 also. In around half of cases it is bilateral [39, 40].

Glaucoma is the main ocular manifestation affecting about 30–70% of patients [41]. Dilated conjunctival and subconjunctival vasculature may also found [39]. CNS and neurological features include epilepsy with seizures that are usually focal but generalized attacks and infantile spasm may also occur [42]. Neurological impairment and stroke like symptoms which may be permanent or transient mainly after minor trauma, it occurs in form hemiparesis or hemianopsia, usually contralateral to port wine nevus [43]. Migraine like headache is no uncommon.

Growth hormone deficiency associated with short stature and abnormal growth curve was also noted [44].

According to above mentioned findings, Sturge-Weber syndrome is classified to three subtypes: type 1 [45], which is the most common classical type that includes port wine nevus with CNS involvement, with or without ocular glaucoma. Type 2 which include patients with port wine nevus without CNS involvement with possible ocular features. Types 3 include CNS involvement without port wine nevus [46].

13.3.5 Ataxia Telangiectasia

Ocular apraxia is the first sign to appear at about 6–18 months of life, the patient showing general dysfunctional cerebellar signs which then developed starting with truncal swaying, involving of extremeties being later. Dysartheria, low muscle tone and weakness also being a result of cerebellar involvement [47]. Extrapyramidal symptoms such as dystonia, chorea and athetosis may also appear [48].

Cutaneous features may present at birth or appear later in life; however, it may never be present [49]. It is mainly cutaneous telangiectasia which involve face, ear, sclera and sometimes in the flexor surface of extremities. Ocular telangiectasia is the most common site [50]. Other cutaneous features include café-au-lait spots, papulosquamous rash and non-infectious granulomas.

70% of patients with ataxia telangiectasia developed primary immunodeficiency, mainly related to abnormal cells signaling, low T and B cells count and antibodies deficiency [51].

Respiratory failure is a great burden in patients with Ataxia telangiectasia; it is responsible for about 50% of adultescence with the disease. The pathophysiology remains unknown [52].

Ataxia telangiectasia is related to highly increase cancer predisposition, with leukemia (T cell acute lymphoblastic leukemia) and lymphoma being the most common associated malignancies. Other solid tumors such as breast, parotid gland, esophagus, stomach and liver was also reported [53, 54].

13.4   Diagnostic Evaluation

The diagnosis of neurocutaneous syndromes is mainly based upon clinical criteria with neuro imaging is helpful in reaching the diagnosis and genetic testing is rarely required except in atypical cases that has not enough manifestations.

Some of the disorders have diagnostic criteria and the others relies more on neuro imaging for confirming the diagnosis.

13.4.1   Neurofibromatosis Type 1

Diagnostic criteria of the consensus conference by The National Institutes of Health (NIH) are highly used in the diagnosis of NF1 [16, 55, 56].

Given their high sensitivity and specify for the disease, a multidisciplinary team composed of neurologist and ophthalmologist [6] is required for examination of these criteria, history of seizures, visual disturbance neurological deficits should also be obtained, the diagnostic criteria of National Institutes of Health (NIH) include the following:

1. Six or more café-au-lait macules larger than 5 mm in diameter [57].
2. Two or more cutaneous/subcutaneous neurofibroma or one plexiform neurofibroma
3. Freckling in the axillary or inguinal region
4. Sphenoid dysplasia or long bone pseudoarthrosis or anterolateral bowing of the tibia
5. Optic pathway glioma (OPG)
6. Positive family history
7. Two or more lisch nodules or two or more choroidal abnormalities [58].

Intracranial neoplasms such as gliomas, schwannomas of cranial nerves, plexiform neurofibroma alongside sphenoid wing dysplasia and cerebral vasculopathy can be confirmed using neuro imaging and helpful in aiding the diagnosis and determine the prognosis [59].

13.4.2   Neurofibromatosis Type 2

The Manchester diagnostic criteria are used in the diagnosis of neurofibromatosis type 2 [60, 61].

And they are summarized in Table 13.1:

Table 13.1 The Manchester diagnostic criteria

Major criteria	Additional criteria
Bilateral vestibular schwannoma	None
Unilateral vestibular schwannoma	Two NF2-associated lesions (meningioma, schwannoma, ependymoma, cataract)
First degree relative with the disease	Unilateral vestibular schwannoma OR two NF2-associated lesions (meningioma, schwannoma, ependymoma, cataract)
Multiple meningioma	Unilateral vestibular schwannoma OR two of the following lesions: schwannoma, ependymoma, cataract

13.4.3   Tuberous Sclerosis

In 1998, the first International Tuberous Sclerosis Complex Consensus Conference was held, due to the variability of the disease, clinical diagnostic criteria were suggested [29].

In 2012, genetic diagnostic criteria were introduced. The identification of pathogenic mutation in TSC1 or TSC2 was recommended as sufficient for definitive diagnosis of tuberous sclerosis regardless the clinical criteria [33, 62].

. However, other TSC1, TSC2 variants effects are not certain and their identification regarded not sufficient for the definitive diagnosis.

Definitive diagnosis is defined as 2 major criteria or 1 major with 2 minor criteria, 1 major or $\geq$2 minor criteria is regarded as possible diagnosis.

MRI is essential for all patients to identify cortical tuberous, subependymal nodules or giant cell astrocytoma and radial migration defects. If not available CT scan or head Ultrasound can be used but they are not sensitive as MRI [63–65].

13.4.4   Sturge-Weber syndrome

Neurological imaging is indicated in two cases, clinically symptomatic patient and in patient with port wine nevus involving v1 distribution of trigeminal nerve [66, 67].

The hallmark of cerebral involvement by Sturge-Weber syndrome is leptomeningeal angiomatosis which is best seen using contrast enhanced MRI. However, post contrast FLAIR sequence was superior in detecting those changes [68, 69].

CT scan is better than MRI in detecting calcification. Dystrophic cortical laminar calcification taking the typical "Tram- Track" appearance which result from calcification involvement along the gyri [70].

Other changes include cerebral atrophy and Choroidal plexus glomus. It is important to know that MRI and CT scan lack sensitivity in neonates and very young infants, another approach include diagnosis depending on history, examination and EEG findings [66, 71] (Fig. 13.1).

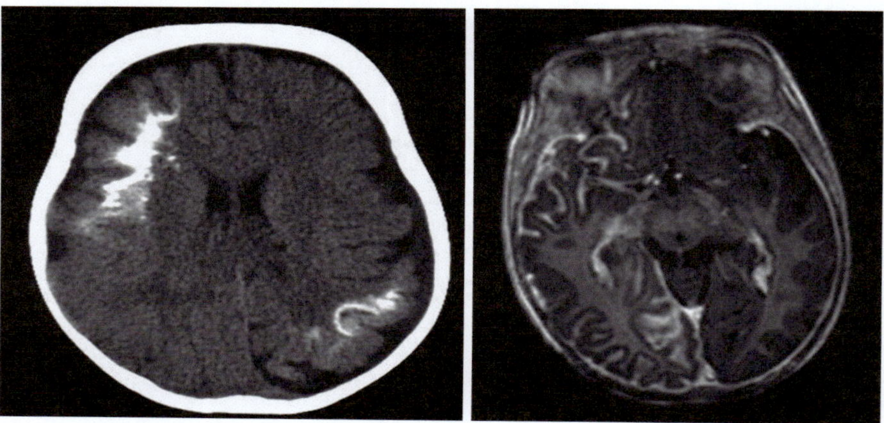

Fig. 13.1 on the left Native CT scan showing Multiple calcification, on the right MRI with gadolinium enhancement showing leptomeningeal angiomatosis [72]

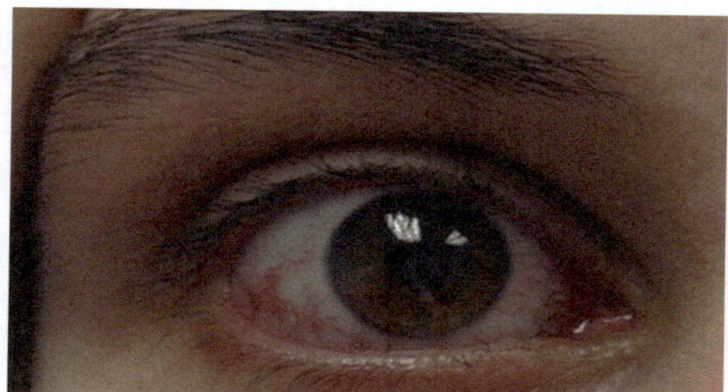

Fig. 13.2 Ocular Telangiectasia in patient with AT [54]

13.4.5   Ataxia Telangiectasia

MRI is the best modality to evaluate patients with ataxia telangiectasia. In the first 2 years of life, neurological imaging is usually negative. Then, cerebellar atrophy, involving the vermis more than cerebellar spheres is the Characteristic finding. It is progressive and correlate the severity of the disease [73]. Hemosiderin depositions may be shown, which sites of telangiectasia [74] is (Fig. 13.2).

13.5   Treatment and Prognosis

The treatment of neurocutaneous syndromes is symptomatic in general and aiming for enhancing quality of life since there is no cure for almost all of these disorders.

In neurofibromatosis type 1, there are new therapies appearing to influence the signaling of the RAS aiming for treatment of cognitive deficit in patients with NF1 [75]. Tumors associated with Neurofibromatosis type 1 and type 2 require surgical resection only if they cause symptoms such as spinal cord tumors or tumors effect visions, otherwise asymptomatic tumors may be left alone without intervention [76]. Treatment for neuropathic pain associated with neurofibromatosis type 2 other than that caused by tumors include gabapentin and pregabalin along with palliative care [76].

The management of TS starting with offering genetic counseling to the affected members and first-degree family relatives. Patients younger than 25 years are recommended to obtain MRI each 1–3 years, to detect the presence of Subependymal giant cell astrocytoma (SEGA) [77]. Surgical resection must be done for large tumors, but small tumors can be treated with mTOR inhibitors which can also be used as neoAdjuvant therapy for large masses prior to surgical resection [63]. Epilepsy treatment and the choice of antiepileptic follows the general rules in other types of epilepsy, everulimus and cannabidiol were shown to be effective in clinical [78].

However, infantile spasm induced by TS in particular shows to be effectively controlled by Vigabatrin which recommended as the first line treatment of infantile spasm and west syndrome induced by TS [79, 80]. ACTH can be used as a second line choice [81].

Neuropsychiatric disorders associated with TS should be treated by appropriate specialist, no specific interventions are existing and every case should be individualized [82]. Large, rapidly growing renal angiolipoma is treated with mTOR inhibitors [83].

Annual monitoring of renal function and blood pressure is recommended. Hypertension is best controlled by ACEI & ARBS [84]. Sirolimus is the first line treatment of pulmonary Lymphangioleiomyomatosis [85]. Topical sirolimus is effective in curing facial angiofibromas but the risk-benefit ratio excludes the systemic usage of mTORI drugs for skin lesions alone [86, 87].

Prophylactic of presymptomatic patients affected with Sturge-Weber syndrome include low dose aspirin and antiepileptic medications is unapproved [88, 89]. Seizures in SWS patients is typically focal, so the preference of drugs selection is targeted against focal seizures [90]. Many reports the benefit of low-dose Aspirin in decreasing number of seizures and stroke like episodes [91, 92].

Like other neurocutaneous syndromes, Ataxia telangiectasia treatment is mainly supportive and no drug show effectiveness in curing all aspects of the disease. Amantadine is found to be efficient in the treatment of ataxia and bradykinesia [93]. Some trails show the effectiveness of betamethasone in improvement of ataxia [94]. Management of immunodeficiency, cancer and pulmonary associated disease should follow the usual guidelines [73].

Multiple Choice Questions

1. **Clinical manifestation of NF1 includes all the following except:**

   (A) Café-au-lait
   (B) sphenoid dysplasia
   (C) lisch nodules
   (D) facial Angiofibroma

Answer:

2. **Neurofibromatosis Type 2 is the commonest among Neurocuatneous syndromes:**

   (A) True
   (B) False

Answer:

3. **The most common presentation of NF2 is:**

   (A) Meningioma
   (B) Schwannoma
   (C) Bilateral vestibular schwannoma
   (D) Ependymoma

Answer:

4. **One of the following is not presenting in tuberous sclerosis:**

   (A) Shagreen patch
   (B) Ungula fibromas
   (C) Cardiac rhabdomyoma
   (D) Optic pathway Glioma

Answer:

5. **Port wine nevus is characteristic finding in Sturge-Weber syndrome:**

   (A) True
   (B) False

Answer:

6. **Percentage of people with Ataxia telangiectasia who develop primary immunodeficiency:**

   (A) 30%
   (B) 50%
   (C) 70%
   (D) 90%

Answer:

7. **The Neurocutaneous syndromes is curable disorders:**

(A) True
(B) False

Answer:

8. **In tuberous sclerosis, the mutation occurs in TSC1 gene encodes for:**

(A) Hamartin protein
(B) neurofibromin protein
(C) Merlin protein
(D) Tuberin protein

Answer:

9. **Neurocutaneous syndromes caused by genetic mutations of certain genes that has inhibition properties over several oncogenes:**

(A) True
(B) False

Answer:

10. **Drug of choice in patient with tuberous sclerosis who has hypertension:**

(A) Beta blockers
(B) Diuretics
(C) Calcium channel blockers
(D) ACI inhibitors

Answer:

References

1. Klar N, Cohen B, Lin D. Neurocutaneous syndromes. Handb Clin Neurol. 2016;135:565–89.
2. Vinken P, Aminoff M. Handbook of clinical neurology. Amsterdam: Elsevier; 2002.
3. Tong J, Hannan F, Zhu Y, Bernards A, Zhong Y. Neurofibromin regulates G protein–stimulated adenylyl cyclase activity. Nat Neurosci. 2002;5(2):95–6.
4. Aoki Y, et al. The RAS/MAPK syndromes: novel roles of the RAS pathway in human genetic disorders. Hum Mutat. 2008;29(8):992–1006.
5. Viskochil D. Review article: genetics of neurofibromatosis 1 and the NF1 gene. J Child Neurol. 2002;17(8):562–70.
6. Anon. Harper's Textbook of Pediatric Dermatology. Wiley; 2019.
7. Awaad YM. Absolute pediatric neurology. Springer Science and Business Media LLC; 2018.
8. Evans DG. Neurofibromatosis type 2. Handb Clin Neurol. 2015;132:87–96.
9. Islam MP, Roach ES. Tuberous sclerosis complex. Handb Clin Neurol. 2015;132:97–109.
10. Moch H, Ohashi R, Gandhi JS, Amin MB. Morphological clues to the appropriate recognition of hereditary renal neoplasms. Semin Diagn Pathol. 2018;35:184–92.

11. Schneider KA. Hereditary cancer syndromes. In: Counseling about cancer strategies for genetic counseling. Wiley; 2011.
12. Hodgson N, Kinori M, Goldbaum MH, Robbins SL. Ophthalmic manifestations of tuberous sclerosis: a review. Clin Exp Ophthalmol. 2016;45:81–6.
13. Nunley KS, Gao F, Albers AC, Bayliss SJ, Gutmann DH. Predictive value of café au lait macules at initial consultation in the diagnosis of neurofibromatosis type 1. Arch Dermatol. 2009;145(8):883–7.
14. Riccardi V. Von Recklinghausen neurofibromatosis. N Engl J Med. 1981;305(27):1617–27.
15. Lubs M, Bauer M, Formas M, Djokic B. Lisch nodules in neurofibromatosis type 1. N Engl J Med. 1991;324(18):1264–6.
16. Anon. Diagnostic assessment and treatment of peripheral nerve tumors. Springer Science and Business Media LLC; 2021.
17. Kurlemann G. Neurocutaneous syndromes. Handb Clin Neurol. 2012;108:513–33.
18. Prada CE, Rangwala FA, Martin LJ, Lovell AM, Saal HM, Schorry EK, Hopkin RJ. Pediatric plexiform neurofibromas: impact on morbidity and mortality in neurofibromatosis type 1. J Pediatr. 2012;160:461–7.
19. Korf BR. Plexiform neurofibromas. Am J Med Genet. 1999;89:31–7.
20. Evans DG, Baser ME, McGaughran J, Sharif S, Howard E, Moran A. Malignant peripheral nerve sheath tumours in neurofibromatosis 1. J Med Genet. 2002;39:311–4.
21. McCaughan JA, Holloway SM, Davidson R, Lam WW. Further evidence of the increased risk for malignant peripheral nerve sheath tumour from a Scottish cohort of patients with neurofibromatosis type 1. J Med Genet. 2007;44:463–6.
22. Tucker T, Wolkenstein P, Revuz J, Zeller J, Friedman JM. Association between benign and malignant peripheral nerve sheath tumors in NF1. Neurology. 2005;65:205–11.
23. Listernick R, Charrow J, Greenwald MJ, Mets M. Natural history of optic pathway tumors in children with neurofibromatosis type 1: a longitudinal study. J Pediatr. 1994;125:63–6.
24. Perilongo G, Moras P, Carollo C, et al. Spontaneous partial regression of low-grade glioma in children with neurofibromatosis-1: a real possibility. J Child Neurol. 1999;14:352–6.
25. Molloy PT, Bilaniuk LT, Vaughan SN, et al. Brainstem gliomas in patients with neurofibromatosis type 1: a distinct clinical entity. Neurology. 1995;45:1897–902.
26. Evans DGR, Huson SM, Donnai D, et al. A clinical study of type 2 neurofibromatosis. Q J Med. 1992;84:603–18.
27. Parry DM, Eldridge R, Kaiser-Kupfer MI, Bouzas EA, Pikus A, Patronas N. Neurofibromatosis 2 (NF2): clinical characteristics of 63 affected individuals and clinical evidence for heterogeneity. Am J Med Genet. 1994;52:450–61.
28. Mautner VF, Lindenau M, Baser ME, et al. The neuroimaging and clinical spectrum of neurofibromatosis. Neurosurgery. 1996;38:880–6.
29. Roach ES, Gomez MR, Northrup H. Tuberous sclerosis complex consensus conference: revised clinical diagnostic criteria. J Child Neurol. 1998;13(12):624–8.
30. Anon. The Phakomatoses. In: Albert and Jakobiec's principles and practice of pediatric neurosurgery. Springer; 2015. p. 7891–924.
31. Neal FD. Non-neurologic manifestations of tuberous sclerosis complex. J Child Neurol. 2004;19(9):690–8.
32. Roach ES, Sparagana SP. Diagnosis of tuberous sclerosis complex. J Child Neurol. 2004;19(9):643–9.
33. Krueger D, Northrup H, Roberds S, Smith K, et al. Tuberous sclerosis complex surveillance and management: recommendations of the 2012 international tuberous sclerosis complex consensus conference. Pediatr Neurol. 2013;49(4):255–65.
34. Curatolo P, Bombardieri R, Jozwiak S. Tuberous sclerosis. Lancet. 2008;372(9639):657–68.
35. Rosser T, Panigrahy A, McClintock W. The diverse clinical manifestations of tuberous sclerosis complex: a review. Semin Pediatr Neurol. 2006;13(1):27–36.
36. Castro M, Shepherd C, Gomez M, Lie J, Ryu J. Pulmonary tuberous sclerosis. Chest. 1995;107(1):189–95.

37. O'Callaghan F, Osborne J. Endocrine, gastrointestinal, hepatic, and lymphatic manifestations of tuberous sclerosis complex. In: Kwiatkowski D, Whittemore V, Thiele E, editors. Tuberous sclerosis complex: genes, clinical features, and therapeutics. Weinheim: Wiley-Blackwell; 2010. p. 369–85.
38. Tallman B, et al. Location of port-wine stains and the likelihood of ophthalmic and/or central nervous system complications. Pediatrics. 1991;87(3):323–7.
39. Piram M, et al. Sturge-Weber syndrome in patients with facial port-wine stain. Pediatr Dermatol. 2012;29(1):32–7.
40. Anon. Rook's textbook of dermatology. Wiley; 2010.
41. Thomas-Sohl KA, et al. Sturge-Weber syndrome: a review. Pediatr Neurol. 2004;30(5):303–10.
42. Fukuyama Y, Tsuchiya S. A study on Sturge-Weber syndrome. Report of a case associated with infantile spasms and electroencephalographic evolution in five cases. Eur Neurol. 1979;18:3.
43. Lin DDM, et al. Dynamic MR perfusion and proton MR spectroscopic imaging in Sturge-Weber syndrome: correlation with neurological symptoms. JMRI. 2006;24(2):274–81.
44. Miller RS, et al. Growth hormone deficiency in Sturge-Weber syndrome. Arch Dis Child. 2006;91(4):340–1.
45. Satyarthee GD, Prabhu M, Moscote-Salazar LR. Sturge Weber Syndrome: review of literature with case illustration. Romanian Neurosurgery. 2017;
46. Roach ES, Delgado MR. Tuberous sclerosis. Dermatol Clin. 1995;13(1):151–61.
47. Hoche F, Seidel K, Theis M, et al. Neurodegeneration in ataxia telangiectasia: what is new? What is evident? Neuropediatrics. 2012;43:119–29.
48. Shaikh AG, Zee DS, Mandir AS, Lederman HM, Crawford TO. Disorders of upper limb movements in ataxia-telangiectasia. PLoS One. 2013;8:e67042.
49. Tavani F, et al. Ataxia-telangiectasia: the pattern of cerebellar atrophy on MRI. Neuroradiology. 2003;45(5):315–9.
50. Greenberger S, et al. Dermatologic manifestations of ataxia-telangiectasia syndrome. J Am Acad Dermatol. 2013;68(6):932–6.
51. Fiorilli M, Businco L, Pandolfi F, Paganelli R, Russo G, Aiuti F. Heterogeneity of immunological abnormalities in ataxia-telangiec-tasia. J Clin Immunol. 1983;3:135–41.
52. Canny GJ, Roifman C, Weitzman S, Braudo M, Levison H. A pulmonary infiltrate in a child with ataxia telangiectasia. Ann Allergy. 1988;61(422–3):66–8.
53. Morrell D, Cromartie E, Swift M. Mortality and cancer incidence in 263 patients with ataxia-telangiectasia. J Natl Cancer Inst. 1986;77:89–92.
54. Rothblum-Oviatt C, Wright J, Lefton-Greif MA, McGrath-Morrow SA, Crawford TO, Lederman HM. Ataxia telangiectasia: a review. Orphanet J Rare Dis. 2016;11:159.
55. Gutmann DH, Aylsworth A, Carey JC, et al. The diagnostic evaluation and multidisciplinary management of neurofibromatosis 1 and neurofibromatosis 2. JAMA. 1997;278(1):51–7.
56. National Institutes of Health consensus development conference statement: neurofibromatosis. Bethesda, Md., USA, July 13–15, 1987. Neurofibromatosis. 1988;1(3):172–8.
57. Anon. Atlas of pediatric brain tumors. Springer; 2016.
58. Anon. Multidisciplinary approach to neurofibromatosis type 1. Springer Science and Business Media LLC; 2020.
59. Nandigam K, Mechtler LL, Smirniotopoulos JG. Neuroimaging of neurocutaneous diseases. Neurol Clin. 2014;32:159–92.
60. Evans DGR, Baser ME, O'Reilly B, et al. Management of the patient and family with neurofibromatosis 2: a consensus conference statement. Br J Neurosurg. 2005;19:5–12.
61. Hannan CJ, Ward CH, Pathmanaban ON, Smith MJ, et al. Multiple meningiomas as a criterion for the diagnosis of neurofibromatosis type 2 and other tumor predisposition syndromes. Neurosurgery. 2022;304
62. Kondo T, Niida Y, Mizuguchi M, Nagasaki Y, Ueno Y, Nishimura A. Autopsy case of right ventricular rhabdomyoma in tuberous sclerosis complex. Legal Med. 2019;36:37–40.

63. Northrup H, Aronow ME, Martina Bebin E, Bissler J, et al. Updated international tuberous sclerosis complex diagnostic criteria and surveillance and management recommendations. Pediatr Neurol. 2021;123:50–66.

64. Inoue Y, Nemoto Y, Murata R, et al. CT and MR imaging of cerebral tuberous sclerosis. Brain and Development. 1998;20:209e221.

65. Kalantari BN, Salamon N. Neuroimaging of tuberous sclerosis: spectrum of pathologic findings and frontiers in imaging. Am J Roentgenol. 2008;190:W304eW309.

66. Boukobza M, et al. "Syndrome de Sturge-Weber. Données actuelles de l'imagerie neuroradiologique" [Sturge-Weber syndrome. The current neuroradiologic data]. J Radiol. 2000;81(7):765–71.

67. Anon. Pediatric brain and spine. Springer Science and Business Media LLC; 2005.

68. Hu J, et al. MR susceptibility weighted imaging (SWI) complements conventional contrast enhanced T1 weighted MRI in characterizing brain abnormalities of Sturge-Weber Syndrome. JMRI. 2008;28(2):300–7.

69. Griffiths PD, et al. Contrast-enhanced fluid-attenuated inversion recovery imaging for leptomeningeal disease in children. AJNR. 2003;24(4):719–23.

70. Smirniotopoulos JG. Neuroimaging of phakomatoses: Sturge-Weber syndrome, tuberous sclerosis, von Hippel-Lindau syndrome. Neuroimaging Clin N Am. 2004;14(2):171–83. vii

71. Ewen JB, et al. Use of quantitative EEG in infants with port-wine birthmark to assess for Sturge-Weber brain involvement. Clin Neurophysiol. 2009;120(8):1433–40.

72. Higueros E, Roe E, Granell E, Baselga E. Sturge-Weber syndrome: a review. Actas Dermosifiliogr. 2017;108(5):407–17.

73. Nissenkorn A, Ben-Zeev B. Ataxia telangiectasia. Handb Clin Neurol. 2015;132

74. Lin DDM, et al. Cerebral abnormalities in adults with ataxia-telangiectasia. AJNR Am J Neuroradiol. 2014;35(1):119–23.

75. Sharif S, et al. Second primary tumors in neurofibromatosis 1 patients treated for optic glioma: substantial risks after radiotherapy. J Clin Oncol. 2006;24(16):2570–5.

76. Tielsch JM. The know, do, and quality gaps in international maternal and child health care interventions. JAMA Pediatr. 2015;169(4):313–4.

77. Anon. Clinical neuroradiology. Springer Science and Business Media LLC; 2019.

78. Thiele EA, Bebin EM, Bhathal H, et al. Add-on cannabidiol treatment for drug resistant seizures in tuberous sclerosis complex: a placebo-controlled randomized clinical trial. JAMA Neurol. 2021;78:285e292.

79. Bombardieri R, Pinci M, Moavero R, Cerminara C, Curatolo P. Early control of seizures improves long-term outcome in children with tuberous sclerosis complex. Eur J Paediatr Neurol. 2010;14:146e149.

80. Chu-Shore CJ, Major P, Camposano S, Muzykewicz D, Thiele EA. The natural history of epilepsy in tuberous sclerosis complex. Epilepsia. 2010;51:1236e1241.

81. O'Callaghan FJ, Edwards SW, Alber FD, et al. Safety and effectiveness of hormonal treatment versus hormonal treatment with vigabatrin for infantil spasms (ICISS): a randomised, multicentre, open-label trial. Lancet Neurol. 2017;16:33e42.

82. Kingswood JC, d'Augeres GB, Belousova E, et al. Tuberous sclerosis registry to increase disease awareness (TOSCA)—baseline data on 2093 patients. Orphanet J Rare Dis. 2017;12:2.

83. Bissler JJ, Kingswood JC, Radzikowska E, et al. Everolimus for angiomyolipoma associated with tuberous sclerosis complex or sporadic lymphangioleiomyomatosis (EXIST-2): a multicentre, randomised, double-blind, placebo-controlled trial. Lancet. 2013;381:817e824.

84. Siroky BJ, Yin H, Dixon BP, et al. Evidence for pericyte origin of TSC-associated renal angiomyolipomas and implications for angiotensin receptor inhibition therapy. Am J Physiol Renal Physiol. 2014;307:F560–70.

85. McCormack FX, Gupta N, Finlay GR, et al. Official American Thoracic Society/Japanese Respiratory Society clinical practice guidelines: lymphangioleiomyomatosis diagnosis and management. Am J Respir Crit Care Med. 2016;194:748–61.

86. Koenig MK, Bell CS, Hebert AA, et al. Efficacy and safety of topical rapamycin in patients with facial angiofibromas secondary to tuberous sclerosis complex: the TREATMENT randomized clinical trial. JAMA Dermatol. 2018;154:773–80.
87. Wataya-Kaneda M, et al. Sirolimus gel treatment vs placebo for facial angiofibromas in patients with tuberous sclerosis complex: a randomized clinical trial. JAMA Dermatol. 2018;154(7):781–8.
88. Ville D, et al. Prophylactic antiepileptic treatment in Sturge-Weber disease. Seizure. 2002;11(3):145–50.
89. Lance EI, et al. Aspirin use in Sturge-Weber syndrome: side effects and clinical outcomes. J Child Neurol. 2013;28(2):213–8.
90. Emedicine.medscape.com. 2018. Sturge-Weber syndrome treatment & management: approach considerations, pharmacologic treatment of seizures, Pharmacologic Treatment of Glaucoma [online]. Available at: https://emedicine.medscape.com/article/1177523-treatment#d8.
91. Udani V, et al. Natural history and magnetic resonance imaging follow-up in 9 Sturge-Weber syndrome patients and clinical correlation. J Child Neurol. 2007;22(4):479–83.
92. Bay MJ, et al. Survey of aspirin use in Sturge-Weber syndrome. J Child Neurol. 2011;26(6):692–702.
93. Nissenkorn A, et al. Movement disorder in ataxia-telangiectasia: treatment with amantadine sulfate. J Child Neurol. 2013;28(2):155–60.
94. Zannolli R, et al. A randomized trial of oral betamethasone to reduce ataxia symptoms in ataxia telangiectasia. Mov Disord. 2012;27(10):1312–6.

Chapter 14
Schizencephaly

Hashim Talib Hashim, Mays Sufyan Ahmad, and Ibrahim Saeed Gataa

Test your learning and check your understanding of this book's contents: use the "Springer Nature Flashcards" app to access questions using ▶ https://sn.pub/YnQHwS
To use the app, please follow the instructions in Chapter 1.

14.1 Introduction

Schizencephaly is defined as "Abnormal slits or clefts in the brain hemispheres" [1]. This cleft can be unilateral or bilateral and it involves the whole thickness of the brain.
There are two types for it [2]:

1. *Type I: Close-lip*: in which the walls of the slits are in contact
2. *Type II: Open-lip*: in which the walls of the slits are separated.

H. T. Hashim
Department of Research, University of Warith Al-Anbiyaa, College of Medicine, Karbala, Iraq

M. S. Ahmad
College of Medicine, University of Baghdad, Baghdad, Iraq

I. S. Gataa (✉)
Oral and Maxillofacial Surgery, University of Warith Al-Anbiyaa, Karbala, Iraq
e-mail: ibraheem@uowa.edu.iq

K. F. AlAli, H. T. Hashim (eds.), *Congenital Brain Malformations*,
https://doi.org/10.1007/978-3-031-58630-9_14

In another study conducted by Paul D. Griffiths, University of Sheffield, UK, a different classification system was used by studying cases using MRI during a 10 y period:

"Schizencephaly 1: Trans-mantle column of abnormal grey matter (polymicrogyria and/or heterotopia) but no evidence of a CSF-containing cleft on MRI.

Schizencephaly (type 2)—CSF-containing cleft present, abutting lining lips of abnormal grey matter opposed.

Schizencephaly (type 3)—CSF-containing cleft present, non-abutting lining lips of abnormal grey matter" [3].

The causes of this malformation are not well known and are mostly attributed to genetic defects like EMX 2 gene and COL4A1 gene [4].

This malformation may be associated with other malformations or defects like microcephaly, absence of the corpus callosum, hydrocephalus or even spine defects.

There is some evidence suggesting that intrauterine infection may contribute to the development of Schizencephaly, these infections include the TORCH infections like cytomegalovirus. Another study suggests heterogeneous etiologies as a cause, many of them causing vascular disruption. In addition, chromosomal anomalies, early parental age and twins increase the risk of having this defect [5].

Pregnant mothers infected with Zika virus, report babies with different defects, schizencephaly one of them [6].

The presentations of these malformations are wide and include seizures, paralysis, abnormal development or developmental delay and others.

14.2   Epidemiology

In California, there was a study conducted from 1985 to 2001, found the prevalence of Schizencephaly is 1.54 per 100,000 [5].

While in the UK, the prevalence is 1.48/100000 births, among 2,567,165 births [7].

14.3   Clinical Presentations of Schizencephaly

Schizencephaly can be presented during birth during the fetal examination at birth or later on. These features and presentations are varying and depend on the severity and the extent of the malformation in the brain tissue. The most suspicious signs and symptoms of Schizencephaly are:

1. Seizures
2. Psychomotor delay or abnormal development
3. Hemiparesis
4. Quadriplegia
5. Dysarthria
6. Cerebral Palsy

7. Hypotonia
8. Mental retardation

These symptoms are mostly presented with different severity depending on the type and the extent of the malformation within the brain and the area involved.

A general neurological examination is very important to assess the neurological deficit and the developmental delay and to guide the management plan.

14.4 Diagnosis

The diagnosis of schizencephaly is not only dependent on the clinical presentations but on the imaging studies and laboratory investigations as follows:

1. MRI: is the investigation of choice to diagnose it.
2. CT: is also an important alternative to confirm the diagnosis.
3. CSF studies
4. MRV: to investigate the vessels overlying the area of schizencephaly.

14.5 Management

The management of schizencephaly consists of managing the symptoms and improving the life quality and preventing neurological damage from progressing. So, it comes in three ways [8]:

1. *Physical therapy:* for hypotonia and muscle weakness and for paralysis.
2. *Occupational therapy*: for the psychomotor delay and mental retardation.
3. *Medical therapy*: for the seizures.
4. *Surgical therapy*: like shunt for hydrocephalus in they come together.

14.6 Complications and Prognosis

The complications of these malformations are dependent on the signs and symptoms of presentations:

1. The child can be a burden on his family with a neurological demise.
2. The child will need continuous care for his needs and special attention for his life and study.
3. The child may continue on physical and occupational therapy for life.
4. The child will be suffering from a psychomotor delay that has a psychological impact on him.
5. Seizures may continue and cause epilepsy.
6. Infections can be serious and may be fatal.

The prognosis of the malformations is highly dependent on the severity and their size of it. Also, the extent of it in the brain tissue and the area of the brain included can determine the prognosis.

14.7 Conclusion

In conclusion, schizencephaly is a slit in the brain's hemisphere that can impact the neurological development of the child. Its presentation and prognosis are highly dependent on the size and extent of it inside the brain tissue. Management of schizencephaly focuses on managing the symptoms and preventing progression.

Multiple Choice Questions
1. **Schizencephaly is:**

   (a) A complicated hydrocephalus
   (b) A slit in the brain hemisphere
   (c) An abnormal development of the pituitary gland
   (d) Absence of corpus colosseum

   Answer: b

2. **The best diagnostic way of schizencephaly is:**

   (a) MRI
   (b) MRV
   (c) CT
   (d) CSF

   Answer: a

3. **The prognosis of schizencephaly is:**

   (a) Good
   (b) Bad
   (c) Depend on the size and severity
   (d) Depend on the management

   Answer: c

4. **Schizencephaly can be managed by:**

   (a) Surgery
   (b) Medical therapy
   (c) Physical and Occupational therapy
   (d) All the above

   Answer: d

5. **The clinical presentation of schizencephaly includes:**

   (a) Epilepsy
   (b) Respiratory failure
   (c) Abnormal limbs' development
   (d) Seizures

   Answer: d

6. **The medical management in schizencephaly is mostly for managing:**

   (a) The seizures
   (b) The hypotonia
   (c) The paralysis
   (d) The hydrocephalus

   Answer: a

7. **There are two types for schizencephaly which are:**

   (a) Right and left defect
   (b) Open and close lip
   (c) Unilateral and bilateral
   (d) Anterior and posterior

   Answer: b

8. **Schizencephaly:**

   (a) Includes the dura matter only
   (b) Includes the partial thickness of the hemispheres
   (c) Includes the full thickness of the hemispheres
   (d) Includes the cranium

   Answer: c

9. **Schizencephaly:**

   (a) Can come with other malformations like microcephaly
   (b) Can be treated prenatally
   (c) Needs no intervention
   (d) Cannot be diagnosed at birth

   Answer: a

10. **Schizencephaly causes:**

    (a) Are infectious in origin
    (b) Are genetic in origin
    (c) Can be caused by genetics or intrauterine infections
    (d) Drugs and radiation are the main causes.

    Answer: c.

References

1. Halabuda A, et al. Schizencephaly—diagnostics and clinical dilemmas. Childs Nerv Syst. 2015;31(4):551–6.
2. Fatterpekar G, Naidich T, Som P. The Teaching Files: Brain and Spine Imaging E-Book. Amsterdam: Elsevier; 2012.
3. Griffiths P. Schizencephaly revisited. Neuroradiology. 2018;60:945–60. https://doi.org/10.1007/s00234-018-2056-7.
4. Tietjen I, Bodell A, Apse K, Mendonza AM, Chang BS, Shaw GM, Barkovich AJ, Lammer EJ, Walsh CA. Comprehensive EMX2 genotyping of a large schizencephaly case series. Am J Med Genet A. 2007;143A(12):1313–6.
5. Curry CJ, Lammer EJ, Nelson V, Shaw GM. Schizencephaly: heterogeneous etiologies in a population of 4 million California births. Am J Med Genet A. 2005;137(2):181–9. https://doi.org/10.1002/ajmg.a.30862.
6. Honein MA, Dawson AL, Petersen EE, et al. Birth defects among fetuses and infants of US women with evidence of possible Zika virus infection during pregnancy. JAMA. 2017;317(1):59–68. https://doi.org/10.1001/jama.2016.19006.
7. Howe DT, Rankin J, Draper ES. Schizencephaly prevalence, prenatal diagnosis and clues to etiology: a register-based study. Ultrasound Obstet Gynecol. 2012;39(1):75–82. https://doi.org/10.1002/uog.9069.E pub 2011 Dec 5.
8. Herrera Ortiz A, Ortiz Sandoval H. Open lip Schizencephaly: a case report. Rev Cuarzo. 2021;26(2):27–9.

Chapter 15
Lissencephaly

Qasim Mehmood, Hafiz Muhammad Iqbal, Saira Naz, and Danish Ali

Test your learning and check your understanding of this book's contents: use the "Springer Nature Flashcards" app to access questions using ▶ https://sn.pub/YnQHwS
To use the app, please follow the instructions in Chapter 1.

15.1 Introduction

Lissencephaly, which means "smooth brain [1–4]," is a spectrum of severe and rare brain malformations characterized by the lack of normal convolutions (folds) in the brain and microcephaly (a few cases) that affects developing fetuses [5]. It is an abnormality of cortical development associated with deficient neuronal migration (the process in which nerve cells move from their place of origin to their permanent location) during embryonic development between 12 and 24 weeks of gestation [2] and abnormal formation of cerebral gyri (the surface of a normal brain is formed by a complex series of folds and grooves) [3]. The folds/bumps are called gyri or convolutions, and the grooves/indentations are called sulci. In children with lissencephaly, the normal convolutions are absent or only partly formed, making the surface of the brain smooth) [5]. Gyri and sulci are important because they increase your brain's surface area (and thus cognitive ability) and separate brain regions [1].

Q. Mehmood (✉) · H. M. Iqbal · S. Naz
King Edward Medical University, Lahore, Pakistan

D. Ali
Rawalpindi Medical University, Rawalpindi, Pakistan

Children with lissencephaly present with mental disabilities and significant developmental delays, which vary from child to child depending on the severity of the brain malformation and the presence of intractable epilepsy [1, 2].

Lissencephaly includes a spectrum of severe brain malformations, including agyria (absent folds), pachygyria (incompletely developed/broad gyri), and subcortical band heterotopia [2, 5–7]. The spectrum of malformations is described by two terms: lissencephaly (LIS = agyria + pachygyria) and subcortical band heterotopia (SBH). LIS's key features are an abnormally thick cortex and the decreased or absent formation of the cerebral gyri. SBH features are a normal cortex with abnormal bands of neurons beneath it; there may be cerebral gyri separated by unusually shallow sulci [5].

Lissencephaly can occur separately (isolated lissencephaly) or as part of syndromes (e.g., Miller-Dieker syndrome, Walker-Warburg syndrome), Miller-Dieker and Baraitser-Winter cerebrofrontofacial syndromes, and X-linked lissencephaly with abnormal genitalia (XLAG) are examples of the multiple congenital anomaly syndromes with LIS [5].

15.2 Types of Lissencephaly

More than 20 types (31 lissencephaly-associated genes) of lissencephaly have been studied, and most of them fall into two main categories: classic lissencephaly (Type 1) and cobblestone lissencephaly (Type 2). Each category has similar symptoms but different genetic mutations [1, 7].

15.2.1 Lissencephaly Type I

Lissencephaly type I is synonymous with lissencephaly, agyria, or classic lissencephaly (LIS1). Subdivisions include isolated lissencephaly sequence (ILS) [8], Miller-Dieker syndrome [8], subcortical band heterotopia, and x-linked lissencephaly [7].

Lissencephaly type 1 (classic lissencephaly) may occur as an isolated abnormality (isolated lissencephaly sequence [ILS]) or in association with certain syndromes (e.g., Miller-Dieker syndrome) [1, 2, 8]. The condition is characterized by agyria or pachygyria causing unusually smooth brain tissue, which results from a neuromigrational arrest between 12 and 16 weeks of gestation [8].

A few patients with classical lissencephaly have severe congenital microcephaly (i.e., a head that is smaller than would be expected), a condition designated as micro-lissencephaly (MLIS) [7]. Abnormalities like seizures, profound intellectual disability, feeding difficulties, growth retardation, and impaired motor abilities may occur. Additional symptoms and physical findings occur if an underlying syndrome is present. Possible causes of isolated lissencephaly, include viral infections, decreased blood flow to the brain during development, or certain genetic factors. Many gene mutations have been implicated in isolated lissencephaly: LIS1, RELN, TUBA1A, NDE1, KATNB1, CDK5, ARX, and DCX. Of these, LIS1 and DCX gene mutations have been most studied [7].

The cortex has four (normally six) layers (a marginal, superficial cellular, cell sparse, and deep cellular layer). The cell sparse layer can appear as a hypodense area and as hyperintensity on computerized tomography (CT) and T2 weighted magnetic resonance (MR) images respectively, especially in the perisylvian region [8].

Macroscopic abnormalities on neuroimaging include agyria, complete pachygyria or mixed agyria/pachygyria, a thick cerebral cortex, a shallow Sylvian fissure due to incomplete opercularisation, and the typical "figure of eight" appearance of the brain, hypoplastic corpus callosum, persistent septum cavum pellucidum, dilatation of the posterior horns of the lateral ventricles, also known as "colpocephaly", probably because of incomplete development of the calcarine gyri and the hippocampi or other adjacent structures, and heterotopias. In some cases, midline calcification not associated with infection can be observed. Importantly the cerebellum is usually normal [8].

15.2.2 Lissencephaly Type II

It is a related brain abnormality, which is also known as cobblestone lissencephaly. It is characterized by decreased normal sulcation, with a bumpy/verrucous cortical surface (thus the term cobblestone lissencephaly), absent in lissencephaly type I. It is due to over-migration (unlike type I lissencephaly, a result of neuronal under-migration) [9]. it is also characterized by associated obstructive hydrocephalus (obstructed flow of the fluid surrounding the brain and spinal cord (cerebrospinal fluid), resulting in increased fluid pressure in the brain) which may lead to abnormal enlargement of the ventricles of the brain, rapid enlargement of the head, and seizures. Lissencephaly type ll is a major manifestation of Walker-Warburg syndrome (see below) [7].

Walker-Warburg syndrome (an autosomal recessive trait, syndrome and its related disorders are now known collectively as muscular dystrophy-dystroglycanopathies) is characterized by lissencephaly type ll in association with retinal dysplasia (abnormal development of the nerve-rich membrane at the back of the eyes), obstructive hydrocephalus, and incomplete development or absence of corpus callosum. Severe growth failure, an unusually small head, seizures, and additional abnormalities of the eyes including a detachment of the retinas, corneal abnormality, small eyes (microphthalmia), and cataracts also typically affect the infant. In some affected infants, there may be occipital encephalocele (abnormal protrusion of the brain through a defect at the back of the skull) [7].

There is an unlayered cortex with extensive ectopia of neuronal and glial cells in the leptomeninges. Changes are seen in the cerebellum as well as the cerebrum, although to a slightly lesser degree [8].

Macroscopically, the brain is predominantly agyric with a somewhat verrucous surface ("cobblestone lissencephaly"), areas of pachygyria and polymicrogyria, the cortex is thickened(but less thick than in type I). Obliteration of the subarachnoid space and consequently hydrocephalus from thick meninges which are also adherent to the cortex. There is also a fusion of the cerebral hemispheres, Myelination is poor, the septum pellucidum and corpus callosum are hypoplastic or absent and the cerebellum is often small and the vermis hypoplastic. Dandy-Walker malformation and occipital cephaloceles are other abnormalities [8]. The extent of the cerebral and cerebellar abnormalities is variable in the syndromes described.

15.3 Epidemiology

15.3.1 Incidence

Lissencephaly is a rare disorder and the incidence is not known [2]. Researchers estimate that it affects about 1 out of every 100,000 babies1(the overall incidence of lissencephaly is estimated at around 1.2 per 100,000 births [7].

15.3.2 Prevalence

Lissencephaly affects fetuses and usually develops during the 12th and 24th weeks of fetal development [1]. A study in the Netherlands estimated the prevalence of lissencephaly around 1.2 per 100,000 births [2]. The only epidemiological data on the prevalence of type I lissencephaly come from The Netherlands, with 11.7 per million births [10]. There is no reliable prevalence data available on type II lissencephaly though most commonly seen in the United Kingdom as Walker Warburg syndrome (personal observations) [8]. With improving imaging technology, the diagnosis and the prevalence of lissencephaly will increase [2].

15.4 Etiology

Lissencephaly may be caused by genetic or non-genetic factors.

15.4.1 Non-Genetic Factors

In rare cases intrauterine viral infections or viral infections in the fetus during the first trimester (the first to twelfth week of pregnancy) [1–4] insufficient blood supply to the baby's brain early in pregnancy [1–4].

For example, Cytomegalovirus (CMV) has been associated with developing lissencephaly. It reduces blood supply to the fetal brain. The severity depends on the gestational age (early infection is more likely to cause lissencephaly because neuronal migration takes place early in the pregnancy) [2].

15.4.2 Genetic Factors

There are two distinct genetic causes of lissencephaly.

X-Linked [3, 4]

Chromosome 17-Linked [3, 4]

With the discovery of deletion 17p13.3 in children with severe LIS and characteristic facial dysmorphism (i.e., Miller-Dieker syndrome) discovery of the genetic causes of LIS began in 1982, and with the subsequent discovery of the two most common causal genes i.e., LIS1 (aka PAFA1H1) and DCX—in 1993 and 1998 [5]. The advancement in molecular genetics has led to the identification of 316 lissencephaly-associated genes (giving an overall diagnostic yield of over 80%), many of which are microtubule structural (tubulin), or microtubule-associated proteins (MAPs), including ACTB, ACTG1, ARX, CDK5, CRADD, DCX, DYNC1H1, KIF2A, KIF5C, LIS1, NDE1, RELN, TUBA1A, TUBA8, TUBB, TUBB2B, TUBB3, TUBG1, VLDLR, etc. [2].

Some of the Better-Studied Genetic Causes Are Listed Below

LIS1

The most studied LIS1 (PAFAH1B1) is located on chromosome 17p13.37 (it encodes platelet-activating factor acetylhydrolase isoform 1B that interacts with microtubule-associated proteins: dynein and dynactin7 (the motor protein linked to neuronal nuclei movement along microtubules) [2, 8]. The mutation or deletion in the LIS1 gene is associated with lissencephaly type 1 i.e., both isolated Lissencephaly syndrome and Miller-Dieker syndrome (MDS infants mostly have mutations in the LIS1 gene but also additional deletions of adjacent genes on chromosome 17, thus resulting in lissencephaly type 1 feature and other craniofacial abnormalities) [2, 7]. The risk of another child with this condition is extremely low because such chromosomal alterations occur randomly and are observed in the child only [7].

DCX (X-Linked Lissencephaly Type 1/XLIS 1 or LISX 1)

DCX is located on the X chromosome. It encodes for the doublecortin protein(a neuronal microtubule-associated protein, essential for neuronal migration). The mutation causes defects in neuronal migration. [2] Males (one X chromosome and one Y chromosome) with DCX mutation are more likely to be severely affected, while females (who have two X chromosomes) with the same mutation have a milder version of the disorder (can be healthy without symptoms) [2].

ARX (X-Linked Lissencephaly Type 2/XLIS 2 or LISX 2)

The ARX gene (also located on the X chromosome, so male infants are typically more severely affected by this mutation than infant females) encodes for the aristaless-related homeobox protein (a transcription factor with an important action in the forebrain and other tissue) [2, 7]. Children with ARX mutation present with other symptoms along with lissencephaly, such as missing sections of their brain (agenesis of the corpus callosum), abnormal genitalia, and severe epilepsy. X-linked forms of lissencephaly can recur in a family because a healthy mother can have the mutation [7].

RELN

It encodes reelin (an extracellular matrix glycoprotein) A mutation of the RELN gene causes Norman-Roberts syndrome (autosomal recessive inheritance pattern), which includes lissencephaly [1, 2]. Other associated features are cerebellar hypoplasia and hippocampal abnormalities.

All three syndromes mentioned in type 2 lissencephaly are considered to be autosomal recessive with reports of more than one affected offspring of consanguineous parents [8].

There are a few reported cases of prenatal ultrasound diagnosis. Ultrasound scanning during pregnancy can be a useful diagnostic tool, especially in those families with a previously affected child because in the second trimester, features such as hydrocephalus, encephaloceles, and microphthalmia, can be detected [8].

15.5 Signs and Symptoms

Lissencephaly appears as multitude of symptoms. There may be short term learning differences, but its severity varies from patient to patient [1]. There may be microcephaly i.e., a smaller-than-normal head size accompanied by Dysphagia i.e., difficulty in eating and swallowing [11].

The patient may feel apparent satiety. Child cannot thrive and there are prolonged periods of growth and development. Mental capabilities are deteriorated, learning differences are frequently seen but cognitive functions are retained, muscle twitches and spasms are seen too [11].

Psychomotor functions like hand-eye coordination are disturbed, there is slow physical development, there are Limb differences prevalent in hands and feet, inability of kids to sit, stand, walk or roll over [11]. Accompanied by seizures or epilepsy, especially during the first 10 months of life [12].

There may be malformations of cortical development including agyria which shows a strong relationship to silver dust exposure prenatally or afterwards commonly seen as bluishness hue to skin, or there may be pachygyria characterized by unusual thickening of cerebral convolutions. The subcortical band heterotopia, also known as double cortex syndrome, in which developmentally the neurons can't reach their proper physiological location in brain is also found [6].

15.6 Diagnosis

Lissencephaly can be diagnosed based on clinical and molecular diagnosis or on histopathological changes. Magnetic resonance imaging (MRI) can also be of profound use. Smooth gyral pattern hints at lissencephaly [13].

Molecular genetics also has helped in the detection of two of the genes: LIS1 (PAFAH1B1) on chromosome 17 and DCX (doublecortin) on the X chromosome involved in pathogenesis [14].

Ventriculomegaly diagnosed in utero is also another hint at the pathology. Some other specific laboratory tests can also help in making the right diagnosis [15].

Electroencephalography (EEG) shows 'major fast dysrhythmia', with abnormally rapid, high-voltage activity, mainly in the alpha and beta frequency bands [16].

15.7 Treatment

Since the insult causing defective neuronal migration leading to lissencephaly occurs in embryonic period so the treatment of lissencephaly is mainly targeted to manage the symptoms and improve caloric intake as no gene specific treatment for lissencephaly is available at present. Interdisciplinary management of LIS patients beginning at the time of diagnosis is crucial to improve survival and the quality of life for such patients. As LIS clinical manifestations vary from patient to patient depending on degree of brain malformations [17]. Therefore, once the diagnosis is established complete evaluation of patient comprising of neurologic, developmental, ophthalmic and feeding evaluation along with head circumference and growth evaluation and consultation from clinical geneticist are important to establish clinical manifestations of LIS in individual patients [18].

Almost all patients of LIS have seizures and therefore anti-convulsant medications are a part of treatment regime for LIS [19]. Feeding problems are also quite common in newborns due to uncoordinated sucking and may require placement of percutaneous endoscopic gastrostomy tube to prevent malnutrition. In children with hypotonia physiotherapy may help to improve mobility and prevent contractures. Fine motor control and oral motor control may improve by occupational therapy. Communication skills of LIS patients are usually poor and they may benefit from speech therapy [20].

Along with treatment of symptoms continuous surveillance is also very important to prevent complications and manage LIS patients. Complications like aspiration pneumonia, foot deformities, scoliosis and epileptic encephalopathy are commonly observed in such patients which not only affects quality of life but also increases the mortality [21].

Genetic testing is not only important for diagnosis but can also be used to predict the rate of recurrence and can also be useful in prenatal testing in high-risk pregnancies. Usually neglected but an important factor for genetic counselling is the genetic status of the parents. Research on some animal models is suggestive that it might be possible to enable neuronal migration postnatally after re-expression of missing gene which may be helpful in controlling seizures and reducing clinical severity [22].

15.8 Prognosis

Prognosis of lissencephaly is poor in general but it varies and is dependent on grade of clinical severity [23]. There are three clinical grades of LIS mild, moderate and severe depending on intellectual disability and epilepsy. Patients having mild grade of LIS are expected to survive to adulthood and have moderate intellectual disability [24]. Patients having moderate LIS have poorly controlled seizures, moderate to severe intellectual disability and reduced life expectancy but they may survive to adulthood while patients having severe LIS have poor survival rate and more than half of them die by 10 years and such patients usually have profound intellectual disability with poorly controlled seizures [25].

Multiple Choice Questions

1. **Lissencephaly is closely related to which metallic toxicity?**

   (a) Mercury
   (b) Silver
   (c) Copper
   (d) Iodine
   (e) Thallium

   Answer: b) Silver

2. **Gyral pattern is lissencephaly is?**

   (a) Smooth
   (b) Irregular
   (c) Nodular
   (d) Patchy

   Answer: a) Smooth

3. **In Utero presentation of lissencephaly is?**

   (a) Microcephaly
   (b) Seizures
   (c) Agyria
   (d) Ventriculomegaly

   Answer: d) Ventriculomegaly

4. **Double cortex syndrome is?**

   (a) Subcortical band heterotopia
   (b) Developmental abnormality
   (c) Related to Cerebral cortex
   (d) All the above

   Answer: d) All the above

5. **Lissencephaly can be diagnosed by all except?**

   (a) CT scan
   (b) MRI
   (c) EEG
   (d) Molecular genetics
   (e) Histological features

   Answer: a) CT scan

6. **A 1-month-old male patient who is diagnosed case of lissencephaly has feeding problems how will be the nutrition of the patient improved?**

   (a) Nasogastric tube placement
   (b) Shifting patient on formula feed

   (c) Parenteral nutrition
   (d) Percutaneous endoscopic gastrostomy tube placement

   Answer: d) percutaneous endoscopic gastrostomy tube placement

7. **Which complication of lissencephaly is associated with high mortality?**

   (a) Aspiration pneumonia
   (b) Epileptic encephalopathy
   (c) Contractures
   (d) Scoliosis

   Answer: a) aspiration pneumonia

8. **Lissencephaly is best managed by:**

   (a) Gastroenterologist
   (b) Neurologist
   (c) Physiotherapist
   (d) Interdisciplinary team management

   Answer: d) interdisciplinary team management

9. **In which clinical grade of lissencephaly patient may have normal intelligent quotient**

   (a) Mild lissencephaly
   (b) Moderate lissencephaly
   (c) Severe lissencephaly
   (d) All of the above

   Answer: a) mild lissencephaly

10. **Which investigation is important not only to establish diagnosis but to predict recurrence as well?**

    (a) CT scan
    (b) Genetic testing
    (c) Measurement of growth parameters
    (d) Ophthalmic evaluation

    Answer: b) genetic testing

References

1. Lissencephaly (Smooth Brain) [Internet]. Cleveland Clinic. [cited 2023 Jan 4]. https://my.clevelandclinic.org/health/diseases/6033-lissencephaly.
2. Kattuoa M, M Das J. Lissencephaly. [Updated 2022 Jul 4]. In: StatPearls [Internet]. Treasure Island, FL: StatPearls Publishing; 2022. https://www.ncbi.nlm.nih.gov/books/NBK560766/.

3. Office of Communications and Public Liaison National Institute of neurological disorders and stroke. Cephalic disorders fact sheet. Maryland: NINDS; 2003. Publication No. 98-433.
4. Cephalic Disorders Fact Sheet | National Institute of Neurological Disorders and Stroke [Internet]. [cited 2023 Jan 8]. https://www.ninds.nih.gov/cephalic-disorders-fact-sheet.
5. Di Donato N, Chiari S, Mirzaa GM, Aldinger K, Parrini E, Olds C, et al. Lissencephaly: expanded imaging and clinical classification. Am J Med Genet A. 2017;173(6):1473–88.
6. Koenig M, Dobyns WB, Di Donato N. Lissencephaly: update on diagnostics and clinical management. Eur J Paediatr Neurol. 2021;35:147–52.
7. Lissencephaly [Internet]. NORD (National Organization for Rare Disorders). [cited 2023 Jan 4]. https://rarediseases.org/rare-diseases/lissencephaly/
8. Pilz DT, Quarrell OW. Syndromes with lissencephaly. J Med Genet. 1996;33(4):319–23.
9. Deng F, Gaillard F. Lissencephaly type II. In: Radiopaedia.org [Internet]. Radiopaedia.org; 2011 [cited 2023 Jan 8]. http://radiopaedia.org/articles/16167.
10. de Rijk-van Andel JF, Arts WFM, Hofman A, Staal A, Niermeijer MF. Epidemiology of Lissencephaly type I. Neuroepidemiology. 1991;10(4):200–4. https://doi.org/10.1159/000110270.
11. Lissencephaly: types, symptoms, causes, diagnosis, treatment [internet]. WebMD WebMD; [cited 2023Jan 28]. https://www.webmd.com/brain/what-is-lissencephaly.
12. Andel JD, Arts WF, Barth PG, Loonen MC. Diagnostic features and clinical signs of 21 patients with lissencephaly type I. Dev Med Child Neurol. 1990;32(8):707–17.
13. Saltzman DH, Krauss CM, Goldman JM, Benacerraf BR. Prenatal diagnosis of lissencephaly. Prenat Diagn. 1991;11(3):139–43.
14. Leventer RJ, Pilz DT, Matsumoto N, Ledbetter DH, Dobyns WB. Lissencephaly and subcortical band heterotopia: molecular basis and diagnosis. Mol Med Today. 2000;6(7):277–84.
15. Holzgreve W, Feil R, Louwen F, Miny P. Prenatal diagnosis and management of fetal hydrocephaly and lissencephaly. Childs Nerv Syst. 1993;9(7):408–12.
16. Gastaut H, Pinsard N, Raybaud CH, Aicardi J, Zifkin B. Lissencephaly (agyria-pachygyria): clinical findings and serial EEG studies. Dev Med Child Neurol. 1987;29(2):167–80.
17. Kattuoa ML, Das MJ. Lissencephaly. In: StatPearls. Treasure Island, FL: StatPearls Publishing; 2022. https://pubmed.ncbi.nlm.nih.gov/32809601/.
18. Hehr U, Uyanik G, Aigner L, et al. DCX-related disorders. 2007 Oct 19 [updated 2019 Feb 7]. In: Adam MP, Everman DB, Mirzaa GM, et al., editors. GeneReviews® [internet]. Seattle: University of Washington, Seattle; 2007.
19. Guerrini R, Sicca F, Parmeggiani L. Epilepsy and malformations of the cerebral cortex. Epileptic Disord. 2003;5(Suppl 2):S9–S26.
20. Dobyns WB. The clinical patterns and molecular genetics of lissencephaly and subcortical band heterotopia. Epilepsia. 2010;51(Suppl 1):5–9. https://doi.org/10.1111/j.1528-1167.2009.02433.x.
21. Okumura A, Hayashi M, Tsurui H, et al. Lissencephaly with marked ventricular dilation, agenesis of corpus callosum, and cerebellar hypoplasia caused by TUBA1A mutation. Brain and Development. 2013;35(3):274–9. https://doi.org/10.1016/j.braindev.2012.05.006.
22. Fry AE, Cushion TD, Pilz DT. The genetics of lissencephaly. Am J Med Genet C Semin Med Genet. 2014;166C(2):198–210. https://doi.org/10.1002/ajmg.c.31402.
23. Di Donato N, Chiari S, Mirzaa GM, et al. Lissencephaly: expanded imaging and clinical classification. Am J Med Genet A. 2017;173(6):1473–88. https://doi.org/10.1002/ajmg.a.38245.
24. Leventer RJ, Cardoso C, Ledbetter DH, Dobyns WB. LIS1 missense mutations cause milder lissencephaly phenotypes including a child with normal IQ. Neurology. 2001;57(3):416–22. https://doi.org/10.1212/wnl.57.3.416.
25. Bahi-Buisson N, Poirier K, Fourniol F, et al. The wide spectrum of tubulinopathies: what are the key features for the diagnosis? Brain. 2014;137(Pt 6):1676–700. https://doi.org/10.1093/brain/awu082.

Chapter 16
Heterotopias

Mrinmoy Kundu, Wireko Andrew Awuah, Jyi Cheng Ng, Helen Huang, Abubakar Nazir, Shehroze Tabassum, Riaz Jiffry, Tulika Garg, Toufik Abdul-Rahman, Debrah Fosuah Anastasia, Aymar Akilimali, Rohan Yarlagadda, and Arda Isik

Test your learning and check your understanding of this book's contents: use the "Springer Nature Flashcards" app to access questions using ▶ https://sn.pub/YnQHwS
To use the app, please follow the instructions in Chapter 1.

M. Kundu
Institute of Medical Sciences and SUM Hospital, Bhubaneswar, India

W. A. Awuah (✉) · T. Abdul-Rahman · D. F. Anastasia
Sumy State University, Sumy, Ukraine

J. C. Ng
Faculty of Medicine and Health Sciences, University of Putra Malaysia, Serdang, Malaysia

H. Huang · R. Jiffry
Royal College of Surgeons in Ireland, University of Medicine and Health Sciences, Dublin, Ireland
e-mail: HelenHuang@rcsi.ie; riazjiffry20@rcsi.com

A. Nazir · S. Tabassum
King Edward Medical University, Lahore, Pakistan

T. Garg
Government Medical College and Hospital, Chandigarh, India

A. Akilimali
Faculty of Medicine, Official University of Bukavu, Bukavu, DR, Congo

R. Yarlagadda
Rowan University School of Osteopathic Medicine, Stratford, NJ, USA

A. Isik
Department of General Surgery, Istanbul Medeniyet University, Istanbul, Turkey

K. F. AlAli, H. T. Hashim (eds.), *Congenital Brain Malformations*, https://doi.org/10.1007/978-3-031-58630-9_16

16.1   Introduction

Heterotopias is a broad term that groups conditions classified by the misplacement and ectopic collection of neurons, primarily attributed to disorders of neuronal migration [1]. Heterotopia is a very heterogeneous disorder, and has risen significantly in neurological conditions such as epilepsy and seizures. Its subtypes are often divided based on clinical characteristics upon imaging with recent studies suggesting that there are biochemical alterations within neuronal networks that give rise to morphological types [2].

Its pathophysiology is believed to be caused by failed neuronal migration to the cortical plates and may appear superficial in white matter [3]. Depending on its location and pattern, heterotopias can be divided into three main groups: subependymal or periventricular, subcortical, and band or double cortex heterotopia [2]. Subependymal can be shown as lesions near the lateral ventricles and can be associated with multiple genetic factors such as Filamin A mutations and ARGEF2 [4]. With very distinct appearances of subependymal nodules in this subtype, it can often be detected on MRI but unfortunately underdiagnosed with prenatal ultrasounds. On the other hand, subcortical heterotopia contains gray matter in deep and subcortical white matter, with further divisions based on its extensions into the white matter [5]. Genetic mutations such as LIS1 and DCX are associated with this type and can often manifest with severe developmental delay in children and have strong associations with epilepsy [6, 7].

Band heterotopia is characterized by gray matter between layers of white matter and is found underneath the cerebral cortex [8]. With a gender predominance in females, band heterotopia is fatal due to its asymptomatic nature and can classically present with seizures. Lissencephaly is linked to heterotopias due to genetic similarities, such as LIS1 and DCX mutations, which frequently explain its developmental patterns [9]. However, the precise mechanism underlying these conditions is unknown, necessitating the need to definitively identify the types of heterotopias and lissencephaly in order to guide treatment guidelines.

16.2   Anatomy and Physiology of the Brain and Gray Matter

The brain may be largely divided into three main defining anatomical sections; cerebrum, brainstem, and cerebellum. [10]. Gray matter (the cerebral cortex) and white matter make up the cerebrum, the front of the brain (Fig. 16.1). The cerebrum, which is the biggest component of the brain, controls temperature as well as initiating and coordinating movement. Speech, judgment, thinking and reasoning, problem-solving, emotions, and learning are all made possible by different regions of the cerebrum [10]. Other functions deal with the senses of sight, sound, touch, and others. The cerebrum and spinal cord are linked by the brainstem, which is in the center of the brain. The cerebellum, sometimes known as the "little brain," is a

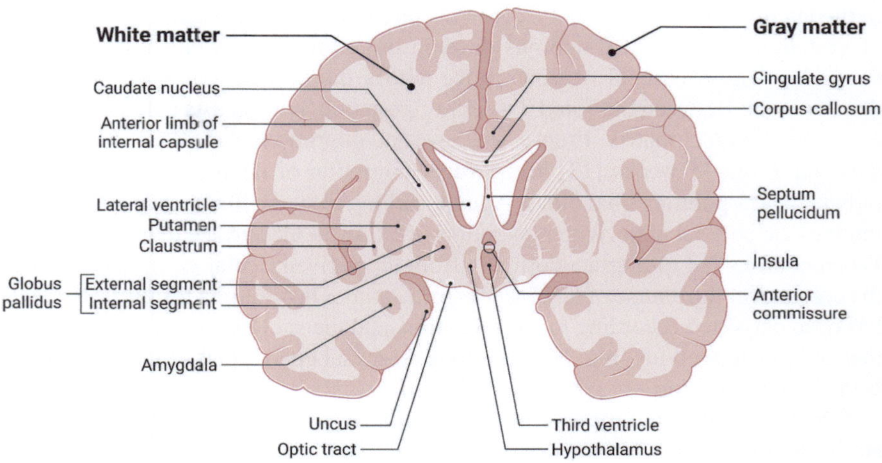

Fig. 16.1 Cross-section of the brain depicting areas of white matter and gray matter (created with Biorender.com)

fist-sized region of the brain situated in the rear of the head, above the brainstem and below the temporal and occipital lobes [10]. The brainstem is made up of the midbrain, the pons, and the medulla. It features two hemispheres, just like the cerebral cortex. While the inner region connects with the cerebral cortex, the outside section includes neurons. In order to maintain posture, balance, and equilibrium, it serves to coordinate voluntary muscle movements.

Gray matter contains a high concentration of neuronal cell bodies, and unlike white matter, its axons are not heavily myelinated [11]. It arises from the ectoderm, which continues to divide into specialized cells until the CNS forms [11]. Gray matter expands throughout development, but after the age of eight, it becomes denser while decreasing in volume, allowing for increased mental processing and intellectual advancement [11]. It also makes up the cerebral cortex, the outermost layer of the brain that surrounds the cerebrum. It is located in the inner portion of the spinal cord and is surrounded by white matter, giving it a horn-like appearance. Gray matter plays an important role in day-to-day functioning as it has an enormous number of neurons, allowing effective information processing. It also allows us to control our movements, emotions, and memories [11].

16.3 Overview of Gray Matter Heterotopias

Gray matter heterotopia (GMH) is characterized by the ectopic location of neurons. It is the most prevalent malformation of cortical development, and it is one of the most frequent congenital causes of familial and early onset epilepsy [12]. GMH occurs due to in utero arrest of radial neuronal migration from the germinal matrix in the lateral ventricle wall to the evolving cerebral cortex between 6 and 16 weeks of gestation [12]. Cortical neurons develop in germinal areas close to the lateral ventricles. These cortical neurons move across the cortical plate during normal development. Between the 7 and 8 weeks of gestation, neuroblasts begin to proliferate in the germinal matrix. From 8 to 25 weeks, migration takes place, with a peak between 8 and 15 weeks [13]. Centrifugal migration of neuroblasts occurs along radial upward-pointing glial fibers. After detaching from the fibers, they stop migrating into the cortical plate, with newer fibers resting on the surface than earlier ones. When neurons fail to migrate normally from the periventricular germinal matrix to the cortex over the course of 8–25 weeks, gray matter heterotopia results [13]. GMH has been classified according to their location, and the subtypes will be discussed in the subsequent sections (Fig. 16.2). Among these, subependymal heterotopia (SEH) is the commonest form of GMH [12, 14].

GMH is usually identified during investigations of epilepsy in children or young adults, and children with neurodevelopmental disorders; it may also appear as an incidental finding [12]. However, the exact pathogenesis and etiology remained unknown. GMH has a female predominance but the underlying reason is yet to be known [15]. The risk factors for developing GMH can be categorized into genetic and epigenetic. The epigenetic causes include hypoxic-ischemic changes, hemorrhages, physical and chemical factors, radiation, thermal injuries, and periventricular leukomalacia [14]. The genetic factors will be discussed in more detail in the following sections. GMH often coexists with other central nervous system developmental disorders. The most common ones are corpus callosum malformation,

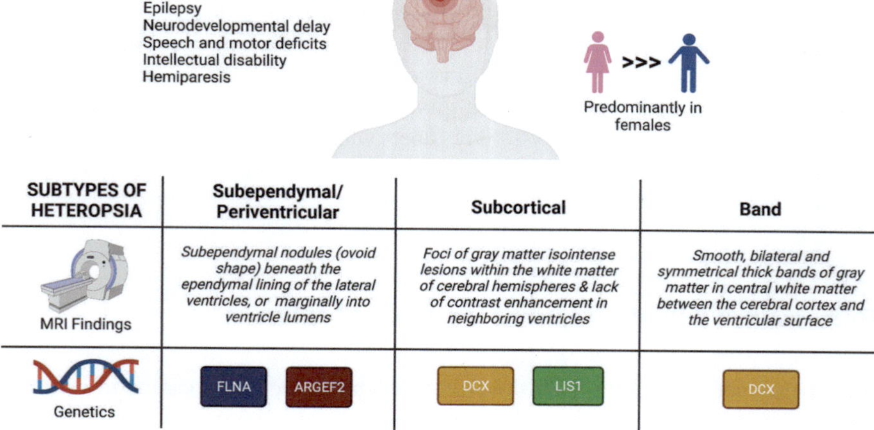

Fig. 16.2 Summary of clinical presentations and subtypes based on MRI findings and genetic risks in Heterotopia

cerebral fissure, arachnoid cyst and disorder of the septum pellucidum and the vault [14, 16] Less frequently, GMH is also associated with Arnold-Chiari malformation, pachygyria, epidermal cyst of the olfactory groove, polymicrogyria, Dandy-Walker syndrome and Hippocampal sclerosis [14].

GMH is generally diagnosed when patients undergo extensive brain imaging to determine the underlying cause of refractory seizures [17]. Although any type of imaging that can produce cross-sectional images of the brain can identify abnormal heterotopic tissue, MRI has shown to be superior to other neuroimaging modalities [18–21]. Following the widespread application of MRI, GMH has become more easily recognized as GMH are difficult to be visualized on CT scan [12]. GMH appears as isointense lesions with gray matter on all MR pulse sequences [22]. The inversion recovery pulse sequences are the most effective in revealing GMH as it demonstrates a clear contrast between gray and white matter [22]. Activation in heterotopic nodules can be shown using functional MRI, which may correspond to any epileptogenic EEG discharges [22, 23]. It is difficult to identify heterotopic gray matter during the antenatal and neonatal period using ultrasound as the echogenicity of gray matter during these periods are similar to the adjacent white matter [24].

16.4 Types of Gray Matter Heterotopias

GMH is classified according to its location and configuration of the ectopic neuronal tissue [25]. Generally, GMH can be divided into focal (nodular) or diffuse heterotopia. Focal heterotopia is further divided according to their location, depending on the lobes involved, and classified according to the extent of hemispheric involvement, into small, medium or large [23]. If the heterotopia occupied less than one-third of a single hemisphere, it is considered as small; if it occupies one- to two-thirds of a hemisphere, it is considered as medium; and if it occupies more than two-thirds of a hemisphere, it is considered as large [23]. In contrast, diffuse heterotopia is defined as bilateral lesions involving more than half of each hemisphere [23]. The location and pattern of the heterotopia is observed to influence the degree of clinical severity [12]. Therefore, defining the type and extent of GMH is useful in outlining the management and predicting patients' prognosis and outcome [12].

16.4.1 Nodular or Focal Heterotopia

Nodular heterotopia is further divided according to their location, depending on the lobes involved, and classified according to the extent of hemispheric involvement, into small, medium or large [23]. If the heterotopia occupied less than one-third of a single hemisphere, it is considered as small; if it occupies one- to two-thirds of a hemisphere, it is considered as medium; and if it occupies more than two-thirds of a hemisphere, it is considered as large [23].

The prevalence of nodular heterotopia is unknown [24]. The exact mechanism of nodular heterotopia formation is unknown, but it was thought to be a result of cell overproduction due to deficiency of stop signal in the germinal periventricular region, and defective neuronal migration due to early transformation of radial glial cells into astrocytes [24].

Subependymal or Periventricular Heterotopia

Subependymal heterotopia (SEH), also known as periventricular heterotopia, is characterized by presence of ectopic gray matter near the wall of the lateral ventricles, beneath the ependyma [25]. Subependymal heterotopia occurred due to arrest in neuronal migration, or failure of apoptosis of clusters of neuroblasts within the periventricular germinal matrix. SEH is associated with female predominance but the underlying reason is yet to be known [15]. The genetic risk factor of SEH includes mutations in Filamin A (FLNA) and ARGEF2 genes. FLNA mutation has been reported in all familial cases, and was found in 25% of the sporadic cases. The FLNA gene is located on chromosome Xq28 [21] and inherited in an autosomal dominant pattern, causing prenatal mortality of male fetuses. Therefore, it may explain the female predominance associated with SEH [14, 15]. In females, SEH manifests clinically in the second decade of life as partial seizures [14]. In contrast, the clinical features in males depend on the pattern of inheritance. X-linked inheritance of SEH in males are associated with other CNS disorders, and thus presenting as developmental delay in childhood affecting their speech [14, 25]. On the other hand, autosomal inheritance in male has similar clinical features with females [14].

The appearance of SEH on MRI include presence of subependymal nodules which are round to ovoid in shape, typically located beneath the ependymal lining of the lateral ventricles, or may protrude marginally into the lumen of the ventricles, disrupting the ventricular outline [12]. SEH may be unilateral or bilateral; the trigone and occipital horns of lateral ventricles were the most common areas where subependymal nodules were found, followed by the body and frontal region of the lateral ventricles [7, 12]. In the prenatal period, SEH often goes undetected because of the poor quality of prenatal ultrasound images, even when targeted scans are used. However, fetal ventriculomegaly can be noticed on ultrasound, raising suspicion of abnormalities, prompting neuropathological evaluation of the fetus's brain [1]. As FLNA-related periventricular nodular heterotopia is associated with vascular abnormalities such as aortic or carotid dissection, patients should have ultrasound of the abdomen and carotid artery done. [26].

Focal Subcortical Heterotopia

Subcortical heterotopia is defined as foci of gray matter within the deep and subcortical white matter [12]. Dysplastic basal ganglia are seen in most cases of subcortical heterotopias. Involvement of parietal lobe and thalamus leads to transient sensory loss by impairing the somatosensory pathway [27]. Subcortical heterotopia may be further divided into the nodular form, which extends from the ventricle to the white matter, the curvilinear form, which extends from the cortex into the underlying white matter, and the mixed form, which consist of both nodular and curvilinear features [12, 27]. On MRI, subcortical heterotopia appears as clusters of isointense gray matter nodules within the white matter of cerebral hemispheres. The sizes of subcortical heterotopia are variable from small to large focal lesions with mass effect but without contrast enhancement [12].

16.4.2 Diffuse Heterotopia

Band or Double Cortex Heterotopia

Band heterotopia is characterized by a symmetrical thick band of gray matter between layers of white matter with smooth inner and outer margin [12]. Band formation underneath the cerebral cortex results from impaired neuronal migration that leads to misplaced neurons [4, 28]. Subcortical band heterotopia (SBH), also known as "double cortex" syndrome, is characterized by the presence of bilateral, heterotopic, symmetrical gray matter between the cortex and ventricles [29]. SBH is different in both morphology and etiology from other forms of subcortical heterotopia, i.e. subcortical nodular heterotopia and subcortical curvilinear heterotopia [30]. The patterns of gyri range from normal to simple, often increased cortical thickness and broad convolutions [31, 32]. Genetic mutations of LIS1 (17p13.3) and DCX (Xq22.3-q23) are associated with the development of SBH [14, 33]. The LIS1 gene is associated with chromosome X and inherited in an autosomal dominant pattern, with a possibility for occipital lobe involvement [14]. The doublecortin (DCX) gene mutation is an X-linked dominant disorder, contributing to a female predominance as male fetuses often died in-utero or developed severe cerebral defects; it is often associated with frontal lobe involvement [14]. Most children with LIS1 mutation have severe developmental delay [14]. Females with band heterotopias may be asymptomatic, or demonstrate mild to severe symptoms, depending on the thickness of the heterotopic band [14, 34]. The most common symptom of band heterotopias, as with other GMH, is seizure. Seizure attacks in band heterotopias may be partial or generalized, or even have atypical presentation with loss of consciousness and drop attacks [12, 14]. Apart from seizure, patients may present with hemiparesis, intellectual disability, behavioral disturbances, language impairment, psychomotor delay, and microcephaly [35]. In the first decade of life, patients may exhibit developmental delay affecting motor and speech [12]. The severity of neurological deficits correlates with the size of heterotopia. Thicker bands of heterotopia have been found to be associated with worse disability and developmental delay [12]. Patients with bilateral SBH almost always present with severe developmental delay and intellectual disability [14]. On MRI, band heterotopia appears as smooth, bilateral and symmetrical thick bands of gray matter located within the central white matter between the cerebral cortex and the ventricular surface [12].

16.5 Subcortical Band Heterotopia's Association with Lissencephaly

Subcortical Band Heterotopia and Lissencephaly encompass a spectrum of severity, as both disorders are related to mutations in the LIS1 and DCX genes [35–42]. Heterozygous females have SCH, but males develop lissencephaly and Scheme [4]. Lissencephaly, or "smooth brain", is the most severe form of neuronal migration disorder. It is caused by mutations in many genes including including platelet-activating factor acetylhydrolase isoform 1b gene (PAFAH1B1, also known as LIS1) [43, 44], and the tubulin-α1a gene (TUBA1A) [45, 46]. Classification analysis has played a vital role to comprehend brain development, and analysis of patients suffering from the similar signs and symptoms has contributed to the identification of the causative genes [47]. However, the exact mechanism for these conditions is unknown and therefore, raises the need to definitively identify the types of heterotopias and lissencephaly to guide treatment guidelines. Lissencephaly were first described as type 1 and type 2 lissencephaly in 1983 by Dambska [48].

16.5.1 Type 1 Lissencephaly

Type 1 lissencephaly is usually referred to as "classical lissencephaly", and its macroscopic hallmarks are reduced gyration and cortical thickening. Upon macroscopic inspection, the brain shows failure of opercularization of the insular areas and poorly developed Sylvian and Rolandic fissures, and the most severe cases manifest failure of primary sulci formation [49]. Instead of the expected six, only four layers of thick and poorly organized cortex are observed upon microscopic examination [50–52]. Abnormality of the LIS1 or DCX genes are found in about 80% of the cases [53–55]. Type 1 lissencephaly has not shown any association with environmental factors. The clinical features of type 1 lissencephaly include early hypotonia, severe mental retardation, feeding problems, epileptic seizures, and limb spasticity [55–59]. Reports of fetal onset of seizures have also been documented [24]. Hypsarrhythmic patterns are also observed on electroencephalography [8, 60]. On MRI, classical lissencephaly usually appears as agyria or pachygyria with thickened cortex. The severe form can be diagnosed with computed tomography (CT), which shows smooth cerebral surface with no opercularization and a distinctive 'figure of eight' appearance [61]. However, mild form may be missed on CT scan. Ultrasound can detect a paucity of gyration after 23 weeks gestation [51, 62].

16.5.2 Type 2 Lissencephaly

Type II lissencephaly was first described by Walker in 1942 [63]. Haltia used the term 'cobblestone cortex' for type II lissencephaly [64]. Massive glial and neuronal ectopia are observed grossly which can be attributed to impaired integrity of the pial–glial barrier [33]. In the absence of muscular dystrophy, Isolated lissencephaly type II is very uncommon [65, 66]. The common pathway which contributes to the development of type 2 Lissencephaly is brain-specific impairment of a-dystroglycan perturbing the glia limitans which results in over migration of the neurons into the subarachnoid space ultimately resulting in deficiency of cortical layers [67]. Type II lissencephaly usually presents with Walker-Warburg Syndrome, Fukuyama Syndrome, muscle-eye-brain disease. Chromosomal analysis and genetic testing are helpful to confirm diagnosis [68, 69]. Electroencephalograms also play a role in the diagnosis of Type II lissencephaly [70]. Prognosis depends upon the severity of the disease, which depends on the type of mutations [71].

16.6 Treatment of Gray Matter Heterotopias

The principal management of GMH is the same as other structural brain disorders causing seizures. Carbamezipine is the medical treatment of choice for GMH patients suffering from focal seizures [72]. Nevertheless, the choice of antiepileptic depends on the drug efficacy, adverse effects, and patients' tolerance. Epilepsy caused by focal heterotopia is usually drug-resistant. In these cases, minimally invasive strategies, such as magnetic resonance-guided laser interstitial thermal therapy (MRgLiTT), and stereoelectroencephalography-guided radiofrequency thermocoagulation (SEEG-RFTC) can be considered [73]. Both are alternative options to open resective surgery in patients with nodular heterotopias [30]. The best determinant of surgical outcome is the ictal onset zone [74–76]. Surgery may not be effective in patients with bilateral involvement [77]. Corpus callosotomy (CC) is a surgical procedure that restricts the spread of epileptogenic activity between both the cerebral hemispheres, performed for SBH with generalized seizures. Supportive management for seizures in GMH includes deep brain stimulation, feeding techniques for infants with poor sucking, physiotherapy to prevent contractures and improve mobility, occupational therapy to enhance fine motor skills, speech therapy, tailored schooling and educational programmes [78]. The RNS® System (NeuroPace, Inc., Mountain View, CA), a responsive neurostimulation device, has been used to treat pharmacoresistant seizures in patients with SEH [79]. The system is also being investigated for its usage in patients with SBH [80].

Multiple Choice Questions

1. **Heterotopia is misplacement of:**

   (a) White matter
   (b) Gray matter
   (c) Dura mater
   (d) Arachnoid mater

   Answer:

2. **Most common clinical presentation of heterotopia is:**

   (a) Amnesia
   (b) Hearing loss
   (c) Ataxia
   (d) Epilepsy

   Answer:

3. **The gold standard imaging used for heterotopia is:**

   (a) CT
   (b) X-ray
   (c) MRI
   (d) PET

   Answer:

4. **Abnormality of the LIS1 or DCX genes causes:**

   (a) Type 1 Lissencephaly
   (b) Type 2 Lissencephaly
   (c) Focal heterotopia
   (d) Subependymal heterotopia

   Answer:

5. **Which is also known as cobblestone cortex:**

   (a) Type 1 Lissencephaly
   (b) Type 2 Lissencephaly
   (c) Focal heterotopia
   (d) Subependymal heterotopia

   Answer:

6. **Which of the following is used in diagnosis of type 2 Lissencephaly:**

   (a) Chromosomal analysis
   (b) Genetic testing
   (c) Both A and B
   (d) CT

   Answer:

7. **What is treatment of choice for GMH patients**

    (a) Prednisone
    (b) Phenobarbital
    (c) Tramadol
    (d) Carbamazepine

    Answer:

8. **The best determinant of surgical outcome in heterotopia is**

    (a) Placement of gray matter
    (b) Extent of surgical resection
    (c) Ictal onset zone
    (d) Involvement of blood vessel

    Answer:

9. **To stop the spread of epileptogenic activity, which is done**

    (a) Temporal lobectomy
    (b) Corpus callosotomy
    (c) Increase in dosage of carbamazepine
    (d) Craniectomy

    Answer:

10. **Which is not a management strategy of drug resistant heterotopia**

    (a) Minimally invasive strategies
    (b) Magnetic resonance-guided laser interstitial thermal therapy (MRgLiTT)
    (c) Whole brain radiotherapy
    (d) Stereoelectroencephalography-guided radiofrequency thermocoagulation (SEEG-RFTC)

    Answer:

11. **Which one is known as "classical lissencephaly"**

    (a) Type 1 lissencephaly
    (b) Type II lissencephaly
    (c) Focal heterotopia
    (d) None of these

    Answer:

References

1. Vriend I, Oegema R. Genetic causes underlying grey matter heterotopia. Eur J Paediatr Neurol. 2021;35:82–92. https://doi.org/10.1016/j.ejpn.2021.09.015.
2. Barkovich AJ. Morphologic characteristics of subcortical heterotopia: MR imaging study. AJNR Am J Neuroradiol. 2000;21(2):290–5.

3. Pang T, Atefy R, Sheen V. Malformations of cortical development. Neurologist. 2008;14(3):181–91. https://doi.org/10.1097/NRL.0b013e31816606b9.

4. Manganaro L, Saldari M, Bernardo S, Aliberti C, Silvestri E. Bilateral subependymal heterotopia, ventriculomegaly and cerebellar asymmetry: fetal MRI findings of a rare association of brain anomalies. J Radiol Case Rep. 2013;7(11):38–45. Published 2013 Nov 1. https://doi.org/10.3941/jrcr.v7i11.1457.

5. Watrin F, Manent JB, Cardoso C, Represa A. Causes and consequences of gray matter heterotopia. CNS Neurosci Ther. 2015;21(2):112–22. https://doi.org/10.1111/cns.12322.

6. Delatycki MB, Leventer RJ. Listen carefully: LIS1 and DCX MLPA in lissencephaly and subcortical band heterotopia. Eur J Hum Genet. 2009;17(6):701–2. https://doi.org/10.1038/ejhg.2008.230.

7. Mahmud R. Subcortical band heterotopia presented with refractory epilepsy and reversible aphasia. Cureus. 2021;13(8):e16990. Published 2021 Aug 8. doi:10.7759/cureus.16990.

8. Leventer RJ, Guerrini R, Dobyns WB. Malformations of cortical development and epilepsy. Dialogues Clin Neurosci. 2008;10(1):47–62. https://doi.org/10.31887/DCNS.2008.10.1/rjleventer.

9. Spalice A, Parisi P, Nicita F, Pizzardi G, Del Balzo F, Iannetti P. Neuronal migration disorders: clinical, neuroradiologic and genetics aspects. Acta Paediatr. 2009;98(3):421–33. https://doi.org/10.1111/j.1651-2227.2008.01160.x.

10. Ackerman S. Major structures and functions of the brain. In: Discovering the Brain. Washington, DC: National Academies Press (US); 1992. https://www.ncbi.nlm.nih.gov/books/NBK234157/.

11. Maldonado KA, Alsayouri K. Physiology, brain [Updated 2021 Dec 27]. In: StatPearls [Internet]. Treasure Island, FL: StatPearls Publishing; 2022. https://www.ncbi.nlm.nih.gov/books/NBK551718/.

12. Donkol RH, Moghazy KM, Abolenin A. Assessment of gray matter heterotopia by magnetic resonance imaging. World J Radiol. 2012;4(3):90–6. https://doi.org/10.4329/wjr.v4.i3.90.

13. Martín Fernández-Mayoralas D, Muñoz Jareño N, Alba Menéndez A, Fernández-Jaén A. Periventricular heterotopias: broadening of the clinical spectrum of the clathrin 1 gene (CLTC) pathogenic variants. Neurologia (Engl Ed). 2021;36(4):327–9. https://doi.org/10.1016/j.nrl.2020.06.008. Epub 2020 Oct 9.

14. Zając-Mnich M, Kostkiewicz A, Guz W, Dziurzyńska-Białek E, Solińska A, Stopa J, Kucharska-Miąsik I. Clinical and morphological aspects of gray matter heterotopia type developmental malformations. Pol J Radiol. 2014;79:502–7. https://doi.org/10.12659/PJR.890549.

15. Raymond AA, Fish DR, Stevens JM, Sisodiya SM, Alsanjari N, Shorvon SD. Subependymal heterotopia: a distinct neuronal migration disorder associated with epilepsy. J Neurol Neurosurg Psychiatry. 1994;57(10):1195–202. https://doi.org/10.1136/jnnp.57.10.1195.

16. Lowenstein DH. Epilepsy after head injury: an overview. Epilepsia. 2009;50(Suppl 2):4–9. https://doi.org/10.1111/j.1528-1167.2008.02004.x.

17. van der Valk PH, Snoeck I, Meiners LC, Des Portes V, Chelly J, Pinard JM, Ippel PF, van Nieuwenhuizen O, Peters AC. Subcortical laminar heterotopia in two sisters and their mother: MRI, clinical findings and pathogenesis. Neuropediatrics. 1999;30(3):155–60. https://doi.org/10.1055/s-2007-973483.

18. Kuzniecky RI. Magnetic resonance imaging in developmental disorders of the cerebral cortex. Epilepsia. 1994;35(Suppl 6):S44–56. https://doi.org/10.1111/j.1528-1157.1994.tb05988.x.

19. Sims J. On hypertrophy and atrophy of the brain. Med Chir Trans. 1835;19:315–80. https://doi.org/10.1177/095952873501900120.

20. Bairamian D, Di Chiro G, Theodore WH, Holmes MD, Dorwart RH, Larson SM. MR imaging and positron emission tomography of cortical heterotopia. J Comput Assist Tomogr. 1985;9(6):1137–9. https://doi.org/10.1097/00004728-198511000-00031.

21. Nowell MA, Grossman RI, Packer R, Hackney DB, Goldberg HI, Bilaniuk LT, Zimmerman RA. Focal cortical dysplasia on magnetic resonance imaging: a case report. J Comput Tomogr. 1988;12(1):61–3. https://doi.org/10.1016/0149-936x(88)90033-1.

22. Mitchell LA, Simon EM, Filly RA, Barkovich AJ. Antenatal diagnosis of subependymal heterotopia. AJNR Am J Neuroradiol. 2000;21(2):296–300.

23. Barkovich AJ, Kjos BO. Gray matter heterotopias: MR characteristics and correlation with developmental and neurologic manifestations. Radiology. 1992;182(2):493–9. https://doi.org/10.1148/radiology.182.2.1732969.

24. Tassi L, Colombo N, Cossu M, Mai R, Francione S, Lo Russo G, Galli C, Bramerio M, Battaglia G, Garbelli R, Meroni A, Spreafico R. Electroclinical, MRI and neuropathological study of 10 patients with nodular heterotopia, with surgical outcomes. Brain. 2005;128(Pt 2):321–37. https://doi.org/10.1093/brain/awh357. Epub 2004 Dec 23.

25. Abdel Razek AA, Kandell AY, Elsorogy LG, Elmongy A, Basett AA. Disorders of cortical formation: MR imaging features. AJNR Am J Neuroradiol. 2009;30(1):4–11. https://doi.org/10.3174/ajnr.A1223. Epub 2008 Aug 7.

26. Chen MH, Walsh CA. FLNA Deficiency. In: Adam MP, Everman DB, Mirzaa GM, et al., editors. GeneReviews®. Seattle, WA: University of Washington, Seattle; 2002. p. 1993–2022. https://www.ncbi.nlm.nih.gov/books/NBK1213/.

27. Rypens F, Sonigo P, Aubry MC, Delezoide AL, Cessot F, Brunelle F. Prenatal MR diagnosis of a thick corpus callosum. AJNR Am J Neuroradiol. 1996;17(10):1918–20.

28. Ekşioğlu YZ, Scheffer IE, Cardenas P, Knoll J, DiMario F, Ramsby G, Berg M, Kamuro K, Berkovic SF, Duyk GM, Parisi J, Huttenlocher PR, Walsh CA. Periventricular heterotopia: an X-linked dominant epilepsy locus causing aberrant cerebral cortical development. Neuron. 1996;16(1):77–87. https://doi.org/10.1016/s0896-6273(00)80025-2.

29. Khoo HM, Gotman J, Hall JA, Dubeau F. Treatment of Epilepsy associated with periventricular nodular heterotopia. Curr Neurol Neurosci Rep. 2020;20(12):59. https://doi.org/10.1007/s11910-020-01082-y.

30. Cossu M, Mirandola L, Tassi L. RF-ablation in periventricular heterotopia-related epilepsy. Epilepsy Res. 2018;142:121–5. https://doi.org/10.1016/j.eplepsyres.2017.07.001. Epub 2017 Jul 3.

31. Kobayashi E, Bagshaw AP, Grova C, Gotman J, Dubeau F. Grey matter heterotopia: what EEG-fMRI can tell us about epileptogenicity of neuronal migration disorders. Brain. 2006;129(Pt 2):366–74. https://doi.org/10.1093/brain/awh710. Epub 2005 Dec 9.

32. Lin Y, Wang Y. Neurostimulation as a promising epilepsy therapy. Epilepsia Open. 2017;2(4):371–87. https://doi.org/10.1002/epi4.12070.

33. Pilz DT, Matsumoto N, Minnerath S, Mills P, Gleeson JG, Allen KM, Walsh CA, Barkovich AJ, Dobyns WB, Ledbetter DH, Ross ME. LIS1 and XLIS (DCX) mutations cause most classical lissencephaly, but different patterns of malformation. Hum Mol Genet. 1998;7(13):2029–37. https://doi.org/10.1093/hmg/7.13.2029.

34. D'Agostino MD, Bernasconi A, Das S, Bastos A, Valerio RM, Palmini A, Costa da Costa J, Scheffer IE, Berkovic S, Guerrini R, Dravet C, Ono J, Gigli G, Federico A, Booth F, Bernardi B, Volpi L, Tassinari CA, Guggenheim MA, Ledbetter DH, Gleeson JG, Lopes-Cendes I, Vossler DG, Malaspina E, Franzoni E, Sartori RJ, Mitchell MH, Mercho S, Dubeau F, Andermann F, Dobyns WB, Andermann E. Subcortical band heterotopia (SBH) in males: clinical, imaging and genetic findings in comparison with females. Brain. 2002;125(Pt 11):2507–22. https://doi.org/10.1093/brain/awf248.

35. Hehr U, Uyanik G, Aigner L, Couillard-Despres S, Winkler J. DCX-related disorders. In: Adam MP, Everman DB, Mirzaa GM, Pagon RA, Wallace SE, LJH B, Gripp KW, Amemiya A, editors. GeneReviews® [internet]. Seattle, WA: University of Washington, Seattle; 2007. p. 1993–2022.

36. Blumcke I, Spreafico R, Haaker G, Coras R, Kobow K, Bien CG, Pfäfflin M, Elger C, Widman G, Schramm J, Becker A, Braun KP, Leijten F, Baayen JC, Aronica E, Chassoux F, Hamer H, Stefan H, Rössler K, Thom M, Walker MC, Sisodiya SM, Duncan JS, McEvoy AW, Pieper T, Holthausen H, Kudernatsch M, Meencke HJ, Kahane P, Schulze-Bonhage A, Zentner J, Heiland DH, Urbach H, Steinhoff BJ, Bast T, Tassi L, Lo Russo G, Özkara C, Oz B, Krsek P, Vogelgesang S, Runge U, Lerche H, Weber Y, Honavar M, Pimentel J, Arzimanoglou A,

Ulate-Campos A, Noachtar S, Hartl E, Schijns O, Guerrini R, Barba C, Jacques TS, Cross JH, Feucht M, Mühlebner A, Grunwald T, Trinka E, Winkler PA, Gil-Nagel A, Toledano Delgado R, Mayer T, Lutz M, Zountsas B, Garganis K, Rosenow F, Hermsen A, von Oertzen TJ, Diepgen TL, Avanzini G, EEBB Consortium. Histopathological findings in brain tissue obtained during epilepsy surgery. N Engl J Med. 2017;377(17):1648–56. https://doi.org/10.1056/NEJMoa1703784.

37. Barkovich AJ, Jackson DE Jr, Boyer RS. Band heterotopias: a newly recognized neuronal migration anomaly. Radiology. 1989;171(2):455–8. https://doi.org/10.1148/radiology.171.2.2468173.

38. Smith AS, Weinstein MA, Quencer RM, Muroff LR, Stonesifer KJ, Li FC, Wener L, Soloman MA, Cruse RP, Rosenberg LH, et al. Association of heterotopic gray matter with seizures: MR imaging. Radiology. 1988;168(1):195–8. https://doi.org/10.1148/radiology.168.1.3132731.

39. Brodtkorb E, Nilsen G, Smevik O, Rinck PA. Epilepsy and anomalies of neuronal migration: MRI and clinical aspects. Acta Neurol Scand. 1992;86(1):24–32. https://doi.org/10.1111/j.1600-0404.1992.tb08049.x.

40. Strauss KA, Puffenberger EG, Huentelman MJ, Gottlieb S, Dobrin SE, Parod JM, Stephan DA, Morton DH. Recessive symptomatic focal epilepsy and mutant contactin-associated protein-like 2. N Engl J Med. 2006;354(13):1370–7. https://doi.org/10.1056/NEJMoa052773.

41. Crino PB, Miyata H, Vinters HV. Neurodevelopmental disorders as a cause of seizures: neuropathologic, genetic, and mechanistic considerations. Brain Pathol. 2002;12(2):212–33. https://doi.org/10.1111/j.1750-3639.2002.tb00437.x.

42. Cepeda C, André VM, Levine MS, Salamon N, Miyata H, Vinters HV, Mathern GW. Epileptogenesis in pediatric cortical dysplasia: the dysmature cerebral developmental hypothesis. Epilepsy Behav. 2006;9(2):219–35. https://doi.org/10.1016/j.yebeh.2006.05.012. Epub 2006 Jul 27.

43. Andres M, Andre VM, Nguyen S, Salamon N, Cepeda C, Levine MS, Leite JP, Neder L, Vinters HV, Mathern GW. Human cortical dysplasia and epilepsy: an ontogenetic hypothesis based on volumetric MRI and NeuN neuronal density and size measurements. Cereb Cortex. 2005;15(2):194–210. https://doi.org/10.1093/cercor/bhh122. Epub 2004 Aug 5.

44. Weerakkody Y, Gaillard F. Band heterotopia. Radiopaediaorg; 2009. https://doi.org/10.53347/rid-6617.

45. Palmini A, Najm I, Avanzini G, Babb T, Guerrini R, Foldvary-Schaefer N, Jackson G, Lüders HO, Prayson R, Spreafico R, Vinters HV. Terminology and classification of the cortical dysplasias. Neurology. 2004;62(6 Suppl 3):S2–8. https://doi.org/10.1212/01.wnl.0000114507.30388.7e.

46. Palmini A, Andermann F, Aicardi J, Dulac O, Chaves F, Ponsot G, Pinard JM, Goutières F, Livingston J, Tampieri D, et al. Diffuse cortical dysplasia, or the 'double cortex' syndrome: the clinical and epileptic spectrum in 10 patients. Neurology. 1991;41(10):1656–62. https://doi.org/10.1212/wnl.41.10.1656.

47. Taylor DC, Falconer MA, Bruton CJ, Corsellis JA. Focal dysplasia of the cerebral cortex in epilepsy. J Neurol Neurosurg Psychiatry. 1971;34(4):369–87. https://doi.org/10.1136/jnnp.34.4.369.

48. Bahi-Buisson N, Souville I, Fourniol FJ, Toussaint A, Moores CA, Houdusse A, Lemaitre JY, Poirier K, Khalaf-Nazzal R, Hully M, Leger PL, Elie C, Boddaert N, Beldjord C, Chelly J, Francis F, SBH-LIS European Consortium. New insights into genotype-phenotype correlations for the doublecortin-related lissencephaly spectrum. Brain. 2013;136(Pt 1):223–44. https://doi.org/10.1093/brain/aws323.

49. González-Morón D, Vishnopolska S, Consalvo D, Medina N, Marti M, Córdoba M, Vazquez-Dusefante C, Claverie S, Rodríguez-Quiroga SA, Vega P, Silva W, Kochen S, Kauffman MA. Germline and somatic mutations in cortical malformations: molecular defects in Argentinean patients with neuronal migration disorders. PLoS One. 2017;12(9):e0185103. https://doi.org/10.1371/journal.pone.0185103.

50. Oegema R, Barkovich AJ, Mancini GMS, Guerrini R, Dobyns WB. Subcortical heterotopic gray matter brain malformations: classification study of 107 individuals. Neurology. 2019;93(14):e1360–73. https://doi.org/10.1212/WNL.0000000000008200. Epub 2019 Sep 4.

51. Di Donato N, Chiari S, Mirzaa GM, Aldinger K, Parrini E, Olds C, Barkovich AJ, Guerrini R, Dobyns WB. Lissencephaly: expanded imaging and clinical classification. Am J Med Genet A. 2017;173(6):1473–88. https://doi.org/10.1002/ajmg.a.38245. Epub 2017 Apr 25.

52. Rakic P. Evolution of the neocortex: a perspective from developmental biology. Nat Rev Neurosci. 2009;10:724–35. https://doi.org/10.1038/nrn2719.P.

53. Francis F, Meyer G, Fallet-Bianco C, Moreno S, Kappeler C, Socorro AC, Tuy FP, Beldjord C, Chelly J. Human disorders of cortical development: from past to present. Eur J Neurosci. 2006;23(4):877–93. https://doi.org/10.1111/j.1460-9568.2006.04649.x.

54. Guerrini R, Dobyns WB, Barkovich AJ. Abnormal development of the human cerebral cortex: genetics, functional consequences and treatment options. Trends Neurosci. 2008;31(3):154–62. https://doi.org/10.1016/j.tins.2007.12.004. Epub 2008 Feb 8.

55. Kato M, Dobyns WB. Lissencephaly and the molecular basis of neuronal migration. Hum Mol Genet. 2003;12 Spec No 1:R89–96. https://doi.org/10.1093/hmg/ddg086.

56. Reiner O, Carrozzo R, Shen Y, Wehnert M, Faustinella F, Dobyns WB, Caskey CT, Ledbetter DH. Isolation of a miller-Dieker lissencephaly gene containing G protein beta-subunit-like repeats. Nature. 1993;364(6439):717–21. https://doi.org/10.1038/364717a0.

57. Shimojima K, Sugiura C, Takahashi H, Ikegami M, Takahashi Y, Ohno K, Matsuo M, Saito K, Yamamoto T. Genomic copy number variations at 17p13.3 and epileptogenesis. Epilepsy Res. 2010;89(2–3):303–9. https://doi.org/10.1016/j.eplepsyres.2010.02.002. Epub 2010 Mar 12.

58. Kumar RA, Pilz DT, Babatz TD, Cushion TD, Harvey K, Topf M, Yates L, Robb S, Uyanik G, Mancini GM, Rees MI, Harvey RJ, Dobyns WB. TUBA1A mutations cause wide spectrum lissencephaly (smooth brain) and suggest that multiple neuronal migration pathways converge on alpha tubulins. Hum Mol Genet. 2010;19(14):2817–27. https://doi.org/10.1093/hmg/ddq182. Epub 2010 May 12.

59. Okumura A, Hayashi M, Tsurui H, Yamakawa Y, Abe S, Kudo T, Suzuki R, Shimizu T, Shimojima K, Yamamoto T. Lissencephaly with marked ventricular dilation, agenesis of corpus callosum, and cerebellar hypoplasia caused by TUBA1A mutation. Brain and Development. 2013;35(3):274–9. https://doi.org/10.1016/j.braindev.2012.05.006. Epub 2012 May 26.

60. Dambska M, Wisniewski K, Sher JH. Lissencephaly: two distinct clinico-pathological types. Brain and Development. 1983;5(3):302–10. https://doi.org/10.1016/s0387-7604(83)80023-0.

61. Curran T, D'Arcangelo G. Role of reelin in the control of brain development. Brain Res Brain Res Rev. 1998;26(2–3):285–94. https://doi.org/10.1016/s0165-0173(97)00035-0.

62. Norman MG, McGillivray B, Kalousek DK, Hill A, Poskitt K. Congenital malformations of the brain: Pathological, embryological, clinical, radiological, and genetic aspects. New York: Oxford University Press; 1995.

63. Fong KW, Ghai S, Toi A, Blaser S, Winsor EJ, Chitayat D. Prenatal ultrasound findings of lissencephaly associated with miller-Dieker syndrome and comparison with pre-and postnatal magnetic resonance imaging. Ultrasound Obstet Gynecol. 2004;24(7):716–23. https://doi.org/10.1002/uog.1777.

64. Dobyns WB, McCluggage CW. Computed tomographic appearance of lissencephaly syndromes. AJNR Am J Neuroradiol. 1985;6(4):545–50. PMID: 3927671; PMCID: PMC8335189.

65. de Rijk-van Andel JF, Arts WF, Barth PG, Loonen MC. Diagnostic features and clinical signs of 21 patients with lissencephaly type 1. Dev Med Child Neurol. 1990;32(8):707–17. https://doi.org/10.1111/j.1469-8749.1990.tb08431.x.

66. Barkovich AJ, Koch TK, Carrol CL. The spectrum of lissencephaly: report of ten patients analyzed by magnetic resonance imaging. Ann Neurol. 1991;30(2):139–46. https://doi.org/10.1002/ana.410300204.

67. Dobyns WB, Curry CJ, Hoyme HE, Turlington L, Ledbetter DH. Clinical and molecular diagnosis of miller-Dieker syndrome. Am J Hum Genet. 1991;48(3):584–94.

68. Dobyns WB, Elias ER, Newlin AC, Pagon RA, Ledbetter DH. Causal heterogeneity in isolated lissencephaly. Neurology. 1992;42(7):1375–88. https://doi.org/10.1212/wnl.42.7.1375.
69. Dobyns WB, Reiner O, Carrozzo R, Ledbetter DH. Lissencephaly. A human brain malformation associated with deletion of the LIS1 gene located at chromosome 17p13. JAMA. 1993;270(23):2838–42. https://doi.org/10.1001/jama.270.23.2838.
70. Patane L, Ghidini A. Fetal seizures: case report and literature review. J Matern Fetal Med. 2001;10(4):287–9. https://doi.org/10.1080/714052746.P.
71. Hakamada S, Watanabe K, Hara K, Miyazaki S. The evolution of electroencephalographic features in lissencephaly syndrome. Brain and Development. 1979;1(4):277–83. https://doi.org/10.1016/s0387-7604(79)80042-x.
72. Xiong L. Analysis on the treatment of gray matter heterotopia Epilepsy. Adv Soc Sci Educ Humanities Res. 2022; https://doi.org/10.2991/assehr.k.220110.162.
73. Wang Y, Xu J, Liu T, Chen F, Chen S, Xie Z, Fang T, Liang S. Magnetic resonance-guided laser interstitial thermal therapy versus stereoelectroencephalography-guided radiofrequency thermocoagulation for drug-resistant epilepsy: a systematic review and meta-analysis. Epilepsy Res. 2020;166:106397. https://doi.org/10.1016/j.eplepsyres.2020.106397. Epub 2020 Jun 15.
74. Choi JY, Krishnan B, Hu S, Martinez D, Tang Y, Wang X, Sakaie K, Jones S, Murakami H, Blümcke I, Najm I, Ma D, Wang ZI. Using magnetic resonance fingerprinting to characterize periventricular nodular heterotopias in pharmacoresistant epilepsy. Epilepsia. 2022;63(5):1225–37. https://doi.org/10.1111/epi.17191. Epub 2022 Mar 28. PMID: 35343593; PMCID: PMC9081261.
75. Acar G, Acar F, Oztura I, Baklan B. A case report of surgically treated drug resistant epilepsy associated with subependymal nodular heterotopia. Seizure. 2012;21(3):223–6. https://doi.org/10.1016/j.seizure.2011.11.002. Epub 2011 Dec 7
76. Li LM, Dubeau F, Andermann F, Fish DR, Watson C, Cascino GD, Berkovic SF, Moran N, Duncan JS, Olivier A, Leblanc R, Harkness W. Periventricular nodular heterotopia and intractable temporal lobe epilepsy: poor outcome after temporal lobe resection. Ann Neurol. 1997;41(5):662–8. https://doi.org/10.1002/ana.410410516.
77. Garcia PA. Surgery for heterotopia: a second look. Epilepsy Curr. 2005;5(5):197–s9. https://doi.org/10.1111/j.1535-7511.2005.00063.x. PMID: 16175224; PMCID: PMC1201644.
78. Hehr U, Uyanik G, Aigner L, Couillard-Despres S, Winkler J. DCX-related disorders. 2007 Oct 19 [updated 2019 Feb 7]. In: Adam MP, Everman DB, Mirzaa GM, Pagon RA, Wallace SE, Bean LJH, Gripp KW, Amemiya A, editors. GeneReviews®. Seattle, WA: University of Washington, Seattle; 1993–2022.
79. Nune G, Arcot Desai S, Razavi B, Agostini MA, Bergey GK, Herekar AA, Hirsch LJ, Lee RW, Rutecki PA, Srinivasan S, Van Ness PC, Tcheng TK, Morrell MJ. Treatment of drug-resistant epilepsy in patients with periventricular nodular heterotopia using RNS® system: efficacy and description of chronic electrophysiological recordings. Clin Neurophysiol. 2019;130(8):1196–207. https://doi.org/10.1016/j.clinph.2019.04.706. Epub 2019 May 9.
80. Gilliam FG, Ssentongo P, Sather M, Kawasawa YI. Case report: PAFAH1B1 mutation and posterior band heterotopia with focal temporal lobe Epilepsy treated by responsive Neurostimulation. Front Neurol. 2021;12:779113. https://doi.org/10.3389/fneur.2021.779113. PMID: 34867768; PMCID: PMC8636682.

Chapter 17
Polymicrogyria

Hossam Tharwat Ali

17.1 Introduction

Polymicrogyria (PMG) is one of the common cortical malformations. As the name implies, it means too many small gyri in the cerebral cortex which occur due to disruption in cortical layers and abnormal folding patterns [1]. The term "polymicrogyria" was first used by Bielschowsky in 1916 for excessive small convolutions in the cerebral or cerebellar cortex. Other used terms include micropolygyri and microgyri [2].

PMG constitutes a wide variety of cortical malformations not only one disease, all of which have in common excessive gyration and histopathological abnormalities [2]. Moreover, clinical manifestations, radiological findings, and pathology are heterogeneous [3]. It usually occurs as a part of multiple congenital anomalies, other brain malformations and/or mental disabilities [4].

Malformations of cerebral cortex development (MCD), or cortical malformations, constitute a remarkable cause of neurological disabilities in addition to their effect on development [2] PMG is considered the most common form of MCD [5].

H. T. Ali (✉)
MBBCH, Qena Faculty of Medicine, South Valley University, Qena, Egypt

© The Author(s), under exclusive license to Springer Nature Switzerland AG 2024
K. F. AlAli, H. T. Hashim (eds.), *Congenital Brain Malformations*,
https://doi.org/10.1007/978-3-031-58630-9_17

It is hard to estimate the statistics on the isolated polymicrogyria. However, there was a study concluded that PMG accounts for approximately 20% of all cortical malformation cases [6]. Moreover, the diagnosis frequency is expected to be higher in line with the use of magnetic resonance imaging in the pediatric field for many conditions such as developmental delay, cerebral palsy, seizures, and multiple congenital anomalies [2].

17.2 Etiology and Molecular Basis

PMG is a common endpoint of heterogeneous factors that include both genetic and acquired causes interfering with certain stages of development of the cerebral cortex [7]. The pathogenesis of PMG has been controversial over the past years. The main debate was over the timing of pathology whether it was before or after neuronal migration and the nature of pathology whether it was destructive or developmental [2]. The time of onset of PMG has not been established, however, more evidence suggests PMG is a developmental pathology that occurs after neuronal migration specifically during cortical maturation and folding [3, 8].

17.2.1 Genetics

PMG has been implicated in both contiguous gene syndromes and single gene defects. In contiguous gene syndromes, deletion or duplication of part of genetic material that contains multiple genes results in a recognizable phenotype of many organs [9]. The most common copy number variant related to PMG is 22q11.2 deletion syndrome which is characterized by cardiac defects, thymus, and parathyroid hypoplasia, dysmorphic facies, and PMG [1]. It is thought that the disrupted fetal vascular development, in this case, causes hypoperfusion and malformations rather than a single gene effect on the cerebral cortex [3]. Other variants include 1p36 deletion in which patients experience intellectual disability, microcephaly, PMG, and distinct facial features [1].

To date, more than 40 genes have been identified to be involved in the pathogenesis of PMG [1]. Inheritance of genes could be autosomal dominant, recessive, or x-linked depending on the mutated genes [2].

Variants in the phosphoinositide-3-kinase (PI3K)—protein kinase B (AKT)—mammalian target of rapamycin (mTOR) has a wide spectrum of phenotypes. Megalencephaly-capillary malformation-polymicrogyria (MCAP) is an entity characterized by early onset megalencephaly and cortical malformations (PMG) in addition to capillary malformations. A heterozygous mutation in PIK3CA gene can activate mTOR pathway. This could be a germline or mosaic variant [10]. It can be de novo or inherited as an autosomal dominant gene [2]. Moreover, PIK3CA was found to be involved in glucose metabolism and this gene is frequently mutated in cancer although it doesn't induce carcinogenesis [10]. PIK3R2 gene mutation can also activate mTOR pathway and results in megancephaly-polymicrogyri-polydactyly-hydrocephalus (MPPH) syndrome [1].

PMG has also been linked with disorders of tubulin genes/pathways [11]. This can result from a heterozygous variant in any of these genes; TUBA1A, TUBB, TUBB2B, TUBB2A, or TUBB3 which encode for different isomers of tubulin protein. Brain malformations include atypical gyration and cerebellar dysplasia. Basal ganglia and pons of the brainstem are also affected [1, 11].

The Na +/K + -ATPase (NKA) ion pump is a transmembrane protein that regulates sodium and potassium active transport. With the aid of one hydrolyzed ATP, it transports 3 sodium ions out of the cell in exchange for 2 potassium ions into the cell. It is composed of a large catalytic alpha subunit and smaller beta and gamma subunits. The human body has 4 isoforms of the alpha subunits encoded by genes ATP1A1–4. ATP1A2 and ATP1A3 encode for alpha-2 and alpha-3 isoforms which are highly expressed in CNS. During fetal life, both are expressed in neuronal tissue while in adult life, only the alpha-3 subunit persists in its expression while alpha-2 is expressed on glial cells [12]. Heterozygous variants of ATP1A2/A3 have been linked to some autosomal dominant neurological conditions e.g. alternating hemiplegia of childhood (AHC), rapid-onset dystonia-parkinsonism (RDP), and cerebellar ataxia-areflexia-progressive optic atrophy (CAPOS). Homozygous variants have been associated with early lethal hydrops fetalis, lethal polymicrogyria, and microcephaly especially in ATP1A2 [13]. Recently, polymicrogyria was observed as a novel phenotype of ATP1A2/A3 heterozygous mutations in about 45% of the included cases [12]. ATP1A3 mutations were found to occur de novo in children of healthy unrelated parents [13]. Severe form of ATP1A2/A3 mutations should be considered in cases with polymicrogyria, epilepsy, and postnatal brain atrophy as vanishing basal ganglia [14].

PTEN (phosphatase and TENsin homolog deletion) variants have been associated with PMG or atypical gyration [11]. PMG has also been linked to mutations in other genes. Mutations in the microcephaly gene WDR62, ion channel genes SCN3A, GRIN1, and GRIN2B have been associated with polymicrogyria recently [12].

17.2.2 Acquired Etiologies

Congenital human cytomegalovirus (HCMV) infection is considered the most common congenital infection in developed countries. It can occur following either primary or non-primary maternal infection [15]. Congenital HCMV has been linked with the occurrence of PMG especially if the infection occurs at 18–24 weeks gestational age [2]. A recent study on a group of children with congenital HCMV suggested that non-primary maternal infection is the predominant etiology for HCMV-caused PMG. All symptomatic cases with PMG were born to seropositive mothers. A drawback was that there were no serological studies before conception to assure that. Hence, a peri-conceptional infection cannot be fully excluded. So, it is highly recommended to have serological tests to assess immunity against HCMV to get more reliable data about its impact on pregnancy [15].

Some studies have reported the presence of vascular abnormalities in association with polymicrogyria [2]. Moreover, frequent localization of polymicrogyria around the area of arterial territories may hypothesize vascular role in PMG pathogenesis [16]. There were some cases reported that suggest fetal cerebral ischemia can disrupt brain development which can be in form of PMG [8]. Ischemic cause of PMG is often suspected when accompanied by areas of necrosis in the distribution of known arteries. However, the timing of the vascular insult especially in humans hasn't been determined [3].

17.3 Pathology

Friede defined PMG pathologically as "an abnormally thick cortex formed by the piling upon each other of many small gyri with a fused surface" [17]. Typically, PMG appears macroscopically as an irregular brain surface, abnormal sulci, and many small gyri in more than 85% of cases (Fig. 17.1). Leptomeninges are abnormal in most patients with some showing glial invasion [18]. The extent of pathology varies widely from unilateral focal or diffuse to diffuse bilateral involvement of the cerebral cortex. The perisylvian areas are the most likely to be involved (Fig. 17.2), on the opposite side, the midline cortex and hippocampus are the most likely to be spared [2]. Ventriculomegaly was found to be present in some cases with PMG or MCD. Generally, the post-mortem threshold for PMG diagnosis based on macroscopic findings is low especially in perinatal cases. The specialist often needs pre- and perinatal imaging plus the clinical details [18].

On microscopic examination, cortical layers appear to be overfolded instead of thickened appearance grossly. There may be associated some brain malformations which can include the brainstem, basal ganglia, cerebellum, neuronal heterotopia, and ventriculomegaly [2]. Microscopic examination can reveal one or more subtypes of PMG but all have the common characteristic features; an abnormal arrangement of cells, abnormal cortical lamination, excessive folding, and fused adjacent gyral surfaces (Fig. 17.1) [3].

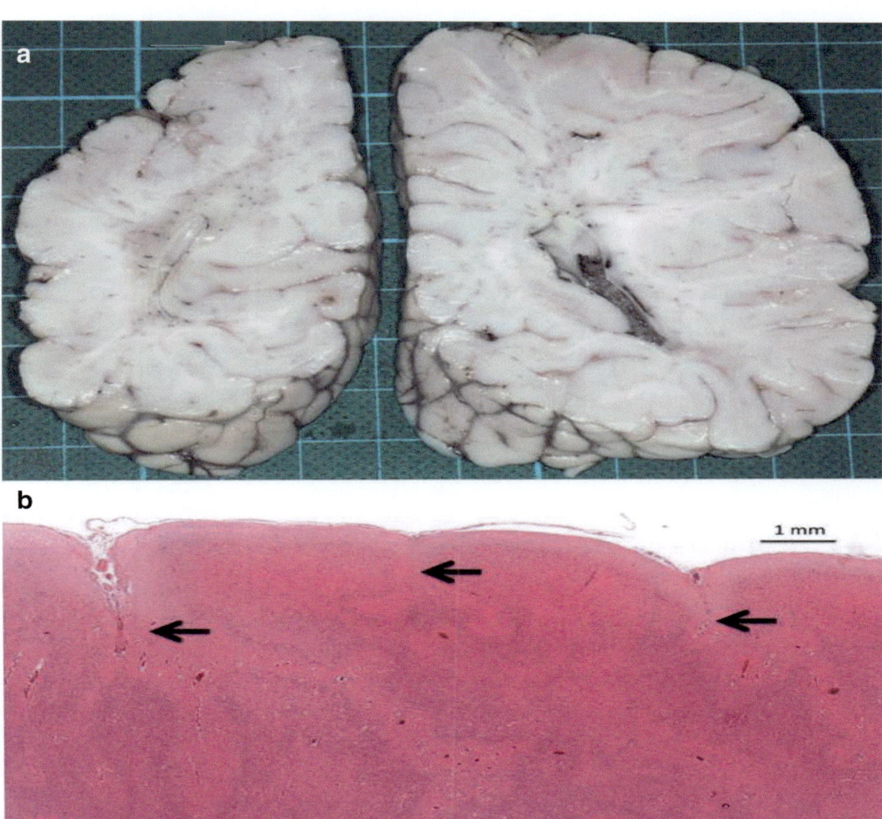

Fig. 17.1 Pathology of PMG in a case of an infant who died from intractable seizures due to extensive right hemisphere PMG. Image (**a**) shows the gross features; a small right hemisphere (on the left of the image) with an impression of a thick cortex and multiple small abnormally-oriented gyri. Image (**b**) shows the microscopic examination with low power using hematoxylin and eosin stain; abnormal layering of the cortex, fusion of the molecular layer (arrows), and deep sulcal branching. Reused with permission from reference [2]

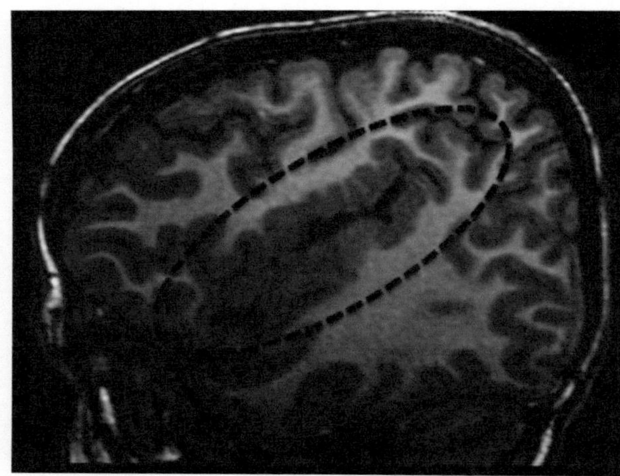

Fig. 17.2 Parasagittal T1-weighted MRI; perisylvian PMG (over folding and apparent thickening), abnormally-oriented and extended Sylvain fissure, and abnormal stippling of grey-white junctions surrounding areas of PMG compared to normal cortical areas. (Reused with permission from reference [2])

17.4 Clinical Features

The clinical manifestations of PMG are largely variable. Clinical features and prognosis of PMG depend on many factors such as the etiology, the load and location of PMG in each case, the presence and effect of complications, and if it is associated with other congenital anomalies weather in the brain or other systems. The diffuse generalized PMG has a worse prognosis than unilateral or bilateral patterns of PMG [2].

17.4.1 Epileptic Seizures

Epilepsy is considered the most common clinical sequelae of PMG which occurs in 65–87% of cases [19]. MCD in general typically presents with seizures. At least 75% of cases of MCD will experience epilepsy [20]. Patients can have any type of seizure from focal or partial or generalized. It can occur in association with jerky movements, twitches, or apneic spells. The time of onset can be any time since birth or day 1 after birth [13]. The prognosis is quite variable, can be seizure free at some point, partially controlled, or frequently resistant (intractable) to multiple antiepileptic drugs. In some reported cases, seizures gradually decrease with age [14]. Status epilepticus has been reported in cases with variants of ATP1A2/A3 who were diagnosed with alternating hemiplegia of childhood (AHC) and familial hemiplegic migraine (FHM) respectively. Thus, cases with PMG due to mutations in ATP1A2/A3 genes could be liable to have status epilepticus [12].

17.4.2 Developmental Delay

Global developmental delay was reported in more than 70% of cases with PMG [2]. Developmental milestones are delayed including intellectual, social, and/or physical. Children can be over 5 years old and have no social smile or head control. Some of them may not have eye contact. Older children can have very delayed speech in form of meaningless words [13].

17.4.3 Motor Affection

Motor system affection occurs in about half of PMG cases [2]. Most symptoms occur due to interruption of corticospinal tracts. Most patients will have moderate to severe motor affection with pyramidal signs [21]. If PMG is unilateral, patients will have hemiplegia or hemiparesis. If bilateral, they will have quadriplegia [2]. Hypotonia was also reported in some cases with bilateral PMG [22].

There was a reported case presented with involuntary mirror movement in the paretic hand and was found to have unilateral polymicrogyria. This indicated ipsilateral projection of the corticospinal tract to the paretic hand from the normal hemisphere. This led to less severe motor affection despite extensive cortical malformations [23].

Recently, some case reports introduced dystonia, which is uncommon for polymicrogyria, as a clinical association with bilateral polymicrogyria. Dystonia was the predominant manifestation for those patients. Clinical severity of dystonia correlated with the finding of PMG on MRI. However, the specific mechanism for dystonia in those patients was unexplained. It could be due to disruption of one or more parts of the motor network; cerebral cortex, basal ganglia, and/or cerebellum. Abnormal inhibitory cortical signals could cause dystonia since most patients have normal cerebellum and basal ganglia. Only a patient has some anatomical abnormality regarding basal ganglia which can have a role in the patient's dystonia [22].

17.4.4 Head Changes

Patients with PMG can present with certain dysmorphic facial characteristics, and hand or feet abnormalities [2]. Abnormal head circumference can be presented with PMG and could be the reason for intrauterine clinical suspicion. Microcephaly was found in around 50% and macrocephaly in around 5% of patients with PMG [2, 13]. Patients with PMG may express dysarthria or language impairment either receptive or expressive types [24].

17.4.5 Other Neurological Changes

PMG could be found with progressive brain atrophy e.g. basal ganglia vanishing and this may raise suspicion for ATP1A3 or ATP1A2 mutations [14]. Ipsilateral brainstem hemi-atrophy was reported in a patient with unilateral PMG. Some cases were reported to have urinary and/or GI disturbance in form of incontinence or irritable bowel [23].

17.4.6 Psychiatric Manifestations

A recent study suggested that all cortical malformations patients, in general, have more risk to develop psychiatric problems than the general population. Around 30% of cases have psychiatric symptoms. Anxiety symptoms, irritability, and agitation were the most found in those patients [20]. Autism spectrum disorder (ASD) was reported in a case with megalencephaly-capillary malformation-polymicrogyria (MCAP) as a result of a somatic mosaic mutation in PIK3CA gene [25].

17.4.7 Other Clinical Manifestations

In cases in which PMG occurs as a result of multiple congenital anomalies, clinical manifestations of other involved organs appear. ATP1A3/A2 variants were found to have liability to experience respiratory disturbance in addition to ECG and cardiac rhythm abnormalities even in conditions other than PMG e.g. AHC [12]. Cardiac lesions can be found in cases of PMG due to 22 q 11 deletion syndrome. Sensorineural hearing loss can be due to congenital cytomegalovirus infection [2].

17.5 Diagnosis

Since PMG starts from as histological abnormalities, the post-mortem histopathological examination is the accurate and gold standard to identify PMG. However, in clinical practice, clinical diagnosis and neuroimaging are almost sufficient [2].

History taking constitutes an essential part of diagnosis specially to identify or exclude acquired or inherited etiologies. Prenatal history of infections, trauma, or any other condition during pregnancy should be thoroughly reviewed. Maternal chronic disease and/or pregnancy-induced conditions should be considered. Family history of similar conditions, any congenital anomaly, metabolic disorders, and/or neurological disturbances e.g. seizures, mental delay, or motor weakness should be taken. If a close relative has neurological symptoms/signs and familial PMG is suspected, MRI should be ordered for both the child and relative [1].

A thorough clinical examination including general, neurological, and other systems examinations should be done. Patients can be micro-, macro-, or normocephalic. Other special facial characters could be found. Other associated musculoskeletal and visceral anomalies raise the suspicion of multiple congenital anomalies or certain genetic syndromes [2].

Genetic testing for known genes should be done. If indicated, family members testing and counseling of the nature of the disease, inheritance mood, and clinical features and complications are a must [1].

17.5.1 Imaging Modalities for PMG

In a minority of cases (5%), PMG can be suspected prenatally using ultrasound examination especially late in gestation. The imaging findings are usually based on microcephaly and/or cortical malformation [1].

Cerebral ultrasonography (cUS) has been used to evaluate brain insults in the pediatric field, especially in cases with congenital infections e.g. HCMV. However, a recent study revealed the low specificity of cUS. Some cases showed transient cortical changes by cUS but a completely normal cerebral magnetic resonance imaging (MRI). So, it is preferable, even for HCMV suspected cases, to evaluate using MRI which also has higher sensitivity than cUS [15].

CT or MRI is generally the best imaging modality for CNS or brain. CT can detect intracranial calcification as seen with HCMV cases. However, CT does not provide the high enough resolution or contrast as MRI to detect changes such as small gyri [1]. CT of PMG cases could reveal only thickened cortex and thus could be misdiagnosed as pachygyria or lissencephaly [2].

MRI is the cornerstone of PMG radiology. Having an appropriate MRI experience, PMG is typically diagnosed using MRI and can be differentiated from other MCD [2]. It also provides clinicians to assess the extent of cortical abnormality and thus the correlated clinical severity and appropriate plan of management e.g. surgery if indicated. MRI remains the best option to look for other brain abnormalities [16]. The appropriate imaging techniques as thin sections and age-specific protocols must be considered to provide the best contrast ratio between grey and white matter and appropriate signal-to-noise ratio [1]. Ultra-high-field (UHF) MRI can provide higher resolution and better clarity to detect abnormalities that cannot be detected using conventional MRI [16].

The most common patterns of PMG are bilateral (more than 50%) or unilateral perisylvian distribution. Others include generalized diffuse or focal involvement of certain lobes or areas such as bilateral frontoparietal, frontal or parietoccipital [2]. PMG can be found with other abnormalities in CNS areas such as ventriculomegaly, grey matter heterotopia, and abnormalities in white matter, brainstem, corpus callosum, or cerebellum (Fig. 17.3) [1].

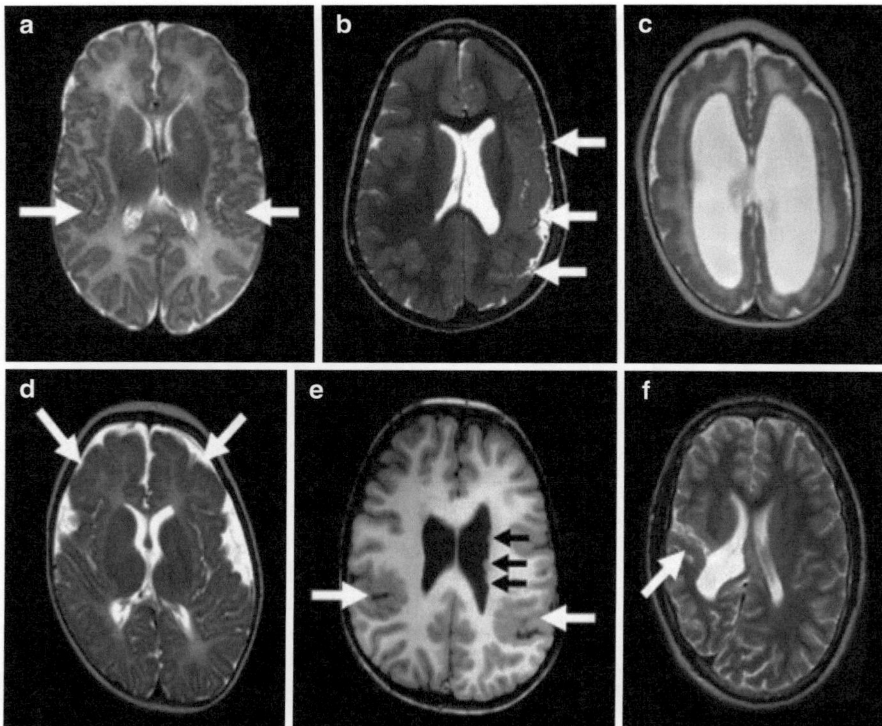

Fig. 17.3 Axial MRI for different subtypes of PMG. All images are either T1- or T2- weighted. Image (**a**) shows bilateral perisylvian microgyri surrounding Sylvian fissure and insula (arrows). Image (**b**) shows extensive unilateral left perisylvian distribution (arrows). Image (**c**) shows bilateral diffuse PMG with ventriculomegaly and periventricular calcifications (low intensity) suggesting congenital HCMV. Image (**d**) shows bilateral frontal PMG with an irregular surface (arrows). Image (**e**) shows bilateral perisylvian PMG (white arrows) and grey matter heterotopia (black arrows). Image (**f**) shows a small-sized right hemisphere and full-thickness cleft lined by PMG (arrow) suggesting SCZ. (Reused with permission from reference [2])

17.6 Management

The incidence of seizures interferes with the daily life of children with PMG. Medical treatment of seizures is often needed in form of a single antiepileptic drug (preferable) or multiple drugs if a single drug failed to control the condition. Adverse effects with higher doses or drug combinations should be taken into consideration. In many cases, the regimen needs to be adjusted according to changes in the type of seizures and age of the child. In other cases, seizures can be refractory and other options may be searched. Ketogenic diet and vagal nerve stimulation are alternatives to antiepileptic drugs [26]. Epilepsy surgery option is controversial. Patients and nurses should be aware of the first aids in case of seizures to prevent serious injuries and/or aspiration [27].

Some cases with PMG may experience some feeding difficulties and they don't get their appropriate caloric need. Increased seizure activity increases the caloric intake of children. A routine visit and follow-up to a nutritionist should be scheduled to maintain the optimal weight for the child, neither over- nor under-weight, to decrease the incidence of complications and mortality. In severe cases, who cannot maintain the appropriate intake, surgical options e.g. gastrostomy may be considered. In case of developmental delay, certain therapists and institutions may help. In case of urinary incontinence, neurogenic bladder, and/or irritable bowel, options of treatment should be provided to keep the bowel and/or bladder habit under control. Psychological counseling of both the child and the family should be a rule [26].

According to the severity of the case, many children may have some restriction in mobility which can complicate the case with many complications e.g. thrombosis, bed sores, liability to infection, urinary retention, and/or constipation. Thus, regular visits from/to therapists and/or nurses should be considered [26].

17.6.1 Surgical Intervention

Seizures due to PMG are often refractory to antiepileptic drugs (AEDs) and hard to achieve the seizure-freedom state. Thus, epilepsy surgery has been considered an option for those cases. In fact, in a certain subset of cases with focal epilepsy, surgery may be superior to AEDs in controlling seizures [27]. PMG cases with epilepsy shouldn't be always excluded from surgical options. Patients with bilateral diffuse PMG may be not good candidates for surgical procedures [28].

Although surgery may be a good option for refractory seizures, it is highly demanding and challenging. Challenges in the case of PMG-associated seizures may include the difficulty of optimally placing the intracranial electrodes due to the nature of PMG. If PMG involves highly functional areas, this may make the decision and outcome of surgery not preferable [19]. The heterogeneous nature of PMG and epileptogenic zones means a meticulous pre-surgical assessment of the specific epileptogenic zones and thus the surgical resection areas [28].

17.7 Differential Diagnosis

PMG should be successfully differentiated from other cortical malformations that may look similar on MRI or low-resolution imaging e.g. CT [2]. Lissencephaly and pachygyria are rare genetic disorders that occur due to failure of neuronal migration resulting in a smooth cortex with absent or coarse gyri and an appearing thick cortex [8]. Both conditions may be misdiagnosed with PMG based on CT (low resolution). However, MRI (or high ultra-field MRI) can easily show the microgyri and microsulci in addition to overfolding of the cerebral cortex in the case of PMG [1].

Schizencephaly (SCZ), which is considered a special pattern of PMG, is character-ized by full-thickness incomplete, or complete cleft lined by PMG. SCZ can be detected with CT or MRI although MRI is preferred [1].

Multiple Choice Questions

1. **Which of the following is correct:**

   (a) PMG occurs only as autosomal dominant
   (b) PMG can be a part of multiple congenital anomalies
   (c) PMG is caused only due to genetic defects
   (d) PMG occurs only with heterozygous variants

   The correct answer is: (b)

2. **In case PMG is suspected, which imaging should be ordered:**

   (a) CT
   (b) Cerebral US
   (c) MRI
   (d) CT Angiography

   The correct answer is: (c)

3. **Seizures associated with PMG:**

   (a) Can be focal seizures
   (b) Always generalized seizures
   (c) Occur only in cases with microcephaly
   (d) Are rare manifestations to occur with PMG

   The correct answer is: (a)

4. **Which of the following variants are more likely to have PMG with ECG changes:**

   (a) PIK3CA
   (b) TUBB
   (c) ATP1A2/3
   (d) PIK3R2

   The correct answer is: (c)

5. **Sensorineural hearing loss co-existence supports which etiology of PMG:**

   (a) X-linked inherited disease
   (b) Fetal cerebral ischemia
   (c) Congenital infection with cytomegalovirus
   (d) 22q11 deletion syndrome

   The correct answer is: (c)

6. **Which of the following is correct regarding PMG pathology:**

   (a) The cortical surface is always irregular and has a cleft macroscopically
   (b) PMG is mostly diagnosed on gross examination
   (c) Excessive folding and abnormal cortical layering are common findings for PMG
   (d) Hippocampus is atrophied in most PMG cases

   The correct answer is: (c)

7. **Which is the most common pattern of distribution of PMG:**

   (a) Unilateral frontal
   (b) Bilateral frontoparietal
   (c) Bilateral perisylvian
   (d) Brainstem and basal ganglia

   The correct answer is: (c)

8. **Which of the following is correct regarding the management of PMG:**

   (a) Surgical intervention is always indicated
   (b) Most PMG requires no medical management
   (c) Epilepsy surgery is always contraindicated in PMG –associated epilepsy.
   (d) AEDs may achieve good control over seizures in some cases.

   The correct answer is: (d)

9. **Conditions that may be misdiagnosed with PMG include:**

   (a) Dandy-Walker syndrome
   (b) Holoprosencephaly
   (c) Lissencephaly
   (d) Chiari malformation

   The correct answer is: (c)

10. **Clinical manifestations of PMG usually include:**

    (a) Dystonia, optic neuritis, and hemiplegia
    (b) Developmental delay, seizures, and microcephaly
    (c) Quadriplegia, seizures, and capillary malformations
    (d) Microcephaly, polydactyly, and neurogenic bladder

    The correct answer is: (b)

11. **Which of the following pathologies can be with PMG:**

    (a) Ventriculomegaly
    (b) Optic nerve atrophy
    (c) Cerebellar cyst
    (d) Hydrocephalus

    The correct answer is: (a)

12. **Which of the following genes has not been linked with PMG:**

    (a) TUBB2B
    (b) ATP1A2
    (c) PIK3R2
    (d) ATP7B

    The correct answer is: (d)

13. **Which step in nervous system development is more likely to be disturbed in PMG pathogenesis:**

    (a) Neural stem cell differentiation
    (b) Neuronal migration
    (c) Synapse remodeling
    (d) Neural crest cells migration

    The correct answer is: (b)

References

1. Stutterd CA, Dobyns WB, Jansen A, Mirzaa G, Leventer RJ. Polymicrogyria overview. In: Gene Review. Seattle, WA: University of Washington, Seattle; 2020.
2. Stutterd CA, Leventer RJ. Polymicrogyria: a common and heterogeneous malformation of cortical development. Am J Med Genet Part C Semin Med Genet. 2014;166(2):227–39.
3. Squier W, Jansen A. Polymicrogyria: pathology, fetal origins and mechanisms. Acta Neuropathol Commun. 2014;2(1):1–16.
4. Ten Donkelaar HJ. Polymicrogyria: the common endpoint of many different aetiological processes. Dev Med Child Neurol. 2016;58(1):7.
5. Klostranec JM, Brinjikji W, Mathur S, Orru E, Andrade DM, Krings T. Cerebral Corticoarterial malformations: a case series of unilateral Polymicrogyria and ipsilateral arterial dysplasia. Clin Neuroradiol. 2020;30(2):389–94.
6. Leventer RJ, Phelan EM, Coleman LT, Kean MJ, Jackson GD, Harvey AS. Clinical and imaging features of cortical malformations in childhood. Neurol Int. 1999;53(4):715–22. https://pubmed.ncbi.nlm.nih.gov/10489031/.
7. Stutterd CA, Brock S, Stouffs K, Fanjul-Fernandez M, Lockhart PJ, McGillivray G, et al. Genetic heterogeneity of polymicrogyria: study of 123 patients using deep sequencing. Brain Commun. 2021;3(1):1–12.
8. Squier W, Jansen A. Abnormal development of the human cerebral cortex. J Anat. 2010;217(4):312–23.
9. Allen AS, Aggarwal V, Berkovic SF, Cossette P, Delanty N, Dlugos D, et al. Diverse genetic causes of polymicrogyria with epilepsy. Epilepsia. 2021;62(4):973–83.
10. Stutterd C, McGillivray G, Stark Z, Messazos B, Cameron F, White S, et al. Polymicrogyria in association with hypoglycemia points to mutation in the mTOR pathway. Eur J Med Genet [Internet]. 2018;61(12):738–40. https://doi.org/10.1016/j.ejmg.2018.06.002.
11. Shao DD, Achkar CM, Lai A, Srivastava S, Doan RN, Rodan LH, et al. Polymicrogyria is associated with pathogenic variants in PTEN. Ann Neurol. 2020;88(6):1153–64.
12. Vetro A, Nielsen HN, Holm R, Hevner RF, Parrini E, Powis Z, et al. ATP1A2-and ATP1A3- associated early profound epileptic encephalopathy and polymicrogyria. Brain. 2021;144(5):1435–50. https://academic.oup.com/brain/article/144/5/1435/6242725.

13. Miyatake S, Kato M, Kumamoto T, Hirose T, Koshimizu E, Matsui T, et al. De novo ATP1A3 variants cause polymicrogyria. Sci Adv. 2021;7(13):eabd2368.
14. Ogawa E, Sakaguchi Y, Enokizono M, Yoshihashi H, Yamada M, Suzuki H, et al. Vanishing basal ganglia in ATP1A3-related polymicrogyria. Am J Med Genet A. 2022;188(2):665–7.
15. Zavattoni M, Lombardi G, Garofoli F, Scalia G, Rizzo A, Angelini M, et al. Neonatal HCMV-related polymicrogyria in seroimmune women: what is the optimal pregnancy management? J Clin Virol [Internet]. 2018;108(September):141–6. https://doi.org/10.1016/j.jcv.2018.10.001.
16. Thompson JE, Castillo M, Thomas D, Smith MM, Mukherji SK. Ultra-high-field MR imaging in Polymicrogyria and epilepsy. Am J Neuroradiol. 1997;18(2):307–12.
17. Friede R. Dysplasias of the cerebral cortex. In: Developmental neuropathology. Cham: Springer; 1989. p. 330–46.
18. Fudyma I, Wadhwani NR, Wadhwani CNR. Histopathology of Polymicrogyria. Pediatr Neurol Briefs. 2015;29(11):25047116.
19. Sculier C, Taussig D, David O, Blustajn J, Ayoubian L, Bonheur J, et al. Focal polymicrogyria in children: contribution of invasive explorations and epileptogenicity mapping in the surgical decision. Seizure [Internet]. 2021;86:19–28. https://doi.org/10.1016/j.seizure.2021.01.010.
20. Ho CSH, Dubeau F, Séguin R, Ducharme S. Prevalence of neuropsychiatric symptoms associated with malformations of cortical development. Epilepsy Behav. 2019;92:306–10. https://doi.org/10.1016/j.yebeh.2019.01.011.
21. Foesleitner O, Nenning KH, Traub-Weidinger T, Feucht M, Bonelli S, Czech T, et al. Assessing corticospinal tract asymmetry in unilateral polymicrogyria. Am J Neuroradiol. 2018;39(8):1536–42.
22. Andelman-Gur MM, Leventer RJ, Hujirat M, Ganos C, Yosovich K, Carmi N, et al. Bilateral polymicrogyria associated with dystonia: a new neurogenetic syndrome? Am J Med Genet A. 2020;182(10):2207–13.
23. Roh CH, Kim DS, Kim GW, Won YH, Ko MH, Seo JH, et al. Motor organization of unilateral polymicrogyria associated with ipsilateral brainstem atrophy—a case report. BMC Neurol [Internet]. 2022;22:1–7. https://doi.org/10.1186/s12883-022-02795-y.
24. Braden RO, Boyce JO, Stutterd CA, Pope K, Goel H, Leventer RJ, et al. Speech, language, and oromotor skills in patients with polymicrogyria. Neurology. 2021;96(14):e1898–912. https://pubmed.ncbi.nlm.nih.gov/33589534/.
25. St John LJE, Rao N. Autism spectrum disorder in a child with megalencephaly-capillary malformation-polymicrogyria syndrome (MCAP). BMJ Case Rep [Internet]. 2021;14(12):e247034. https://pubmed.ncbi.nlm.nih.gov/34969807/.
26. Turkelson SL, Martin C. Management of the child with polymicrogyria. J Neurosci Nurs. 2009;41(5):251–60.
27. Cossu M, Pelliccia V, Gozzo F, Casaceli G, Francione S, Nobili L, et al. Surgical treatment of polymicrogyria-related epilepsy. Epilepsia. 2016;57(12):2001–10.
28. Jalloh I, Cho N, Nga VDW, Whitney R, Jain P, Al-Mehmadi S, et al. The role of surgery in refractory epilepsy secondary to polymicrogyria in the pediatric population. Epilepsia. 2018;59(10):1982–96.

Chapter 18
Encephaloclastic Lesions of the Central Nervous System

Abbas Mohammad

18.1 Introduction

18.1.1 Overview

Destructive lesions of the central nervous system (CNS) also known as encephalomalacia. refer to pathological conditions characterized by the destruction or damage of cells and tissues in the brain or spinal cord. These lesions can result from various causes, including infections, autoimmune disorders, trauma, tumors, or degenerative diseases.

Infections such as bacterial, viral, and fungal infections can lead to destructive lesions in the CNS. Examples include meningitis, encephalitis, or brain abscesses. Autoimmune disorders like multiple sclerosis can cause destructive lesions due to the immune system attacking the myelin sheath, resulting in the destruction of nerve cells. Trauma to the CNS, such as brain or spinal cord injuries, can also lead to destructive lesions.

A. Mohammad (✉)
College of Medicine, Thi Qar University, Al-Nassiryah, Iraq

© The Author(s), under exclusive license to Springer Nature Switzerland AG 2024
K. F. AlAli, H. T. Hashim (eds.), *Congenital Brain Malformations*,
https://doi.org/10.1007/978-3-031-58630-9_18

Tumors in the CNS can be benign or malignant and can give rise to destructive lesions through compression and infiltration of surrounding tissues. Primary CNS tumors, like gliomas or meningiomas, and metastatic tumors from other parts of the body can cause such lesions. Additionally, degenerative diseases like Alzheimer's disease and Parkinson's disease can lead to progressive destructive lesions in the CNS.

The manifestations and consequences of CNS lesions depend on their location, size, and underlying cause. Common symptoms may include neurological deficits like motor or sensory impairments, cognitive dysfunction, seizures, and changes in behavior or personality. The specific symptoms experienced by an individual can vary widely depending on the affected area of the CNS.

Treatment for destructive lesions of the CNS aims to manage the underlying cause, alleviate symptoms, and prevent further damage. The approach may vary depending on the specific condition but can involve medication, surgery, radiation therapy, or rehabilitation. Medications may include antibiotics for infections, corticosteroids to reduce inflammation, or immunosuppressive drugs for autoimmune disorders. Surgical interventions may be necessary to remove tumors or alleviate pressure caused by lesions.

Rehabilitation therapies such as physical therapy, occupational therapy, and speech therapy can be crucial to improve function and quality of life for individuals affected by CNS lesions.

18.1.2 Historical Background

The recognition and understanding of encephaloclastic lesions have evolved over time, with significant contributions from various researchers and advances in medical science.

The earliest recorded documentation of encephaloclastic lesions can be traced back to ancient Egypt. The Edwin Smith Papyrus, dating back to around 1700 BCE, describes cases of head injuries and their consequences, including the softening of brain tissue. However, the understanding of the underlying mechanisms and the term "encephalomalacia" as we know it today came much later.

In the mid-nineteenth century, Claude Bernard, a French physiologist, made important observations on the process of encephalomalacia. He noted that the brain tissue surrounding a clot or hematoma undergoes necrosis and liquefaction, leading to the formation of a cavity. This finding laid the foundation for the concept of encephaloclastic lesions and their association with traumatic brain injuries.

Recognition of encephaloclastic lesions expanded further in the late 19th and early 20th centuries. German pathologist Rudolf Virchow described the necrotic changes that occur in the brain tissue following various insults, including cerebral hemorrhage, infarction, and trauma. He categorized these changes as "softening" and emphasized the importance of understanding the underlying causes and anatomical variations.

Advances in diagnostic imaging techniques in the twentieth century, such as computed tomography (CT) and magnetic resonance imaging (MRI), revolutionized the recognition and diagnosis of encephaloclastic lesions. CT scans, initially introduced in the 1970s, allowed for the visualization of brain tissue abnormalities and the detection of areas of encephalomalacia with greater precision. MRI imaging, introduced in the 1980s, further improved the ability to identify and characterize encephaloclastic lesions, enabling more accurate diagnosis and treatment planning.

Encephaloclastic lesions can arise from various causes, including traumatic brain injury, vascular disorders, infections, tumors, and ischemic events. Their recognition and identification are vital for appropriate management and prognosis assessment in patients with brain injuries or related conditions.

In modern medical literature, the term "encephalomalacia" is widely used to describe the softening and necrosis of brain tissue observed in different clinical scenarios. It has become an integral part of neuropathology and is recognized as an important pathological entity.

In conclusion, the historical background and recognition of encephaloclastic lesions have evolved over time, from ancient Egyptian texts to the contributions of Claude Bernard and Rudolf Virchow. The advancements in diagnostic imaging techniques, particularly CT and MRI, have revolutionized the identification and understanding of these lesions. Encephaloclastic lesions are now recognized as important pathological findings associated with various insults to the central nervous system.

18.2   Epidemiology

Destructive Central Nervous System (CNS) lesions refer to pathological conditions that involve the destruction or damage of brain and spinal cord tissues. These lesions can be caused by various factors, including trauma, ischemia, infections, tumors, and degenerative diseases.

Estimating the exact prevalence and incidence of destructive CNS lesions can be challenging due to differences in study populations, diagnostic criteria, and data collection methods across different studies. However, several studies have provided insights into the frequency of these conditions.

One study conducted by Al-Sharbati et al. (2017) examined the prevalence of CNS lesions in a population of patients who underwent brain imaging. The study found that 8.3% of the individuals had some form of destructive CNS lesions, with tumors being the most common cause.

Another population-based study by Brown et al. (2016) aimed to estimate the incidence of CNS lesions among older adults. The study reported an average annual incidence rate of 35 cases per 100,000 person-years for destructive CNS lesions. The most frequent causes of these lesions in this study were ischemic stroke and brain tumors.

Regarding specific types of destructive CNS lesions, studies have shown varying prevalence and incidence rates. For example, a systematic review conducted by Stienen et al. (2015) focused on malignant brain tumors. They reported an overall incidence rate of 6.02 cases per 100,000 person-years for malignant primary brain tumors.

It is important to note that the prevalence and incidence rates can differ based on factors such as age, gender, geographic location, and other underlying risk factors for CNS lesions.

18.3 Pathophysiology

Encephaloclastic lesions refer to the destruction or loss of brain tissue. The pathophysiology of encephaloclastic lesions can vary depending on the underlying cause.

1. Ischemia and Hypoxia: Ischemia and hypoxia-induced encephaloclastic lesions primarily occur due to the deprivation of vital nutrients and oxygen to brain tissue. The brain relies heavily on oxygen and glucose for energy metabolism, and any disruption to this supply can lead to cellular dysfunction and damage.

   During ischemic conditions, such as stroke or cerebral artery blockage, blood flow to certain brain regions is compromised. This causes a reduction in the delivery of oxygen and nutrients, leading to energy depletion and the accumulation of toxic byproducts. Ischemia triggers a cascade of events, including altered cellular metabolism, activation of inflammatory responses, and the generation of reactive oxygen species, ultimately resulting in tissue injury.

   Hypoxia, on the other hand, refers specifically to a decrease in the availability of oxygen to the brain cells. Hypoxic conditions can arise from various causes, such as respiratory distress, cardiac arrest, or as a secondary effect of severe ischemia. The lack of oxygen impedes vital cellular processes, impairing the synthesis of adenosine triphosphate (ATP) and disrupting ion gradients across cell membranes. This leads to disruption in neuronal signaling, cell death, and subsequent formation of encephaloclastic lesions. These encephaloclastic lesions typically manifest as areas of tissue necrosis, characterized by the loss of neurons, glial cells, and associated structures. The extent of damage and lesion formation is dependent on the duration and severity of ischemia or hypoxia, as well as the specific brain regions affected.

2. Traumatic Brain Injury (TBI): TBI can also result in the development of encephaloclastic lesions. These lesions commonly occur in areas directly affected by the injury and are characterized by tissue necrosis and loss of neural elements.

   When a traumatic brain injury occurs, it often involves a combination of primary and secondary injury mechanisms. The primary injury is the immediate mechanical damage that occurs upon impact, such as tissue deformation, bleeding, and axonal shearing. The secondary injury processes are the complex cascades of biochemical and cellular events that develop after the initial trauma, leading to further damage and inflammation.

Following the primary injury, various secondary injury mechanisms contribute to the formation of encephaloclastic lesions. These include:

(a) Excitotoxicity: The primary injury triggers excessive release of excitatory neurotransmitters like glutamate. This excess glutamate overstimulates receptors on neighboring neurons, leading to an influx of calcium ions and triggering a cascade of events that can cause cell death and lesion formation.

(b) Inflammatory response: TBI induces an inflammatory response, involving the release of inflammatory molecules and activation of immune cells. This response can cause further cellular damage and contribute to the development of encephaloclastic lesions.

(c) Oxidative stress: Traumatic brain injury promotes the generation of reactive oxygen species, leading to oxidative stress. Increased oxidative stress can damage cellular components and exacerbate tissue injury.

(d) Disruption of blood-brain barrier: TBI can cause disruption of the blood-brain barrier, leading to the infiltration of immune cells and substances that further contribute to brain tissue damage.

These secondary injury mechanisms collectively lead to the formation of encephaloclastic lesions, characterized by tissue necrosis and loss of neural architecture.

3. Inflammation: Inflammation plays a significant role in the development of encephaloclastic lesions following brain injury. The inflammatory response triggered by traumatic brain injury (TBI) can lead to tissue damage and the formation of these lesions. Here is an explanation of how inflammation causes encephaloclastic lesions,

(a) Immune cell activation: Following TBI, immune cells, such as microglia and macrophages, are activated in response to injury. These cells release pro-inflammatory molecules, including cytokines, chemokines, and reactive oxygen species. The excessive release of these inflammatory mediators can result in damage to brain tissue and the formation of encephaloclastic lesions.

(b) Blood-brain barrier disruption: Inflammation can contribute to the breakdown of the blood-brain barrier (BBB). The BBB normally regulates the entry of substances into the brain, but when it becomes compromised following TBI, immune cells and inflammatory molecules can infiltrate the brain. This infiltration can exacerbate tissue damage, leading to the formation of encephaloclastic lesions.

(c) Excitotoxicity and inflammation: Excitotoxicity, characterized by excessive release of glutamate and subsequent neuronal overactivation, can contribute to inflammation after TBI. This excitotoxicity-induced inflammation can further damage brain tissue and lead to the formation of encephaloclastic lesions.

4. Excitotoxicity: is a process that occurs when excessive activation of certain glutamate receptors leads to neuronal damage or death. It can indeed contribute to the development of encephaloclastic lesions. The mechanisms of how excitotoxicity can cause encephaloclastic lesions including:

   (a) Glutamate receptors: Glutamate is the primary excitatory neurotransmitter in the brain, and it acts on specific receptors called NMDA receptors and AMPA receptors. Excessive activation of these receptors can occur in various neurodegenerative conditions and lead to excitotoxicity.

   (b) Calcium influx: When NMDA receptors are excessively stimulated, a large amount of calcium ions enter the neurons. This influx of calcium disrupts cellular homeostasis and triggers a cascade of events that ultimately result in cell death.

   (c) Oxidative stress: Excessive calcium influx not only disrupts cellular processes but also triggers the generation of reactive oxygen species (ROS) within the neurons. ROS, including free radicals, can cause oxidative damage to cellular components, leading to further neuronal injury and the formation of encephaloclastic lesions.

5. Metabolic Disorders: Metabolic disorders can lead to encephaloclastic lesions through various mechanisms. Some metabolic disorders affect energy metabolism, neurotransmitter synthesis, or cellular processes, which can result in neuronal damage and the formation of encephaloclastic lesions. The mechanism of how metabolic disorders can cause encephaloclastic lesions including:

   (a) Mitochondrial dysfunction: Mitochondria are crucial for energy production in neurons, and dysfunction of these organelles can result in metabolic disorders. Impaired mitochondrial function can lead to a deficiency in ATP production, increased oxidative stress, and disrupted cellular processes, ultimately contributing to encephaloclastic lesions.

   (b) Disrupted neurotransmitter metabolism: Several metabolic disorders can impair the synthesis, transport, or metabolism of neurotransmitters such as dopamine, serotonin, or GABA. Imbalances in neurotransmitter levels can disrupt normal neuronal function, leading to neuronal damage and the formation of encephaloclastic lesions.

   (c) Accumulation of toxic metabolites: In certain metabolic disorders, the body fails to metabolize certain substances properly, leading to the accumulation of toxic byproducts. These toxic metabolites can have harmful effects on neurons, disrupt cellular processes, and contribute to the development of encephaloclastic lesions.

       The examples for Metabolic disorders that cause encephaloclastic disorders including:

       • Maple syrup urine disease (MSUD): MSUD is an inherited metabolic disorder characterized by the accumulation of branched-chain amino acids (BCAAs) in the blood and tissues. Elevated levels of BCAAs can lead to neurotoxicity, resulting in neuronal damage and encephaloclastic lesions.

- Wilson disease: Wilson disease is an autosomal recessive disorder that impairs the liver's ability to metabolize copper, leading to its accumulation in various organs, including the brain. Excess copper promotes oxidative stress and disrupts neurotransmitter synthesis, causing neuronal damage and the formation of encephaloclastic lesions.
- Leigh syndrome: Leigh syndrome is a severe neurodegenerative disorder affecting the mitochondrial energy production system. Various mitochondrial defects, such as deficiencies in the electron transport chain enzymes, result in impaired ATP production and increased oxidative stress. This energy crisis leads to neuronal damage and the development of encephaloclastic lesions.

18.4   Predisposing and Risk Factors

The causes of encephaloclastic disorders can vary, the followings are some commonly identified risk factors associated with encephaloclastic disorders,

1. Genetic factors: Many encephaloclastic disorders have a genetic basis and are caused by mutations in specific genes or chromosomal abnormalities. These abnormalities including:

   (a) Genetic Mutations: Mutations in specific genes have been associated with encephaloclastic disorders. These mutations can alter the structure or function of proteins involved in brain development, neuronal signaling, or synaptic transmission. For example, mutations in genes such as GABRB3, CHD2, SYNGAP1, and DNM1 have been implicated in different forms of epileptic encephalopathies. These mutations can disrupt normal brain development, leading to neuronal dysfunction and eventual brain damage.

   (b) De Novo Mutations: Many encephaloclastic disorders are caused by de novo mutations. These mutations spontaneously occur in the individual affected by the disorder, rather than being inherited from their parents. De novo mutations can arise during the formation of sperm or egg cells or early embryonic development. Studies have identified a significant number of de novo mutations in individuals with various encephaloclastic disorders, highlighting their role in disease predisposition.

   (c) Inherited Genetic Variants: In addition to de novo mutations, inherited genetic variants can also contribute to the predisposition for encephaloclastic disorders. These variants can affect genes involved in neuronal development, synaptic function, or cellular metabolism, among others. Certain genetic variants may act as susceptibility factors, increasing the risk of developing encephaloclastic disorders when combined with other genetic or environmental factors.

2. Prenatal exposures: Certain prenatal exposures, such as maternal infections, exposure to toxins, or maternal substance abuse, may increase the risk of encephaloclastic disorders. These factors including:

   (a) Maternal Infections: Infections during pregnancy, such as maternal viral or bacterial infections, can increase the risk of encephaloclastic disorders in the offspring. Pathogens like rubella, cytomegalovirus, and toxoplasmosis can cross the placenta and infect the developing brain, leading to inflammation and damage. Studies have shown that prenatal exposure to these infections is associated with an increased risk of encephaloclastic disorders, including intellectual disabilities and epilepsy

   (b) Teratogenic Substances: Prenatal exposure to certain teratogenic substances can also predispose individuals to encephaloclastic disorders. These substances include alcohol, drugs (such as cocaine and methamphetamine), and certain medications (e.g., antiepileptic drugs). Exposure to these substances during critical periods of fetal brain development can disrupt neuronal growth, migration, and synapse formation, leading to long-term brain abnormalities and cognitive impairments

   (c) Maternal Nutritional Deficiencies: Inadequate maternal nutrition during pregnancy can impact fetal brain development and increase the risk of encephaloclastic disorders. Lack of essential nutrients, such as folic acid, iron, iodine, and omega-3 fatty acids, can negatively affect brain development and function. Studies have linked maternal nutritional deficiencies to an increased risk of neurodevelopmental disorders, including encephaloclastic disorders

3. Perinatal complications: Adverse events during the perinatal period, including birth asphyxia, premature birth, or neonatal infections, have been associated with an increased risk of encephaloclastic disorders. These complications occur during the perinatal period, encompassing the time from the 28th week of gestation to the first week after birth which including:

   (a) Birth Asphyxia: Birth asphyxia refers to a condition where the baby does not receive enough oxygen before, during, or immediately after birth. This can occur due to various reasons, such as umbilical cord problems, placental dysfunction, or prolonged labor. Birth asphyxia can result in brain damage and increase the risk of encephaloclastic disorders like cerebral palsy. Studies have shown a significant association between birth asphyxia and cerebral palsy, suggesting the role of perinatal hypoxia in encephaloclastic disorders.

   (b) Prematurity: Premature birth, defined as birth before 37 weeks of gestation, can lead to encephaloclastic disorders due to the immaturity of the baby's brain. The risk of brain damage increases with decreasing gestational age and birth weight. Premature infants are more prone to brain bleeding (intraventricular hemorrhage), white matter injury, and other brain abnormalities, which can contribute to long-term neurodevelopmental impairments.

(c) Neonatal Infections: Infections acquired shortly after birth, such as meningitis or sepsis, can cause inflammation and damage to the developing brain. Neonatal infections can result from exposure to maternal pathogens during delivery or from hospital-acquired infections. These infections can increase the risk of encephaloclastic disorders, including cognitive impairments, epilepsy, and cerebral palsy

4. Infections: Certain infections during pregnancy or early infancy, such as cytomegalovirus, rubella, or toxoplasmosis, can lead to encephaloclastic disorders. Inflammatory processes and direct damage caused by pathogens can contribute to the development of such disorders. These infections including:

(a) Bacterial Infections: Bacterial infections, such as meningitis, can lead to encephaloclastic disorders by causing inflammation and damage to the brain tissue. Meningitis is an infection that affects the meninges, the protective membranes surrounding the brain and spinal cord. It can be caused by various bacteria, including Streptococcus pneumoniae, Neisseria meningitidis, and Haemophilus influenzae. Inflammatory processes triggered by bacterial infections can result in neuronal injury, cognitive impairments, and long-term neurological sequelae

(b) Viral Infections: Viral infections can also predispose individuals to encephaloclastic disorders. For example, certain viruses like herpes simplex virus (HSV), cytomegalovirus (CMV), and Zika virus have been associated with neurologic complications, including encephalitis, microcephaly, and brain malformations. Viral infections during pregnancy or in the early postnatal period can have detrimental effects on the developing brain, leading to long-term neurodevelopmental impairments

(c) Parasitic Infections: Some parasitic infections, such as toxoplasmosis and malaria, have been linked to encephaloclastic disorders. Toxoplasmosis, caused by the parasite Toxoplasma gondii, can lead to congenital neurologic abnormalities and cognitive impairments. Malaria, caused by Plasmodium parasites, can result in cerebral malaria, a severe form of the disease associated with brain damage and long-term neurological sequelae

5. Metabolic disorders: Inherited metabolic disorders, such as mitochondrial diseases or lysosomal storage disorders, are known to increase the risk of encephaloclastic disorders. These metabolic disorders can disrupt normal cellular metabolism and lead to toxic accumulation of substances in the brain, resulting in neuronal injury and cognitive impairments. These factors including

(a) Lysosomal Storage Disorders: Lysosomal storage disorders (LSDs) are a group of inherited metabolic disorders characterized by defective lysosomal function. These disorders lead to the accumulation of various substances, such as lipids, proteins, and carbohydrates, within the lysosomes. Over time, this accumulation can result in neurodegeneration and encephaloclastic disorders. Examples of LSDs include Gaucher disease, Niemann-Pick disease, and Tay-Sachs disease. These disorders often present with progressive cognitive decline, motor impairments, and other neurological symptoms

(b) Mitochondrial Disorders: Mitochondrial disorders are a group of genetic disorders that affect the function of mitochondria, the cellular organelles responsible for energy production. Defects in mitochondrial metabolism can lead to a variety of neurological symptoms, including seizures, developmental delay, and encephaloclastic disorders. Mitochondrial encephalomyopathies, such as Leigh syndrome and MELAS (mitochondrial encephalomyopathy, lactic acidosis, and stroke-like episodes) syndrome, are characterized by progressive brain damage and can result in severe neurological disability

(c) Peroxisomal Disorders: Peroxisomal disorders are a group of genetic conditions characterized by impaired peroxisome function. These disorders can lead to the accumulation of toxic substances and oxidative stress within the cells, including the brain. Disorders, such as Zellweger syndrome and adrenoleukodystrophy, can cause encephaloclastic disorders with symptoms such as developmental regression, seizures, and intellectual disabilities.

18.5 Classification of Encephaloclastic Disorders

Encephaloclastic disorders can be classified in various ways. One common classification is based on the affected structures in the CNS, such as the brain or spinal cord

1. Neurodegenerative Disorders: are a group of chronic and progressive conditions characterized by the gradual loss of structure and function in different regions of the central nervous system (CNS). These disorders pose significant challenges for patients, caregivers, and healthcare professionals. This group including:

   (a) Alzheimer's Disease (AD): it is the most prevalent neurodegenerative disorder and is characterized by the accumulation of beta-amyloid plaques and tau tangles in the brain. It leads to memory loss, cognitive decline, and behavioral changes. The amyloid cascade hypothesis proposes that the accumulation of beta-amyloid triggers an inflammatory response, contributing to neurodegeneration.

   (b) Parkinson's Disease (PD): it is characterized by the degeneration of dopaminergic neurons in the substantia nigra, leading to motor symptoms such as tremors, rigidity, and bradykinesia. The primary pathological hallmark of PD is the presence of Lewy bodies, aggregated alpha-synuclein protein. Advances in understanding the genetic and environmental risk factors have shed light on the underlying mechanisms of PD pathology

   (c) Huntington's Disease (HD): it is an autosomal dominant disorder caused by the expansion of CAG repeats in the huntingtin gene. This results in the accumulation of mutant huntingtin protein, leading to neuronal dysfunction and death. HD primarily affects the basal ganglia, resulting in involuntary movements, cognitive decline, and psychiatric disturbances. Research has explored the potential of gene silencing and gene editing techniques as potential therapeutic approaches for HD (Ross et al., 2014).

(d) Amyotrophic Lateral Sclerosis (ALS): it affects both upper and lower motor neurons, leading to progressive muscle weakness, spasticity, and eventually, paralysis. The exact cause of ALS remains unclear, but studies have identified genetic mutations, oxidative stress, and excitotoxicity as potential contributors. Advances in understanding the molecular mechanisms have paved the way for potential disease-modifying therapies in the future.

In conclusion, Neurodegenerative disorders present a significant burden on individuals, families, and society as a whole. Understanding the underlying pathology and mechanisms driving these disorders is crucial for developing effective treatment strategies. Ongoing research and advancements in genetics, neuroimaging, and therapeutic approaches provide hope for better management and potential disease-modifying interventions for individuals affected by neurodegenerative disorders.

2. Neuroinflammatory disorders: are a group of conditions characterized by inflammation in the central nervous system (CNS). These disorders involve a dysregulated immune response, resulting in neurodegeneration and various neurological symptoms. This group including:

(a) Multiple Sclerosis (MS): is an autoimmune disorder characterized by inflammation, demyelination, and axonal damage in the CNS. The immune system mistakenly attacks the myelin sheath, disrupting the transmission of nerve signals. This leads to a wide range of symptoms, including muscle weakness, impaired coordination, and fatigue. Advances in understanding the role of immune dysregulation and neuroinflammation have paved the way for disease-modifying therapies in

18.6 MS Management

Guillain-Barre Syndrome (GBS): is an acute inflammatory disorder that affects peripheral nerves. It is often preceded by an infection, triggering an abnormal immune response that damages the nerves. Symmetrical muscle weakness, tingling, and loss of reflexes are characteristic symptoms of GBS. The immune-mediated nature of GBS has led to the use of immunomodulatory treatments, such as intravenous immunoglobulin and plasmapheresis, to reduce inflammation and promote nerve regeneration

Neuromyelitis Optica (NMO): also known as Devic's disease, is an autoimmune disorder primarily affecting the optic nerves and spinal cord. It is characterized by severe optic neuritis and myelitis, leading to visual impairment, paralysis, and loss of sensation. The discovery of aquaporin-4 antibodies, targeting water channels in astrocytes, has revolutionized the diagnosis and management of NMO. Immunosuppressive therapies have shown efficacy in preventing relapses and delaying disability progression in NMO.

Autoimmune Encephalitis (AE): it encompasses a group of disorders caused by an immune response targeting neuronal antigens. Common symptoms include cognitive impairment, seizures, and psychiatric disturbances. Various autoantibodies, such as anti-NMDA receptor antibodies, are associated with different subtypes of AE. Early recognition, immunotherapy, and tumor removal, if present, play crucial roles in the management of AE

In conclusion, Neuroinflammatory disorders result from an aberrant immune response in the CNS, leading to inflammation, demyelination, and neuronal damage. Understanding the etiology and underlying mechanisms of these disorders is essential for the development of effective therapeutic strategies. Ongoing research, including the identification of specific autoantibodies and advancements in immunomodulatory treatments, offers hope for improved management and outcomes for individuals affected by neuroinflammatory disorders.

1. Neurovascular Disorders: they are a group of conditions characterized by abnormalities in the blood vessels supplying the brain and/or the spinal cord. These disorders can disrupt the normal blood flow, leading to various neurological symptoms and potentially life-threatening complications. This group including:

    (a) Ischemic Stroke: it occurs when a blood vessel supplying the brain becomes blocked, resulting in inadequate blood flow and oxygen delivery to brain tissue. Common causes include the formation of a blood clot (thrombus) or a traveling clot (embolus) from another part of the body. Symptoms may include sudden weakness or numbness, difficulty speaking, and vision problems. Early intervention through thrombolytic therapy or mechanical clot retrieval can help restore blood flow and reduce disability

    (b) Hemorrhagic Stroke: Hemorrhagic stroke, less common than ischemic stroke, involves bleeding within the brain. This can be caused by the rupture of a weakened blood vessel, such as an aneurysm or arteriovenous malformation (AVM). Symptoms may include severe headache, nausea, and altered consciousness. Management involves controlling bleeding, relieving pressure on the brain, and addressing underlying causes. Surgical interventions, such as aneurysm clipping or endovascular coiling, may be required

    (c) Cerebral Aneurysm: is an abnormal bulge in the wall of a brain artery, increasing the risk of rupture and subsequent bleeding into the brain. The exact cause is often unclear, but factors such as high blood pressure, smoking, and family history contribute to its development. The rupture of an aneurysm can lead to a subarachnoid hemorrhage, causing sudden, severe headache, neck stiffness, and loss of consciousness. Prompt intervention using coiling or surgical clipping is crucial to prevent further bleeding

    (d) Arteriovenous Malformation (AVM): is an abnormal connection between arteries and veins that bypasses the capillary network. The flow of blood through these malformed vessels can exert high pressure, potentially leading to hemorrhage, seizures, or neurological deficits. Treatment options for AVMs include endovascular embolization, stereotactic radiosurgery, and surgical resection, depending on the size, location, and patient's condition

In conclusion, neurovascular disorders pose significant risks to individuals' neurological well-being and functional independence. Prompt recognition, accurate diagnosis, and appropriate management are fundamental for favorable outcomes. Advances in intervention techniques, such as minimally invasive procedures and personalized treatment plans, hold promise for improved patient care.

2. Traumatic Brain (TBIs) and Spinal Cord Injury (SCIs): are devastating conditions that can result from various external forces. These injuries often have life-altering consequences, affecting physical, cognitive, and emotional well-being. These including:

   (a) Traumatic Brain Injuries: it occurs when an external force causes damage to the brain. Common causes include falls, motor vehicle accidents, and sports-related injuries. Mild TBIs, also known as concussions, may present with symptoms such as confusion, headaches, and memory problems. Severe TBIs can lead to prolonged unconsciousness, cognitive impairment, and motor deficits. Acute management involves stabilization, monitoring, and early intervention, while rehabilitation focuses on maximizing functional recovery

   (b) Spinal Cord Injuries: they involve damage to the spinal cord, resulting in varying degrees of motor and sensory loss. These injuries often result from accidents, falls, or sports-related incidents. The level and extent of injury determine the functional consequences. Incomplete injuries may retain some motor or sensory function below the injury level, while complete injuries result in total loss of function. Acute management includes immobilization, surgical interventions, and rehabilitation, which focuses on optimizing physical functioning and quality of life.

   In conclusion, Traumatic brain and spinal cord injuries are debilitating conditions with far-reaching physical, cognitive, and emotional consequences. Timely and appropriate medical interventions, along with comprehensive rehabilitation, are essential for optimizing patient outcomes.

18.7 Clinical Presentation

1. Neurological Deficits: Encephaloclastic disorders can cause a variety of neurological deficits, such as motor impairments, sensory disturbances, and coordination difficulties. These deficits often result from the destruction of specific brain regions responsible for motor control, sensory processing, or coordination.

(a) Motor deficiency: encephaloclastic disorders can lead to various motor deficiencies due to brain damage or degeneration of motor-related structures. These deficiencies including

- Motor Coordination Impairments: Encephaloclastic disorders can result in motor coordination impairments, affecting the ability to perform smooth and coordinated movements. Ataxia is a motor coordination disorder characterized by unsteady movements, disturbed balance, and lack of coordination.
- Muscle Weakness and Spasticity: Encephaloclastic disorders can lead to muscle weakness or spasticity, resulting in difficulties with voluntary movements. Muscle weakness refers to a reduction in muscle strength, while spasticity refers to increased muscle tone and stiffness. Cerebral palsy (CP) is a neurodevelopmental disorder often associated with encephaloclastic processes and is characterized by muscle weakness, spasticity, and impaired motor control.
- Loss of Voluntary Movement: Encephaloclastic disorders can result in loss of voluntary movement due to damage to the motor cortex or corticospinal tracts. This can lead to conditions like hemiplegia or quadriplegia, involving paralysis or weakness of one side or all four limbs, respectively

(b) Sensory disturbances: Encephaloclastic disorders can give rise to various sensory disturbances due to damage to sensory-related structures in the brain. These sensory disturbances including

- Sensory Processing Impairments: Encephaloclastic disorders can lead to disruptions in sensory processing, resulting in difficulties with interpreting and integrating sensory information. Sensory processing disorder (SPD) is a condition where individuals have difficulties organizing and responding to incoming sensory information.
- Changes in Pain Perception: Encephaloclastic disorders can result in altered pain perception. Some individuals may experience heightened or diminished pain sensitivity compared to typical individuals.
- Visual Impairments: Encephaloclastic disorders can cause visual impairments, including reduced visual acuity, visual field deficits, or abnormal visual processing. Cortical visual impairment (CVI) is a condition where there is damage or dysfunction of the visual pathways in the brain, leading to visual difficulties.

(c) Coordination difficulties: Encephaloclastic disorders can often manifest with coordination difficulties due to the damage or dysfunction of motor-related structures in the brain. These difficulties including:

- Ataxia: Ataxia refers to a lack of coordination or unsteady movements. It can result from damage to the cerebellum or its connections. The cerebellum plays a crucial role in coordinating voluntary movements.

- Dysmetria: it is characterized by errors in judging the distance, speed, or amplitude of movements. It can result from cerebellar dysfunction.
- Hypotonia: it refers to decreased muscle tone or reduced resistance to passive movement. It can occur when there is damage to the motor areas in the brain.
- Dyspraxia: also known as developmental coordination disorder, is a condition characterized by difficulties in planning and executing coordinated motor movements. While it can be associated with various developmental disorders, it can also occur in encephaloclastic disorders due to damage to motor planning areas.

2. Cognitive Impairment: Cognitive deficits are frequently observed in individuals with encephaloclastic disorders. These may include difficulties with memory, attention, executive functions, language, and judgment. The severity of cognitive impairment varies depending on the extent and location of brain tissue damage. Several studies have explored the effects of encephaloclastic disorders on cognitive function. For example, a study by Smith et al. (2018) examined cognitive outcomes in individuals with traumatic brain injury (TBI), a common cause of encephaloclastic disorders. The study found that TBI can lead to persistent cognitive impairments, including difficulties with attention, memory, and executive functioning. Another study by Rossi et al. (2016) investigated the cognitive effects of stroke, which can also result in encephaloclastic changes in the brain. The researchers found that stroke survivors often experience cognitive deficits, particularly in areas such as language, attention, and visuospatial skills.

   Furthermore, infections such as encephalitis or meningitis can also cause encephaloclastic damage and lead to cognitive impairment. A study by van der Meche et al. (2019) demonstrated that individuals who had experienced encephalitis had a higher risk of cognitive impairments, including problems with memory, attention, and information processing. These studies, along with others in the field, provide evidence for the potential cognitive impairments associated with encephaloclastic disorders. However, it's important to note that the specific extent and nature of cognitive impairment can vary depending on factors such as the cause and severity of the disorder, as well as individual differences.

3. Seizures: Seizures are a common manifestation of encephaloclastic disorders. Disruption of brain tissue can lead to abnormal electrical activity, resulting in seizures of varying types and frequencies. Seizures may present as convulsions, altered consciousness, or unusual physical and sensory sensations. The seizure can occur different groups of encephaloclastic disorders. Neuroinflammatory Disorders and Seizures such as autoimmune encephalitis or multiple sclerosis, can lead to encephaloclastic changes in the brain. Seizures can be a prominent feature of these conditions. Neurocutaneous Disorders such as tuberous sclerosis complex (TSC) or Sturge-Weber syndrome (SWS) are known to cause encephaloclastic changes in the brain, often resulting in seizures. Structural Abnormalities like neurocysticercosis, structural brain abnormalities resulting from the parasitic infection can contribute to the occurrence of seizures.

4. Behavioral Changes: Many individuals with encephaloclastic disorders experience significant changes in behavior and emotions. This can manifest as irritability, aggression, apathy, impulsivity, depression, or anxiety. Personality changes and emotional instability are also frequently reported.

   Cognitive and behavioral dysfunction including impairments in memory, attention, executive function, language, and social cognition.

   Psychiatric symptoms such as mood disorders, psychosis, anxiety, and behavioral disinhibition. For example, in frontotemporal dementia (FTD), a subtype of neurodegenerative disorder, behavioral changes like disinhibition, apathy, and compulsive behaviors are common.

   Emotional disturbances, such as emotional lability, irritability, and aggression. These changes can occur in various disorders, including traumatic brain injury (TBI) and neurodevelopmental disorders.

5. Communication Problems: Damage to specific brain regions responsible for language processing can lead to communication difficulties. Expressive language impairments, receptive language deficits, and difficulty with speech production or comprehension may arise. Language impairments, including difficulties with understanding (receptive language) and expressing (expressive language) thoughts and ideas. Aphasia, which refers to the loss or impairment of language, can occur in different forms depending on the location and extent of brain damage. Speech and Articulation Problems affecting the production of clear and intelligible speech. Dysarthria, a motor speech disorder characterized by weak, imprecise, or slurred speech, can occur due to damage to the nerves or muscles involved in speech production.

   Social communication difficulties, impacting the ability to engage in effective communication, understand social cues, and maintain appropriate social interactions. Autism spectrum disorders (ASD), for example, involve significant challenges in social communication skills.

6. Autonomic Dysfunction: Damage to the autonomic nervous system can result in dysregulation of various bodily functions. Symptoms may include alterations in heart rate, blood pressure, sweating, temperature control, and bowel or bladder function.

   Autonomic dysregulation refers to the impaired function of the autonomic nervous system, which can manifest in various ways such as dysautonomia, orthostatic hypotension, gastrointestinal dysfunction, and abnormal pupillary responses.

   Cardiovascular abnormalities such as abnormal heart rate variability, cardiac arrhythmias, and cardiovascular autonomic neuropathy.

   Respiratory dysfunction caused by central respiratory centers, leading to respiratory dysfunction such as central sleep apnea, hypoventilation, and respiratory failure.

In conclusion, encephaloclastic disorders are associated with a range of debilitating symptoms that significantly impact brain function and quality of life. The specific symptoms experienced vary depending on the location and extent of brain tissue damage. Early identification and management of these disorders are crucial for mitigating the impact on individuals' physical, cognitive, and emotional well-being.

18.8   Differential Diagnosis

Differential diagnoses for encephaloclastic lesions can vary depending on several factors such as the patient's medical history, clinical presentation, and imaging finding:

Infarction: Ischemic stroke or cerebral infarction can lead to necrotic brain tissue. It can be caused by a blockage in blood vessels supplying the brain, resulting in tissue death. Distinguishing between infarction and encephaloclastic disorders can be challenging as both conditions involve necrotic brain tissue. However, there are some characteristic features and diagnostic criteria that can help differentiate between the two (Table 18.1)

Traumatic brain injury: Severe head trauma can cause areas of necrosis within the brain tissue. The extent and location of the lesions depend on the severity and mechanism of injury. There are some points to distinguish between traumatic brain injury and Encephaloclastic disorders (Table 18.1).

Brain abscess: A localized collection of infectious material (pus) within the brain can lead to necrosis. It is usually caused by bacteria but can also be fungal or parasitic in origin (Table 18.1).

Neoplasms: Certain brain tumors, such as glioblastoma multiform, can exhibit areas of necrosis within the tumor mass (Table 18.1).

Vasculitis: Inflammatory conditions affecting blood vessels in the brain can lead to areas of necrosis. Conditions like granulomatosis with polyangiitis or primary angiitis of the central nervous system can cause encephaloclastic lesions (Table 18.1).

Radiation necrosis: Following radiation therapy for brain tumors, necrotic areas can develop within the irradiated brain tissue. It is a known side effect of radiation treatment. (Table 18.1).

Table 18.1 The differential diagnosis of encephaloclastic disorders

Variable	Encephaloclastic disorders	Infarction	Traumatic brain injury	Brain abscess	Neoplasm	Vasculitis	Radiation necrosis
Cause	A broader category of brain tissue destruction that can occur due to various causes, including trauma, infections, neoplasms, or radiation. Occurs due to a disruption of blood supply to the brain, leading to tissue death	Occurs due to a disruption of blood supply to the brain, leading to tissue death	Occurs due to an external force or trauma to the head, resulting in brain tissue damage	Is a localized infection within the brain parenchyma, usually caused by bacteria, fungi, or parasites	Abnormal growths of cells in the brain, which can be benign or malignant (cancerous)	Inflammation of blood vessels, including those in the brain caused by autoimmune diseases, infections, or drug reactions	Tissue damage that occurs as a result of radiation therapy for brain tumors – It typically occurs months to years after radiation treatment
Risk factors	Risk factors and etiologies including head trauma history, presence of infection, or previous radiation therapy	Risk factors such as hypertension, diabetes, smoking, and atherosclerosis	Men are more likely to get a TBI than women. They are also more likely to have serious TBI. Adults aged 65 and older are at the greatest risk for being hospitalized and dying from a TBI	Arises from a contiguous focus of infection, such as an ear or sinus infection, or from hematogenous spread from a distant site		Age, race, inherited syndromes that increase the risk of brain tumor, exposure to radiation	Exposure to radiation therapy for brain tumors

Clinical Presentations	Depend on the specific etiology, and symptoms may range from subtle cognitive deficits to focal neurological deficits or signs of infection	Including sudden onset focal neurological deficits, such as weakness or speech difficulties	Include symptoms like headache, dizziness, confusion, memory problems, altered consciousness, or focal neurological deficits. Include symptoms like headache, dizziness, confusion, memory problems, altered consciousness, or focal neurological deficits	Clinical presentation includes symptoms such as headache, fever, focal neurological deficits, altered mental status, and signs of increased intracranial pressure	Clinical presentation may include symptoms such as headache, seizures, focal neurological deficits (e.g., weakness, sensory changes), cognitive impairments, or changes in behavior	Include symptoms such as headache, cognitive impairments, focal neurological deficits, seizures, or signs of systemic inflammation	Include focal neurological deficits, cognitive impairments, seizures, or signs of increased intracranial pressure
Imaging studies	Imaging findings may vary depending on the underlying cause. For example, traumatic encephaloclastic lesions may show signs of contusion or hemorrhage, while infectious lesions may exhibit inflammatory changes or abscess formation	CT scan or MRI may show a focal area of restricted diffusion (indicating ischemia) along with corresponding perfusion abnormalities	Like CT scan or MRI may reveal specific findings associated with TBI, such as contusions, hemorrhages, diffuse axonal injury, or skull fractures	Imaging studies, particularly MRI with contrast, can reveal a well-circumscribed lesion with a rim-enhancing pattern, surrounded by edema	Imaging studies, particularly MRI with contrast, can reveal the presence of a space-occupying lesion with variable enhancement patterns, perilesional edema, mass effect, and sometimes necrosis or hemorrhage	Imaging studies, such as MRI or angiography, can reveal the presence of vessel wall thickening, narrowing, or aneurysms in affected areas	Radiological findings often show a well-demarcated, non-enhancing lesion with surrounding edema, which may mimic tumor recurrence. Advanced imaging techniques like perfusion MRI or PET scans can demonstrate decreased blood flow or glucose metabolism within the lesion.

(continued)

Table 18.1 (continued)

Variable	Encephaloclastic disorders	Infarction	Traumatic brain injury	Brain abscess	Neoplasm	Vasculitis	Radiation necrosis
Diagnosis	The diagnosis typically involves a combination of clinical assessment, imaging studies, laboratory tests, and sometimes biopsy or culture analysis	The diagnosis is based on clinical symptoms, imaging findings, and exclusion of other causes	Diagnosis is based on a combination of clinical assessment, imaging findings, and the presence of a history of head trauma	Diagnostic confirmation involves analyzing the aspirated pus or biopsy of the abscess wall to identify the causative organism	Definitive diagnosis often requires a biopsy or surgical resection of the tumor, followed by histopathological examination	Diagnosis often requires a combination of clinical evaluation, laboratory tests (e.g., blood tests, inflammatory markers), imaging studies, and sometimes a biopsy of affected tissue	Definitive diagnosis often requires a combination of clinical assessment, imaging studies, and sometimes biopsy or advanced imaging techniques

18.9   Diagnostic Workup

The diagnosis workup for encephaloclastic disorders typically involves a combination of medical history evaluation, physical examination, neuroimaging, and laboratory tests. Encephaloclastic disorders refer to conditions characterized by the destruction or degeneration of brain tissue.

1. Medical history evaluation: During the medical history evaluation for encephaloclastic disorders, a healthcare provider may typically ask questions related to the following aspects:

   (a) Symptoms: The healthcare provider may inquire about the specific symptoms experienced, their onset, duration, and progression. Symptoms commonly associated with encephaloclastic disorders may include developmental delays, seizures, cognitive impairment, motor dysfunction, and behavioral changes.

   (b) Family history: A thorough assessment of the patient's family history is important, as certain genetic factors can contribute to the development of encephaloclastic disorders. The healthcare provider may ask about any known neurological disorders or conditions among family members.

   (c) Medical history: The healthcare provider will review the patient's medical records, including any previous diagnoses, medical procedures, or treatments. They may inquire about any known medical conditions, infections, or exposure to toxins that could potentially contribute to encephaloclastic disorders.

   (d) Developmental milestones: In the case of pediatric patients, the healthcare provider may ask about the patient's developmental milestones, such as when they achieved motor skills, language skills, and other milestones.

   (e) Medications and supplements: The healthcare provider may ask about any medications, supplements, or herbal remedies that the patient is currently taking or has taken in the past, as certain medications or toxins can potentially contribute to encephaloclastic disorders.

2. Physical examination: During the physical examination for encephaloclastic disorders, a healthcare provider, typically a neurologist, may perform the following assessments:

   (a) Neurological assessment: The healthcare provider will evaluate the patient's overall neurological function. This may include assessing muscle strength, reflexes, coordination, balance, and sensory function. They may use various tests such as the mini-mental state examination (MMSE) to assess cognitive function.

   (b) Cranial nerve examination: The healthcare provider will assess the function of the cranial nerves, which are responsible for various sensory and motor functions in the head and neck. This examination may include assessing vision, hearing, facial movements, and swallowing.

(c) Motor function assessment: The healthcare provider will evaluate the patient's motor function, including muscle strength, tone, and coordination. They may ask the patient to perform specific movements and observe for any abnormalities.

(d) Sensory examination: The healthcare provider will assess the patient's sensory function, including touch, pain, temperature, and proprioception. They may use tools such as a pinprick or a tuning fork to evaluate sensory responses.

(e) Reflex examination: The healthcare provider will test the patient's reflexes, such as the knee jerk reflex, to assess the integrity of the spinal cord and peripheral nerves.

(f) Gait and coordination assessment: The healthcare provider will observe the patient's gait (walking pattern) and coordination to identify any abnormalities that may suggest underlying neurological issues.

3. Neuroimaging: Neuroimaging plays a crucial role in the diagnosis and evaluation of encephaloclastic disorders. It helps visualize the brain's structure and function, allowing healthcare professionals to identify any abnormalities or changes that may be indicative of these disorders. Several neuroimaging techniques are commonly used:

(a) Magnetic Resonance Imaging (MRI): MRI findings in encephaloclastic disorders can vary depending on the underlying cause and the stage of the disease. However, there are some common features that can be observed in these disorders. The following are the key MRI findings seen in encephaloclastic disorders:

   • Tissue Destruction: MRI typically shows areas of tissue destruction or loss in the affected regions of the brain. This can be visualized as areas of abnormal signal intensity on T1-weighted and T2-weighted images. The extent and location of tissue loss depend on the underlying cause.
   • Cystic Changes: In chronic encephaloclastic disorders, cystic changes may develop within the destroyed brain tissue. These cystic spaces can be seen as areas of fluid-filled cavities on MRI images. They often have hypointense signal intensity on T1-weighted images and hyperintense signal intensity on T2-weighted images.
   • Wall Enhancement: In some cases, the cystic spaces may show wall enhancement after contrast administration. This enhancement is typically seen as an increased signal intensity along the inner lining of the cystic wall on post-contrast T1-weighted images. It indicates active inflammation or ongoing pathological processes.
   • Mass Effect: Encephaloclastic disorders can cause mass effect due to tissue destruction and cyst formation. This can result in displacement or compression of adjacent brain structures, leading to midline shift, ventricular compression, or herniation. These mass effect features can be

visualized on MRI and help in assessing the severity and extent of brain damage.

- Diffusion-Weighted Imaging (DWI): DWI is a specialized MRI technique that can provide information about the movement of water molecules within the brain tissue. In encephaloclastic disorders, DWI may show areas of restricted diffusion, indicating ischemic or necrotic brain tissue. Restricted diffusion is typically seen as hyperintense signal intensity on DWI images and hypointense signal intensity on apparent diffusion coefficient (ADC) maps.
- Perilesional Edema: Surrounding the areas of tissue destruction, there may be perilesional edema visible on MRI. This edema appears as hyperintense signal intensity on T2-weighted and fluid-attenuated inversion recovery (FLAIR) images. The extent of perilesional edema can provide additional information about the inflammatory response and severity of the disease.

(b) Tomography (CT) Scan: In encephaloclastic disorders, CT scan findings may vary depending on the specific condition and stage of the disease. Some common findings observed on CT scans include:

- Volume loss: Encephaloclastic disorders often result in the loss of brain tissue, leading to visible volume loss on CT scans. This can manifest as areas of decreased density or atrophy in affected regions.
- Cortical thinning: In certain encephaloclastic disorders, such as hemimegalencephaly, cortical thinning or abnormal thickening may be observed on CT scans.
- Ventricular enlargement: As a consequence of volume loss and tissue destruction, ventricular enlargement or hydrocephalus may be seen on CT scans.
- Calcifications: In some cases, calcifications may be present within the affected brain tissue. These calcifications can appear as hyperdense areas on CT scans

(c) Single-Photon Emission Computed Tomography (SPECT): SPECT is a nuclear medicine imaging technique that uses radioactive tracers to evaluate blood flow and metabolic activity in the brain. It can be helpful in the diagnosis and assessment of encephaloclastic disorders by providing functional information about the affected brain regions. Specific SPECT findings in encephaloclastic disorders may vary depending on the underlying condition and stage of the disease. However, here are some general observations:

- Hypoperfusion: Encephaloclastic disorders often lead to decreased blood flow in the affected areas of the brain. SPECT can show regions of hypoperfusion, indicating reduced blood flow and metabolic activity.
- Asymmetric perfusion: In certain encephaloclastic disorders, such as hemimegalencephaly or focal cortical dysplasia, SPECT may reveal

asymmetric perfusion patterns. This can help in localizing the areas of abnormal brain tissue.

- Hyperperfusion: In some cases, encephaloclastic disorders can cause hyperperfusion in certain brain regions. This increased blood flow can be seen on SPECT images.
- Functional abnormalities: SPECT can provide functional information about the affected brain regions, such as changes in glucose metabolism or neurotransmitter activity. These abnormalities can help in understanding the pathophysiology of encephaloclastic disorders.

(d) Positron Emission Tomography (PET) Scan: Positron Emission Tomography (PET) scan is another nuclear imaging technique used to evaluate brain function and metabolism in various neurological disorders, including encephaloclastic disorders. PET scan findings in encephaloclastic disorders can provide valuable information about the functional abnormalities associated with these conditions. Here are some general findings observed in PET imaging:

- Hypometabolism: PET scans often reveal areas of reduced cerebral glucose metabolism (hypometabolism) in the affected regions of the brain. This indicates decreased activity and function of the damaged or non-functioning tissue.
- Focal or Diffuse Abnormalities: Depending on the specific encephaloclastic disorder, PET findings can show either focal (localized) or diffuse (widespread) abnormalities in cerebral metabolism. These abnormalities can help in determining the extent and severity of tissue damage.
- Asymmetric Patterns: PET imaging may exhibit asymmetric patterns of metabolic abnormalities, indicating uneven distribution of affected brain regions. This can aid in differentiating encephaloclastic disorders from other conditions that may present with similar symptoms.
- Amyloid Deposition: In certain encephaloclastic disorders, such as Alzheimer's disease, PET scans can detect the deposition of amyloid plaques in the brain. Amyloid PET imaging utilizes specific radiotracers to visualize the accumulation of amyloid-beta protein, which is a characteristic feature of Alzheimer's disease.

4. Laboratory tests:

Laboratory tests play a crucial role in the diagnostic workup of encephaloclastic disorders. While the specific tests can vary depending on the suspected underlying cause. Complete Blood Count (CBC) can help identify any abnormalities in the blood cells, such as anemia or infection, which may contribute to encephaloclastic disorders. It provides information about red blood cells, white blood cells, and platelets. Cerebrospinal fluid (CSF) analysis can provide valuable information about the presence of infection, inflammation, or other abnormalities in the central nervous system. It may include measuring the levels of glucose, proteins, and performing cell count and differential. Specific antibody testing for specific infectious agents causing encephaloclastic disorders to identify the causative organism. This can include serological tests, such as enzyme immunoassays or immunofluorescence assays, to detect antibodies against specific pathogens. Genetic testing In some cases, genetic testing may be necessary to identify specific gene mutations associated with certain encephaloclastic disorders, such as certain types of leukodystrophies or lysosomal storage disorders. Metabolic testing for metabolic disorders that can cause encephaloclastic changes. Metabolic testing, such as measuring plasma amino acids, organic acids, or acylcarnitine profiles, can help identify metabolic abnormalities that contribute to the disorder.

5. Electroencephalogram (EEG): An EEG is a non-invasive test that measures the electrical activity of the brain using electrodes placed on the scalp. It can provide valuable information about brain function and help in the diagnosis and management of various neurological disorders, including encephaloclastic disorders. In encephaloclastic disorders, the findings on an EEG can vary depending on the extent and location of the brain tissue damage. However, some common EEG findings in these disorders may include:

   (a) Slow Background Activity: The background activity of the EEG may appear slower than normal, with a decrease in the frequency and amplitude of the brainwaves.
   (b) Focal or Generalized Epileptiform Discharges: Epileptiform discharges, such as spikes, sharp waves, or slow waves, may be observed in specific brain regions or throughout the entire EEG recording.
   (c) Burst Suppression Pattern: A burst suppression pattern is characterized by alternating periods of high-amplitude bursts of activity and periods of low or no activity.
   (d) Periodic Discharges: Periodic discharges, such as periodic sharp waves or periodic complexes, may be present in the EEG.

6. Biopsy: Biopsy is a procedure that involves the removal of a small sample of tissue for microscopic examination. While biopsies are not as common in diagnosing encephaloclastic disorders compared to other diagnostic methods, in certain cases, they can provide valuable insights into the underlying pathology. Biopsy findings in encephaloclastic disorders including the followings:

   (a) Tissue Damage and Cellular Changes: Biopsies from affected brain tissue can reveal evidence of tissue damage, including loss of neurons, gliosis (reactive astrocytosis), and presence of infiltrating immune cells. These findings help in confirming the presence of encephaloclastic pathology.
   (b) Inflammatory Reaction: Depending on the underlying cause of the disorder, biopsies can show signs of inflammation, such as increased immune cell infiltration, activation of microglia, and presence of cytokines or other inflammatory markers. These findings can provide crucial information about the nature and extent of the inflammatory response.

(c) Infectious Agents: In cases where encephaloclastic disorders are caused by infections, biopsies may reveal the presence of specific infectious agents. These can include bacteria, viruses, fungi, or parasites. Identification of the specific pathogen can help guide appropriate treatment strategies.

(d) Secondary Changes: Biopsies can also indicate secondary changes, such as vascular abnormalities, necrosis, or presence of amyloid deposits. These findings can provide additional insights into the complex nature of encephaloclastic disorders and their associated pathologies

It is important to note that the specific diagnostic workup may vary depending on the suspected underlying cause of the encephaloclastic disorder. A multidisciplinary approach involving neurologists, radiologists, geneticists, and other specialists may be necessary to establish an accurate diagnosis and guide appropriate treatment.

18.10 Treatment Strategies

The treatment strategies for encephaloclastic disorders depend on the underlying cause and the specific symptoms and complications present in each individual case.

1. Symptomatic Management: Symptomatic management for encephaloclastic disorders focuses on alleviating symptoms and enhancing the quality of life for affected individuals. It aims to address specific symptoms associated with brain tissue damage or dysfunction. While the specific management strategies may vary depending on the type and severity of the disorder, here are some common approaches:

   (a) Pain Management: Pain management plays a crucial role in addressing the chronic pain often associated with encephaloclastic disorders. While the specific approach may vary depending on the individual's needs and the nature of their condition, the common strategies employed in pain management including:

   - Non-Opioid Analgesics: Non-opioid analgesics are often utilized as the first line of treatment for mild to moderate pain in encephaloclastic disorders. These include medications like acetaminophen (such as Tylenol) and nonsteroidal anti-inflammatory drugs (NSAIDs) such as ibuprofen or naproxen. These medications help reduce pain and inflammation.
   - Opioid Analgesics: In cases of severe or refractory pain, opioids may be considered under close supervision. Opioid analgesics, such as morphine or oxycodone, can help manage severe pain. However, their use requires careful monitoring due to the potential for side effects, tolerance, and dependency. They should only be prescribed and managed by healthcare professionals experienced in pain management.
   - Adjuvant Medications: Adjuvant medications are often used alongside analgesics to enhance pain relief in encephaloclastic disorders. These

may include antidepressants, anticonvulsants, or medications like gabapentin or pregabalin, which have shown efficacy in neuropathic pain management. Adjuvant medications can help target specific pain mechanisms and provide additional pain relief.

- Physical and Occupational Therapy: Physical and occupational therapy can play a crucial role in pain management for individuals with encephaloclastic disorders. These therapies focus on improving physical functioning, reducing disability, and enhancing overall quality of life. They may include exercises, stretches, manual techniques, assistive devices, and ergonomic modifications to promote optimal mobility and minimize pain.
- Complementary Therapies: Complementary therapies can be used alongside conventional pain management approaches to provide additional relief. These may include acupuncture, massage therapy, transcutaneous electrical nerve stimulation (TENS), or relaxation techniques. While their effectiveness can vary, some individuals find these approaches beneficial in managing their pain

(b) Seizure Control: Seizure control is a critical aspect of managing encephaloclastic disorders, as seizures are a common manifestation of these conditions. Effective seizure control aims to reduce the frequency, duration, and severity of seizures, while also minimizing adverse effects of antiepileptic medications and optimizing the individual's quality of life. The key points regarding seizure contro are:

- Antiepileptic Medications: Antiepileptic drugs (AEDs) are the primary treatment for seizure control in encephaloclastic disorders. AEDs work by modulating neuronal excitability and preventing or reducing abnormal electrical activity in the brain. The specific choice of AED depends on various factors, including the type of seizures, patient characteristics, potential drug interactions, and comorbidities.
- Selection of Antiepileptic Medications: In choosing an appropriate AED, healthcare professionals consider the specific seizure type, as different AEDs may have different efficacies against certain seizure types. They also take into account factors such as the patient's age, overall health, potential side effects, and drug interactions. Close monitoring and regular follow-up are crucial to assess the effectiveness and adjust the dosage or switch medications as needed.
- Individualized Approach: Seizure control is highly individualized, as different patients may respond differently to various AEDs. It may take time to find the most effective medication and dosage for each individual. Regular follow-up appointments allow for monitoring the response to treatment, evaluating seizure control, and adjusting the management plan when necessary.
- Potential Combination Therapy: In some cases, combination therapy involving two or more AEDs may be necessary to achieve optimal sei-

zure control. The choice to combine medications is based on the individual's specific needs and the seizure type being targeted. The goal is to find the most effective combination while minimizing side effects and drug interactions.

- Regular Monitoring and Adjustments: Seizure control requires ongoing monitoring to assess the response to treatment and make necessary adjustments. This may involve determining appropriate drug dosages, monitoring AED blood levels, considering potential drug interactions, and evaluating for any emerging side effects. Regular communication with the healthcare team is essential to ensure effective seizure control

(c) Cognitive and Behavioral Support: Cognitive and behavioral support is an important component of managing encephaloclastic disorders. These disorders can often lead to cognitive impairment and behavioral changes that significantly impact an individual's daily functioning and quality of life. Cognitive and behavioral interventions aim to optimize cognitive function, address emotional and behavioral challenges, and enhance overall well-being. This including:

- Cognitive Rehabilitation: Cognitive rehabilitation programs are designed to address cognitive impairments resulting from encephaloclastic disorders. These programs utilize various techniques and strategies to improve cognitive function, including attention, memory, executive function, and problem-solving skills. Rehabilitation may involve individual or group sessions, computer-based training programs, compensatory strategies, and environmental modifications to facilitate optimal cognitive functioning. Occupational therapists, neuropsychologists, or other qualified professionals often lead these interventions.
- Speech Therapy: Speech therapy, also known as speech-language pathology, can help individuals with encephaloclastic disorders improve their communication skills. Speech therapists work on speech production, language comprehension, reading, and writing skills. They may employ specific techniques tailored to the individual's needs, such as articulation exercises, language-based activities, or augmentative and alternative communication methods.
- Behavioral Therapy: Behavioral therapy or counseling can assist individuals in managing emotional and behavioral challenges associated with encephaloclastic disorders. These therapies focus on addressing mood changes, anxiety, social difficulties, impulsivity, and other behavioral issues that may arise. Techniques such as cognitive-behavioral therapy (CBT), mindfulness-based approaches, or positive behavior supports may be employed to develop coping strategies, enhance emotional regulation, and improve overall well-being.
- Occupational Therapy: Occupational therapy aims to improve an individual's ability to perform daily activities and maximize their independence. Occupational therapists help individuals develop skills necessary for self-care, work, leisure, and community participation. They may

focus on physical rehabilitation, training in the use of adaptive devices, sensory integration techniques, and environmental modifications to enhance functional capacity.

(d) Symptomatic Treatment of Movement Disorders: Symptomatic treatment of movement disorders aims to manage motor symptoms associated with encephaloclastic disorders, such as dystonia, tremors, or chorea. The specific treatment approach may vary depending on the type and severity of the movement disorder, and the individual's needs. Here are key points regarding symptomatic treatment:

- Medications: Various medications can be used to manage movement disorders in encephaloclastic disorders. The choice of medication depends on the specific motor symptoms being targeted. Examples of medications commonly used include:

  - Muscle Relaxants: Medications that help relax muscles, such as baclofen or benzodiazepines, may be prescribed to reduce muscle stiffness and spasticity associated with movement disorders.
  - Botulinum Toxin Injections: Botulinum toxin injections, such as onabotulinumtoxinA (Botox), can be helpful in treating focal dystonias or focal spasticity. The toxin blocks the release of acetylcholine, which reduces muscle contractions and involuntary movements.
  - Dopamine-Depleting Agents: Dopamine-depleting agents like tetrabenazine may be used to manage hyperkinetic movement disorders, such as chorea or Huntington's disease. These medications help reduce excessive dopamine activity in the brain, leading to a decrease in abnormal movements.

- Physical Therapy: Physical therapy plays an essential role in managing movement disorders. Physical therapists can provide targeted exercises and techniques to improve mobility, balance, and coordination. They may focus on strengthening weak muscles, stretching tight muscles, and improving overall motor function. Physical therapy helps individuals optimize their physical capabilities and minimize movement limitations.
- Occupational Therapy: Occupational therapy can help individuals with movement disorders adapt their daily activities and enhance their functional independence. Occupational therapists provide strategies and interventions to improve fine motor skills, develop compensatory techniques, and employ adaptive equipment or assistive devices that assist in daily tasks. Occupational therapy aims to enable individuals to maintain optimal functionality and participate in meaningful activities.
- Surgical Interventions: In some cases where medication and therapy are insufficient, surgical interventions may be considered. Deep brain stimulation (DBS) is a surgical procedure that involves implanting electrodes in specific brain regions to modulate abnormal neuronal activity. DBS has shown effectiveness in managing certain movement disorders like dystonia or essential tremors

2. Immunomodulatory Therapy: Immunomodulatory therapy is an approach that aims to modulate the immune system's response in encephaloclastic disorders, including those caused by autoimmune reactions. By regulating the immune response, this therapy aims to reduce inflammation, immune-mediated tissue damage, and slow down the progression of the disorder. The Immunomodulatory therapy including the followings:

   (a) Corticosteroids: Corticosteroids, such as prednisone or methylprednisolone, are commonly used in the initial treatment of autoimmune encephaloclastic disorders. They have potent anti-inflammatory properties and suppress the immune system's inflammatory response. Corticosteroids can help reduce inflammation, alleviate symptoms, and stabilize the condition. However, long-term use of corticosteroids may carry certain potential side effects and risks.

   (b) Immunosuppressants: When corticosteroids alone are not sufficient or to minimize their long-term use, immunosuppressant medications may be employed. These medications target specific parts of the immune system to modulate the immune response and reduce inflammation. Commonly used immunosuppressants include azathioprine, mycophenolate mofetil, methotrexate, or cyclophosphamide. They may be used as monotherapy or in combination with corticosteroids.

   (c) Biological Therapies: Biological therapies, or biologics, are a newer class of immunomodulatory medications that specifically target certain immune cells, cytokines, or signaling pathways involved in autoimmune reactions. For example, monoclonal antibodies such as rituximab, tocilizumab, or natalizumab are used to reduce specific immune cell populations or neutralize specific cytokines. These therapies are often reserved for more severe or refractory cases.

   (d) Plasma Exchange (Plasmapheresis): In certain cases, plasma exchange may be considered as an immunomodulatory intervention. Plasma exchange involves removing the patient's blood plasma, which contains circulating antibodies or immune mediators, and replacing it with donor plasma or suitable substitutes. This procedure helps remove harmful immune factors and reduce the overall autoimmune response.

   (e) Individualized Approach and Monitoring: Immunomodulatory therapy is highly individualized and tailored to each patient's specific needs. The choice of therapy depends on the underlying condition, disease severity, patient characteristics, and potential risks. Regular monitoring is necessary to assess treatment response, manage potential side effects, and adjust treatment strategies accordingly

3. Supportive Care: Supportive care plays a crucial role in managing encephaloclastic disorders by providing general medical care, addressing symptoms, preventing complications, and promoting overall well-being. Supportive care focuses on maintaining quality of life, managing comorbidities, and ensuring optimal physical and emotional support for individuals with these disorders. Supportive care including the followings:

(a) General Medical Care: Supportive care involves providing comprehensive general medical care to individuals with encephaloclastic disorders. This includes regular monitoring of vital signs, management of comorbidities (such as hypertension, diabetes, or infections), preventive care (such as vaccinations), and coordination of overall healthcare needs.

(b) Nutrition and Hydration: Ensuring adequate nutrition and hydration is essential for individuals with encephaloclastic disorders. Supportive care may involve dietary guidance, ensuring proper calorie intake, hydration management, and addressing any swallowing difficulties or feeding challenges that may arise.

(c) Preventing Complications: Supportive care aims to prevent complications commonly associated with encephaloclastic disorders. By promoting activities that reduce the risk of infection, such as proper hygiene and immunizations, and implementing appropriate strategies to prevent pressure ulcers, falls, or other potential complications, healthcare professionals can help maintain the individual's overall well-being.

(d) Comfort and Pain Management: Supportive care involves addressing pain and ensuring the individual's comfort. This may involve the use of non-opioid or opioid analgesics to manage pain, implementing physical comfort measures, and utilizing complementary therapies (such as massage, heat therapy, or relaxation techniques) to enhance comfort.

(e) Psychosocial and Emotional Support: Individuals with encephaloclastic disorders often experience emotional and psychosocial challenges. Supportive care includes providing emotional support, counseling, and access to mental health resources. It also involves promoting social interactions, facilitating engagement in meaningful activities, and addressing the needs of family members and caregivers.

(f) Caregiver Support: Supportive care extends to family members and caregivers, recognizing their role in providing care and addressing their needs. This may involve caregiver education, respite care services, support groups, or counseling, to help caregivers effectively cope with the challenges associated with supporting individuals with encephaloclastic disorders

4. Disease-Specific Treatments:

(a) Stroke: it is a neurological conditions characterized by a sudden loss of blood flow to the brain, resulting in the destruction of brain tissue. The treatment of stroke involves a multi-disciplinary approach that focuses on preventing further damage, restoring blood flow to the affected area, and promoting recovery. Here are some common disease-specific treatments for stroke in encephaloclastic disorders including:

- Thrombolytic Therapy: Thrombolytic therapy, also known as clot-busting therapy, is one of the primary treatments for acute ischemic stroke. It involves the administration of medication, such as intravenous tissue plasminogen activator (tPA), to dissolve the blood clot that is blocking the blood vessels in the brain. This treatment should be initiated within a specific time window after the onset of symptoms to maximize its effectiveness. The guidelines and recommendations for thrombolytic therapy vary depending on the specific country or medical association. You can refer to the American Heart Association/American Stroke Association (AHA/ASA) guidelines for acute ischemic stroke for more information.

- Endovascular Thrombectomy: Endovascular thrombectomy is a minimally invasive procedure performed to remove the blood clot causing an acute ischemic stroke. It involves using specialized catheters and tools to physically remove or break up the clot, restoring blood flow to the affected area. This treatment is generally recommended for patients who have a large vessel occlusion and meet specific criteria. The guidelines from various medical associations, such as AHA/ASA, provide detailed recommendations on patient selection and procedural considerations for endovascular thrombectomy

- Neuroprotective Agents: Neuroprotective agents are medications or approaches aimed at minimizing cell death and preventing further neurological damage after a stroke. These agents may include drugs that target specific pathways involved in cell injury, such as antioxidants, anti-inflammatory drugs, and agents that regulate excitatory neurotransmitters. However, it's important to note that the effectiveness of neuroprotective agents in stroke treatment is still under investigation, and no specific neuroprotective agent has been widely approved for routine clinical use. Further research is required to establish their efficacy and safety

- Rehabilitation Therapy: Rehabilitation therapy plays a crucial role in the recovery and improvement of function after a stroke. It involves various interventions, such as physical therapy, occupational therapy, speech and language therapy, and cognitive rehabilitation. These therapies are tailored to the individual's specific impairments and aim to promote recovery, restore function, and enhance quality of life. Rehabilitation therapy should be initiated as soon as possible after the acute phase of stroke and continued for an extended period to maximize the potential for recovery.

- Secondary Prevention: Once a stroke has occurred, it is crucial to implement measures to prevent future strokes. Secondary prevention measures may include lifestyle modifications, such as adopting a healthy diet, engaging in regular physical activity, managing hypertension, controlling diabetes, quitting smoking, and reducing alcohol consumption. In some cases, antiplatelet medications, such as aspirin or clopidogrel, may be prescribed to prevent blood clots from forming and further narrowing the blood vessels in the brain.

(b) Traumatic Brain Injury: TBI refers to a brain injury caused by an external force, such as a blow or jolt to the head. The treatment of TBI aims to stabilize the patient, prevent further injury, and promote recovery of brain function. There are some disease-specific treatments for TBI, including:

- Emergency Medical Care: Immediately after a traumatic brain injury, it is crucial to provide emergency medical care. This involves ensuring an adequate airway, stabilizing vital signs, and preventing secondary brain injury. Secondary brain injury can result from factors such as increased intracranial pressure, hypoxia, and hypotension. These complications should be aggressively managed to improve patient outcomes. The Brain Trauma Foundation provides guidelines on the management of severe TBI and can serve as a reference for emergency medical care
- Surgical Intervention: In certain cases of TBI, surgical intervention may be necessary to address complications, such as intracranial bleeding, hematomas, or skull fractures. Dependent on the specific TBI subtype, surgical treatments may include craniotomy, craniectomy, hematoma evacuation, or decompressive craniectomy. The decision to perform surgery is made by the neurosurgeon based on the patient's clinical condition and imaging findings. Guidelines from the Brain Trauma Foundation and the American Association of Neurological Surgeons provide detailed recommendations for surgical management
- Pharmacological Intervention: Pharmacological treatment in TBI aims to manage and prevent secondary complications and promote recovery. Medications may be used to control seizures (antiepileptic drugs), reduce intracranial pressure (osmotic diuretics like mannitol or hypertonic saline), manage pain, and address mood disorders. However, the use of pharmacological interventions in TBI is complex and should be tailored to the individual patient's needs. The Brain Trauma Foundation guidelines provide recommendations for pharmacological treatments in TBI
- Rehabilitation Therapy: Rehabilitation is an essential component of TBI treatment and focuses on maximizing functional recovery and quality of life. Rehabilitation programs may include physical therapy, occupational therapy, speech and language therapy, cognitive rehabilitation, and psychological support. These therapies help individuals regain motor skills, relearn cognitive abilities, improve communication, and address emotional and behavioral changes. The duration and intensity of rehabilitation depend on the severity of the injury and the individual's progress. The American Congress of Rehabilitation Medicine offers guidelines on rehabilitation strategies for individuals with moderate to severe TBI
- Long-Term Support and Care: TBI can have lasting effects on individuals and their families. Long-term support and care play a vital role in managing the consequences of TBI. This may include assistance with daily activities, vocational rehabilitation, psychological counseling, and community support services. Support groups and counseling services can also provide emotional support to individuals with TBI and their families.

(c) Autoimmune Encephalitis: it refers to a group of disorders characterized by inflammation in the brain due to an immune response against neuronal proteins. The treatment of autoimmune encephalitis aims to control the inflammation, suppress the immune system, and manage associated symptoms. There are some disease-specific treatments for autoimmune encephalitis including:

- Immunotherapy: Immunotherapy plays a crucial role in the treatment of autoimmune encephalitis. It involves the use of medications that modulate the immune system to reduce inflammation and target the specific autoimmune response. The two primary types of immunotherapy used are corticosteroids and intravenous immunoglobulin (IVIg).

  - Corticosteroids: High-dose corticosteroids, such as methylprednisolone or prednisone, are often the first-line treatment for autoimmune encephalitis. They work by suppressing the immune response and reducing inflammation. The duration and dosage of corticosteroid therapy vary depending on the severity of symptoms and the individual patient's response.
  - Intravenous Immunoglobulin (IVIg): IVIg is derived from pooled human plasma containing antibodies that can regulate the immune system. IVIg therapy is a common second-line treatment option for autoimmune encephalitis, especially when corticosteroids are ineffective or not well-tolerated. It can modulate the immune response and potentially reduce autoantibody levels.
  - Other immunotherapy options that may be considered include plasma exchange (plasmapheresis), which removes autoantibodies from the blood, and immunosuppressive agents such as rituximab or cyclophosphamide. The choice of immunotherapy is based on the specific type of autoimmune encephalitis, individual patient factors, and response to treatment. The guidelines published by the Autoimmune Encephalitis Alliance and the Neurocritical Care Society provide detailed recommendations for immunotherapy in autoimmune encephalitis.

- Symptom Management: Autoimmune encephalitis can present with a variety of symptoms, including cognitive impairment, seizures, movement disorders, and psychiatric symptoms. Symptom management is an important aspect of treatment to improve the quality of life for affected individuals. Treatment strategies may include antiepileptic medications to control seizures, medications to manage movement disorders or psychiatric symptoms, and supportive care to address cognitive and behavioral issues. Multidisciplinary care teams, including neurologists, psychiatrists, and rehabilitation specialists, work together to provide comprehensive symptom management.
- Tumor Removal: In cases of autoimmune encephalitis associated with an underlying tumor, tumor removal is an important part of the treatment plan. Tumors, such as ovarian teratomas or small-cell lung cancer, can trigger the autoimmune response leading to encephalitis. Surgical

removal or other appropriate treatments for the tumor can help alleviate symptoms and prevent further immune-mediated damage. Close collaboration between neurologists, oncologists, and other specialists is necessary for the management of tumor-associated autoimmune encephalitis.

- Long-Term Monitoring and Support: Autoimmune encephalitis requires long-term monitoring and support to manage the chronic effects of the condition. Regular follow-up visits with healthcare providers are essential to assess treatment response, adjust medications, and manage any potential relapses or complications. Supportive care, including cognitive rehabilitation, occupational therapy, and psychological support, is often beneficial to address the functional and psychological consequences of autoimmune encephalitis.

(d) Huntington's Disease: is a genetic neurodegenerative disorder characterized by the progressive loss of neurons in certain regions of the brain. Unfortunately, there is currently no cure for HD. However, there are several disease-specific treatments available that aim to manage symptoms, slow disease progression, and improve quality of life. There are some disease-specific treatments for Huntington's disease, including:

- Medications for Symptomatic Treatment:

  - Tetrabenazine: Tetrabenazine is commonly used to treat chorea, which is an involuntary movement characteristic of HD. It works by reducing dopamine activity in the brain. Tetrabenazine has been approved by the U.S. Food and Drug Administration (FDA) for the treatment of chorea associated with HD.
  - Antipsychotic Medications: Antipsychotic medications such as risperidone, olanzapine, or quetiapine may be prescribed to manage psychiatric symptoms, including psychosis, agitation, and irritability. These medications should be carefully monitored due to the risk of adverse effects, especially in individuals with HD

- Physical and Occupational Therapy:

  - Physical Therapy: Physical therapy can help manage motor symptoms, improve balance, maintain muscle strength, and facilitate mobility. Therapists may recommend exercises, stretching, and assisted devices to aid in movement and reduce the risk of falls.
  - Occupational Therapy: Occupational therapy can assist individuals with HD in maintaining their independence and improving their ability to perform daily activities. Therapists focus on strategies to adapt the environment, recommend assistive devices, and teach compensatory techniques to address difficulties with activities of daily living.

- Speech and Swallowing Therapy: Speech therapy can be beneficial for individuals with HD who experience communication difficulties, including slurred speech (dysarthria) or difficulty organizing and producing speech (apraxia of speech). Speech therapists can provide exercises and techniques to improve speech intelligibility, swallowing function, and overall communication skills.

- Psychological and Psychiatric Support:

  - Counseling and Psychotherapy: HD can have significant psychological and emotional impact. Counseling and psychotherapy can help individuals and their families cope with the emotional challenges associated with HD, including depression, anxiety, and grief.
  - Support Groups: Joining HD support groups can provide a supportive environment, information sharing, and a sense of community among individuals and families affected by HD.

- Experimental and Investigational Treatments: Participating in clinical trials provides access to emerging treatments and interventions for HD. Clinical trials investigate new medications, gene therapies, and potential disease-modifying treatments. The Huntington's Disease Society of America and other research organizations provide information on ongoing clinical trials

  These are some examples for Disease-Specific Treatments in encephaloclastic disorders.

5. Multidisciplinary Care: Multidisciplinary care is an approach that involves a team of healthcare professionals from different specialties working collaboratively to provide holistic and comprehensive care for individuals with encephaloclastic disorders. This approach recognizes that these disorders often involve complex medical, physical, cognitive, and psychological needs that require expertise from various disciplines. There are some details about multidisciplinary care in encephaloclastic disorders:

(a) Composition of the Multidisciplinary Team:

- Neurologist: A neurologist specializes in diagnosing and managing conditions affecting the nervous system, including encephaloclastic disorders. They coordinate and oversee the overall care plan, provide medical interventions, and monitor disease progression.
- Neurosurgeon: A neurosurgeon may be involved in the surgical management of encephaloclastic disorders, such as tumor removal or invasive procedures to relieve pressure on the brain.
- Rehabilitation Specialist: Rehabilitation specialists, such as physiatrists or rehabilitation therapists, play a crucial role in addressing physical, cognitive, and functional impairments. They design and implement rehabilitation programs to optimize recovery, improve mobility, and enhance functional independence.

- Psychologist/Psychiatrist: Mental health professionals provide psychological and psychiatric support to address emotional, behavioral, and cognitive aspects associated with encephaloclastic disorders. They may provide counseling, cognitive-behavioral therapy, or psychotropic medications as needed.
- Speech and Language Therapist: Speech and language therapists work with individuals who experience communication difficulties, speech disorders, or swallowing difficulties due to encephaloclastic disorders. They develop individualized therapy plans to improve speech intelligibility and swallowing function.
- Occupational Therapist: Occupational therapists help individuals optimize their ability to perform activities of daily living and adapt to functional limitations caused by encephaloclastic disorders. They focus on promoting independence, enhancing vocational skills, and modifying the environment to accommodate specific needs.
- Physical Therapist: Physical therapists specialize in evaluating and treating physical impairments, promoting mobility, and maximizing physical function. They design exercise programs, prescribe assistive devices, and provide strategies to improve gait, balance, and overall physical abilities.

(b) Coordination and Collaboration:

- Regular Team Meetings: The multidisciplinary team holds regular team meetings to discuss individual cases, review progress, and develop coordinated care plans. These meetings allow for effective communication, sharing of expertise, and optimization of the care plan.
- Care Plan Development: The team collaboratively develops an individualized care plan tailored to the specific needs of the individual with an encephaloclastic disorder. The care plan integrates various interventions, therapies, and medical treatments to address the physical, cognitive, and psychological aspects of the condition.

(c) Continuity of Care:

- Long-Term Monitoring and Follow-up: The multidisciplinary team provides ongoing monitoring, follow-up, and adjustments to the care plan as needed to address changes in the condition or evolving needs of the individual.
- Transitioning of Care: The team ensures a smooth transition of care across different stages of the encephaloclastic disorder, such as transitioning from acute hospital care to rehabilitation services or from pediatric to adult care.

Multidisciplinary care in encephaloclastic disorders is essential to provide comprehensive and well-coordinated care, optimize functional outcomes, and improve the overall quality of life for individuals affected by these conditions.

18.11 Prognosis and Outcomes

The prognosis of encephaloclastic disorders, which encompass a range of neurological conditions, can vary widely depending on the underlying cause, disease severity, individual factors, and available treatment options. It is important to note that each encephaloclastic disorder has its own unique prognosis. The prognosis of encephaloclastic disorders depend on the following factors:

1. Underlying Cause and Disease Progression: The prognosis of encephaloclastic disorders is influenced by the underlying cause. Some disorders, such as traumatic brain injury, stroke, or autoimmune encephalitis, may have a more acute onset with potential for recovery and improved outcomes if appropriate interventions are initiated promptly. On the other hand, progressive neurodegenerative disorders like Alzheimer's disease, Huntington's disease, or amyotrophic lateral sclerosis (ALS) generally have a more gradual and irreversible decline in function.
2. Disease Severity: The severity of the encephaloclastic disorder at the time of diagnosis or presentation can affect the prognosis. Severe cases may have more significant impairments, reduced functional abilities, and a poorer outlook. However, it is essential to consider that each individual's response to treatment and disease progression can still vary within a given severity category.
3. Treatment and Management: The availability and effectiveness of treatments can have a significant impact on prognosis. Certain encephaloclastic disorders, such as autoimmune encephalitis, may respond well to immunotherapy, leading to symptom improvement and disease stabilization. In contrast, neurodegenerative disorders typically lack curative treatments, and management often aims to slow disease progression, alleviate symptoms, and improve quality of life.
4. Age and Individual Factors: Age at onset and overall health status can influence prognosis. Younger individuals may have better adaptive capacities and response to treatment, while older individuals might experience more challenges in managing functional impairments alongside age-related changes. Other individual factors, such as genetic factors, comorbidities, lifestyle, and social support, can also impact prognosis.
5. Variability in Prognosis: It is crucial to recognize that the prognosis can vary even within a specific encephaloclastic disorder. Factors such as the specific type or subtype of the disorder, disease progression patterns, and individual variations in response may lead to heterogeneity in outcomes

18.12 Future Directions and Research

Encephaloclastic disorders encompass a wide range of neurological conditions that continue to be an active area of research. Ongoing studies and future directions are aimed at advancing our understanding of disease mechanisms, improving diagnostic methods, developing novel treatments, and enhancing patient care. There are some general areas of focus and emerging research directions in the field of encephaloclastic disorders,

1. Biomarkers and Imaging Techniques: Future advancements in biomarkers and imaging techniques hold significant promise for the diagnosis, monitoring, and treatment evaluation of encephaloclastic disorders. Researchers are constantly exploring new approaches to improve the accuracy, sensitivity, and specificity of these diagnostic and prognostic tools. There are some key areas of focus and emerging research in biomarkers and imaging techniques for encephaloclastic disorders including:

   (a) Genetic Biomarkers:

      • Genetic Profiling: Advances in genomics and high-throughput sequencing technologies are enabling comprehensive genetic profiling in encephaloclastic disorders. Researchers are identifying and validating genetic variants associated with specific disorders, allowing for more accurate diagnosis and prognosis. Whole-exome sequencing and genome-wide association studies have yielded important insights into the genetic architecture of these disorders
      • Biomarkers of Disease Progression: Researchers are exploring genetic markers associated with disease progression and severity. This includes identifying genetic factors that modulate the rate of neurodegeneration or predict the onset of clinical symptoms. These markers have the potential to inform prognosis and guide personalized management strategies

   (b) Fluid-based Biomarkers:

      • Cerebrospinal Fluid Biomarkers: Researchers are investigating specific biomarkers in cerebrospinal fluid (CSF) that can aid in the diagnosis and monitoring of encephaloclastic disorders. For example, in Alzheimer's disease, amyloid beta and tau protein levels in CSF have been studied as potential biomarkers of pathology and disease progression [1]. Similar efforts are underway to identify CSF biomarkers for other neurodegenerative disorders.
      • Blood-based Biomarkers: The development of blood-based biomarkers is an active area of research. Researchers are examining blood-based markers that can provide insights into disease pathology, track disease progression, and potentially be used for early detection or therapeutic monitoring. These blood-based biomarkers may include protein levels, microRNA profiles, or other molecular signatures associated with specific encephaloclastic disorders

   (c) Neuroimaging Techniques:

      • Advanced Magnetic Resonance Imaging (MRI): Novel MRI techniques, such as functional MRI (fMRI), diffusion tensor imaging (DTI), and magnetic resonance spectroscopy (MRS), can provide valuable information about brain structure, connectivity, and metabolic changes in encephaloclastic disorders. These techniques enable the detection of subtle alterations in brain structure and function, aiding in early diagnosis and monitoring of disease progression.

- Positron Emission Tomography (PET): PET imaging allows for the visualization and quantification of specific molecular processes in the brain, such as amyloid deposition or neurotransmitter activity. Radioligands specific to certain encephaloclastic disorders can provide valuable information for diagnosis, disease staging, and evaluating treatment response.
- Molecular Imaging: Advancements in molecular imaging techniques, including optical imaging and molecular MRI, enable the visualization and quantification of specific biochemical processes, protein aggregates, or inflammation markers in the brain. These techniques may contribute to a better understanding of disease mechanisms and facilitate the development of targeted therapies

(d) Artificial Intelligence (AI) and Machine Learning: The integration of AI and machine learning techniques in biomarker analysis and imaging interpretation has the potential to enhance diagnostic accuracy, predict disease progression, and optimize treatment stratification. AI algorithms can be trained to detect subtle imaging patterns, identify biomarker profiles, and develop predictive models for patient outcomes

2. Precision Medicine and Personalized Therapeutics: Future advancements in precision medicine and personalized therapeutics hold significant promise for improving outcomes in encephaloclastic disorders. Precision medicine aims to tailor medical interventions to an individual's unique genetic, molecular, and clinical profile, enabling more targeted and effective treatments. There are some key areas of focus and emerging research in the field of precision medicine for encephaloclastic disorders including:

(a) Genetic Profiling and Stratification:

- Genomic Sequencing: Advances in genomics, including whole-exome sequencing and whole-genome sequencing, allow for comprehensive genetic profiling in encephaloclastic disorders. Researchers are identifying specific genetic variants associated with different conditions, enabling more accurate diagnosis and prognosis. Genetic information can guide treatment decisions, facilitate informed genetic counseling, and inform family screening efforts.
- Phenotype-Genotype Correlations: Researchers are working to establish stronger correlations between genetic mutations and specific clinical phenotypes in encephaloclastic disorders. This information helps refine subtyping of disorders, predict disease progression, and personalize treatment approaches.

- Pharmacogenomics: Pharmacogenomics investigates how an individual's genetic makeup affects their response to medications. In encephaloclastic disorders, identifying genetic biomarkers that influence drug metabolism, drug efficacy, or drug toxicity can guide personalized treatment selection and dosing.

(b) Targeted Therapies:

- Disease-Modifying Treatments: Precision medicine aims to develop and optimize disease-modifying treatments specific to different encephaloclastic disorders. Researchers are investigating novel therapeutic targets based on genetic and molecular abnormalities associated with these disorders. Examples include gene therapies, RNA-based therapies, and targeted small molecule drugs designed to interfere with specific disease mechanisms.
- Immunotherapies: Improved understanding of autoimmune mechanisms in encephaloclastic disorders enables the development of personalized immunotherapies. These treatments aim to restore immune tolerance, suppress aberrant immune responses, or target specific autoantibodies involved in autoimmune encephalitis
- Repurposing Existing Medications: Precision medicine approaches involve identifying existing medications that may have therapeutic benefits in specific encephaloclastic disorders. By leveraging knowledge of disease mechanisms and genetic profiles, researchers can explore new uses for approved drugs and improve treatment options.

(c) Non-pharmacological Interventions:

- Lifestyle and Environmental Interventions: Precision medicine recognizes the importance of environmental and lifestyle factors in treatment and disease management. Researchers are investigating how personalized interventions, such as exercise regimens, dietary modifications, stress reduction techniques, and cognitive training, can complement pharmacological treatments and support overall well-being in encephaloclastic disorders.
- Patient-Centered and Supportive Care: Precision medicine also emphasizes patient-centered approaches to care. This includes addressing individual preferences, values, and goals of care when tailoring treatment plans. Supportive care measures, including psychological support, educational resources, and access to support groups, are integral components of personalized care

3. Disease Modification and Neuroprotective Strategies: Future advancements in disease modification and neuroprotective strategies hold great potential for improving outcomes in encephaloclastic disorders. These strategies aim to slow the progression of disease, protect neurons from damage, and promote neuronal

survival. There are key areas of focus and emerging research in the field of disease modification and neuroprotection for encephaloclastic disorders including.

(a) Pathogenesis and Disease Mechanisms:

- Improved Understanding: Ongoing research seeks to enhance our understanding of the underlying disease mechanisms and pathogenesis of encephaloclastic disorders. This includes investigating genetic factors, protein misfolding, immune dysregulation, oxidative stress, and inflammation pathways specific to each disorder.
- Biomarker Development: The identification and validation of reliable biomarkers associated with disease progression, such as genetic markers, neuroimaging markers, or fluid-based biomarkers, can aid in monitoring disease course, assessing therapeutic response, and selecting appropriate intervention strategies.

(b) Gene Therapies:

- Gene Replacement Therapy: Researchers are investigating the use of gene therapy approaches to deliver functional copies of mutated genes in monogenic encephaloclastic disorders. This strategy aims to correct the genetic defect and restore normal protein function.
- Gene Silencing: Techniques such as antisense oligonucleotides, small interfering RNA (siRNA), or clustered regularly interspaced short palindromic repeats (CRISPR) hold promise for selectively silencing or modifying disease-related genes, thereby reducing the production of toxic proteins or restoring normal gene expression.

(c) Neuroprotective Strategies:

- Anti-inflammatory Approaches: In inflammatory encephaloclastic disorders, modulating the immune response and reducing neuroinflammation are important therapeutic targets. Researchers are investigating anti-inflammatory agents, immunomodulatory drugs, and strategies to promote immune tolerance for neuroprotection
- Oxidative Stress Mitigation: Targeting oxidative stress pathways may help protect neurons from damage. Antioxidant therapies, such as small molecules or natural compounds, are being explored as potential neuroprotective interventions.
- Protein Misfolding and Aggregation Inhibition: Strategies aimed at preventing or reducing the accumulation and aggregation of misfolded proteins associated with various encephaloclastic disorders, such as Alzheimer's disease or prion diseases, are being explored. This includes the development of small molecules, peptides, or antibodies that can inhibit protein misfolding and aggregintervent.

(d) Combination Therapies:

- Synergistic Approaches: Researchers are investigating the potential benefits of combining different therapeutic modalities and drug classes to target multiple pathological processes simultaneously. Combination therapies may include pharmacological agents, gene-based therapies, drug repurposing, or immunomodulation approaches.

- Personalized Treatment Strategies: Precision medicine approaches aim to tailor treatment strategies to an individual's unique genetic, molecular, and clinical profile. Personalized combinations of therapies can be designed based on disease subtype, genetic factors, stage of disease, and specific pathogenic mechanisms

4. Development of Innovative Therapies: The future development of innovative therapies in encephaloclastic disorders holds great promise for improving treatment outcomes. Researchers are exploring novel approaches, technologies, and interventions to target the underlying disease mechanisms and provide effective therapies. There are key areas of focus and emerging research in the field of innovative therapies for encephaloclastic disorders including:

(a) Gene Therapies:

- Gene Editing: Gene editing technologies, such as CRISPR-Cas9, hold promise for precise modifications of disease-causing genetic mutations. Researchers are exploring the use of gene editing tools to correct or modify mutant genes associated with various encephaloclastic disorders.
- RNA-based Therapies: RNA-based therapies, including antisense oligonucleotide (ASO) approaches or RNA interference (RNAi) strategies, are being investigated to target disease-related genes, reduce the production of toxic proteins, or modulate gene expression

(b) Cell-based Therapies: this including stem cell-based therapies, Researchers are exploring the use of stem cells, such as induced pluripotent stem cells (iPSCs) or neural stem cells, for cell replacement or regeneration in encephaloclastic disorders. These therapies aim to replace damaged or lost cells, promote tissue repair, and enhance functional recovery

(c) Small Molecule Drug Development:

- Targeted Therapies: Small molecules that selectively target specific disease pathways or abnormal protein aggregates associated with encephaloclastic disorders are being investigated. These targeted therapies aim to modulate disease progression, reduce toxic protein accumulation, or enhance neuronal resilience.
- Drug Repurposing: Researchers are exploring the potential of repurposing existing medications approved for other indications to treat encephaloclastic disorders. This approach allows for faster translation into clinical use and leverages knowledge about safety and tolerability profiles of already approved drugs

(d) Emerging Technologies:

- Nanomedicine: Nanotechnology offers promising potential in delivering therapeutics across the blood-brain barrier and targeting specific brain regions. Researchers are exploring nano-enabled drug delivery systems, such as nanoparticles or liposomes, to enhance the efficacy and precision of therapeutic interventions in encephaloclastic disorders.

- Optogenetics and Neuromodulation: Optogenetics involves using light-sensitive proteins to selectively control and modulate neuronal activity. Researchers are exploring the potential of optogenetics and neuromodulation techniques to restore neural circuitry function and improve symptoms in encephaloclastic disorders.

(e) Combination Therapies or Synergistic Approaches: Researchers recognize the potential benefits of combining multiple therapeutic modalities, such as gene therapies, small molecules, or cell-based interventions. Combination therapies tailored to specific disease mechanisms offer the potential for enhanced efficacy and comprehensive.

5. Understanding Disease Mechanisms and Pathways: Understanding the underlying disease mechanisms and pathways is crucial for the development of effective diagnostic tools and targeted therapeutic interventions. In recent years, significant progress has been made in unraveling the complexity of encephaloclastic disorders, thanks to advancements in various fields such as genetics, neuroimaging, and molecular biology.

(a) Genetic Studies: Genetic studies have contributed extensively to our understanding of encephaloclastic disorders. Many disorders have a genetic basis, and identifying causative genetic mutations can provide valuable insights into disease mechanisms. Whole-exome sequencing and genome-wide association studies (GWAS) have been instrumental in identifying genetic variants associated with encephaloclastic disorders. These studies have highlighted genes involved in key biological pathways, such as neuroinflammation, apoptosis, synaptic plasticity, and energy metabolism.

(b) Animal Models: Animal models, especially transgenic and knockout mice, have played a vital role in studying disease mechanisms in encephaloclastic disorders. By selectively manipulating specific genes associated with the disorders, researchers can gain a better understanding of the underlying molecular pathways and observe phenotypic changes. Animal models also enable the testing of potential therapeutic interventions.

(c) Neuroimaging Techniques: Advancements in neuroimaging techniques, such as magnetic resonance imaging (MRI), functional MRI (fMRI), positron emission tomography (PET), and diffusion tensor imaging (DTI), have revolutionized our ability to study encephaloclastic disorders non-invasively. These imaging tools can help visualize structural and functional abnormalities in the brain, facilitating the identification of affected brain regions and pathways. Additionally, neuroimaging can aid in monitoring disease progression and treatment response.

(d) Molecular and Cellular Studies: Studying the molecular and cellular mechanisms underlying encephaloclastic disorders can provide valuable insights into disease pathogenesis. Techniques like immunohistochemistry, transcriptomics, proteomics, and metabolomics have been used to analyze brain tissue samples from affected individuals. These studies have revealed dysregulation in various cellular processes, including inflammation, oxidative stress, mitochondrial dysfunction, and excitotoxicity.

(e) Pathway Analysis: Pathway analysis techniques, such as gene set enrichment analysis (GSEA) and network analysis, have proven useful in identifying key pathways and biological processes affected in encephaloclastic disorders. By integrating data from various omics studies, researchers can decipher the interconnectedness of genes, proteins, and metabolites involved in disease pathogenesis. This approach helps uncover the underlying molecular mechanisms and potential therapeutic targets

Multiple Choice Questions

1. **Which of the following is a genetic factor associated with encephaloclastic disorders?**

   (A) Inflammatory processes
   (B) Excitotoxicity
   (C) Metabolic abnormalities
   (D) Genetic mutations

2. **Which of the following is a characteristic feature of encephaloclastic disorders?**

   (A) Excessive production of cerebrospinal fluid
   (B) Progressive degeneration of brain tissue
   (C) Impaired blood flow to the brain
   (D) Deficiency of myelin sheath in nerve fibers

3. **Which of the following is NOT considered an encephaloclastic disorder?**

   (A) Alzheimer's disease
   (B) Huntington's disease
   (C) Cerebral palsy
   (D) Traumatic brain injury

4. **Which of the following is a characteristic feature of encephaloclastic disorders?**

   (A) Rapidly progressive cognitive decline
   (B) Seizures as the predominant symptom
   (C) Inflammation of the brain tissue
   (D) Preservation of brain volume

5. **Which of the following is a genetic encephaloclastic disorder characterized by the expansion of CAG trinucleotide repeats?**

   (A) Alzheimer's disease
   (B) Huntington's disease
   (C) Multiple sclerosis
   (D) Parkinson's disease

6. **A 45-year-old male presents with progressive cognitive decline, personality changes, and choreiform movements. On examination, he exhibits involuntary jerky movements and impaired coordination. His father had a similar presentation in his 40 s. Genetic testing reveals an expansion of CAG trinucleotide repeats. Which of the following is the most likely diagnosis?**

   (A) Alzheimer's disease
   (B) Huntington's disease
   (C) Multiple sclerosis
   (D) Parkinson's disease

7. **Which of the following conditions is characterized by the destruction or degeneration of brain tissue?**

   (A) Encephalitis
   (B) Epilepsy
   (C) Encephalomalacia
   (D) Encephalopathy

8. **A 45-year-old female presents with progressive memory loss, personality changes, and difficulties with coordination and balance. Neurological examination reveals ataxia and dysarthria. MRI scan shows multiple bilateral areas of cavitation in the cerebral hemispheres. Which of the following is the most likely diagnosis?**

   (A) Alzheimer's disease
   (B) Multiple sclerosis
   (C) Encephaloclastic leukoencephalopathy
   (D) Creutzfeldt-Jakob disease

9. **A 65-year-old male presents with sudden weakness on the right side of his body, slurred speech, and confusion. He has a history of hypertension and diabetes. CT scan reveals a large area of necrotic brain tissue with surrounding edema. Which of the following is the most likely diagnosis?**

   (A) Encephalitis
   (B) Epilepsy
   (C) Encephalomalacia
   (D) Encephalopathy

10. **Which of the following investigations is commonly used in the diagnosis of encephaloclastic disorders?**

    (A) Electrocardiogram (ECG)
    (B) Magnetic Resonance Imaging (MRI)
    (C) Complete Blood Count (CBC)
    (D) Liver Function Test (LFT)

11. **A 50-year-old male presents to the emergency department with sudden onset confusion, severe headache, and weakness on the right side of his body. On examination, he has right-sided facial droop and hemiparesis. The patient's medical history is significant for poorly controlled hypertension. A computed tomography (CT) scan of the head is performed, which reveals an area of hypodensity in the left frontal lobe. Which of the following is the most likely diagnosis?**

    (A) Ischemic stroke
    (B) Encephalitis
    (C) Traumatic brain injury
    (D) Encephaloclastic disorder

12. **A 45-year-old male is diagnosed with an encephaloclastic disorder. Which of the following factors is the most significant predictor of prognosis in this patient?**

    (A) Age at onset
    (B) Duration of symptoms
    (C) Specific etiology
    (D) Treatment response

13. **Which of the following factors is most commonly associated with the development of encephaloclastic disorders?**

    (A) Genetic predisposition
    (B) Environmental toxins
    (C) Infectious diseases
    (D) Traumatic brain injury.

14. **Which of the following treatment modalities is commonly used in the management of encephaloclastic disorders?**

    (A) Antiviral medications
    (B) Surgery
    (C) Chemotherapy
    (D) Physical therapy

15. **A 35-year-old female presents with a sudden onset of seizures, confusion, and severe headache. Physical examination reveals neck stiffness and fever. Lumbar puncture is performed, and cerebrospinal fluid analysis shows increased white blood cells and elevated protein levels. Which diagnostic test would be most helpful in confirming the diagnosis of encephaloclastic disorder in this patient?**

    (A) Electroencephalography (EEG)
    (B) Magnetic Resonance Imaging (MRI)
    (C) Polymerase Chain Reaction (PCR)
    (D) Brain Biopsy

16. **A 50-year-old male presents with progressive cognitive decline, personality changes, and difficulty with movement coordination. On physical examination, the patient exhibits rigidity and bradykinesia. MRI of the brain reveals bilateral symmetric atrophy of the caudate nucleus. Which of the following conditions is most likely responsible for these findings?**

    (A) Alzheimer's disease
    (B) Huntington's disease
    (C) Parkinson's disease
    (D) Multiple sclerosis

17. **A 60-year-old male presents with progressive memory loss, personality changes, and difficulty with language. Neurological examination reveals bilateral frontal lobe dysfunction. Neuroimaging shows significant atrophy in the frontal and temporal lobes. What is the most likely classification of this encephaloclastic disorder?**

    (A) Cortical degeneration
    (B) Subcortical degeneration
    (C) Multifocal encephalopathy
    (D) Global encephalopathy

18. **Which of the following classifications is most likely for an encephaloclastic disorder characterized by sudden-onset focal neurological deficits and neuroimaging findings of a well-defined, circumscribed area of brain tissue necrosis?**

    (A) Ischemic infarction
    (B) Traumatic brain injury
    (C) Infectious encephalitis
    (D) Neoplastic infiltration

19. **Which of the following treatment approaches is most commonly used for managing encephaloclastic disorders associated with brain tissue necrosis?**

    (A) Surgical resection
    (B) Antibiotic therapy

(C) Radiation therapy
(D) Supportive care

20. **What is the approximate prevalence of encephaloclastic disorders worldwide?**

(A) 1 in 1000 individuals
(B) 1 in 10,000 individuals
(C) 1 in 100,000 individuals
(D) 1 in 1000,000 individuals

21. **A 45-year-old male presents to the emergency department with sudden onset of severe headache, confusion, and left-sided weakness. He has a history of hypertension and diabetes. On examination, he has a decreased level of consciousness, left-sided facial droop, and weakness in the left upper and lower limbs. The patient's symptoms developed rapidly over the past few hours. Neuroimaging reveals an area of infarction in the right middle cerebral artery territory. What is the most likely clinical manifestation of this patient's encephaloclastic disorder?**

(A) Hemiparesis
(B) Ataxia
(C) Visual disturbances
(D) Memory loss

22. **A 65-year-old female is admitted to the hospital with a sudden onset of right-sided weakness and difficulty speaking. She has a past medical history of atrial fibrillation and hypertension. Imaging studies reveal an acute ischemic stroke involving the left middle cerebral artery territory. The patient receives timely treatment with thrombolytic therapy. What is the most significant factor influencing the prognosis of this patient's encephaloclastic disorder?**

(A) Age of the patient
(B) Past medical history
(C) Timeliness of treatment
(D) Severity of neurological deficits

23. **A 25-year-old female presents with progressive muscle weakness, difficulty walking, and frequent falls. On examination, she has bilateral lower limb weakness and increased deep tendon reflexes. The neurologist suspects a possible encephaloclastic disorder. To further evaluate the patient, which electrophysiological test would be most appropriate?**

(A) Nerve Conduction Studies (NCS)
(B) Electromyography (EMG)
(C) Electroencephalogram (EEG)
(D) Visual Evoked Potential (VEP)

24. **A 40-year-old male presents with a sudden onset of confusion, seizures, and altered consciousness. The neurologist suspects a possible encephaloclastic disorder. Which blood test would be most useful in the initial evaluation of this patient?**

    (A) Complete Blood Count (CBC)
    (B) Liver Function Tests (LFTs)
    (C) Creatine Kinase (CK) levels
    (D) Genetic TTestin

25. **Encephaloclastic disorders are a group of neurological conditions characterized by the destruction of brain tissue. Which of the following statements regarding the epidemiology of encephaloclastic disorders is most accurate?**

    (A) Encephaloclastic disorders are more common in children than in adults.
    (B) Encephaloclastic disorders have a higher prevalence in males than in females.
    (C) Genetic factors play a minimal role in the development of encephaloclastic disorders.
    (D) Encephaloclastic disorders are primarily caused by infectious agents.

26. **A 45-year-old female presents with a sudden onset of severe headache, nausea, and vomiting. On examination, she has a decreased level of consciousness and exhibits signs of focal neurological deficits, including right-sided weakness and speech difficulties. Imaging studies reveal a large area of brain tissue destruction in the left frontal lobe. Which of the following clinical manifestations is most likely associated with this condition?**

    (A) Visual disturbances
    (B) Memory loss and confusion
    (C) Hemiparesis and aphasia
    (D) Sleep disturbances and excessive daytime sleepiness

27. **A 65-year-old male presents with progressive cognitive decline, memory loss, and behavioral changes over the past year. Imaging studies reveal bilateral atrophy and significant loss of brain tissue in the temporal lobes. Which of the following treatment options is most appropriate for managing this patient's condition?**

    (A) Antipsychotic medications
    (B) Antibiotics
    (C) Surgical resection of the affected brain tissue
    (D) Symptomatic management and supportive care

28. **Which of the following represents a potential future direction for the management of encephaloclastic disorders?**

    (A) Stem cell therapy

   (B) Psychotherapy
   (C) Nonsteroidal anti-inflammatory drugs (NSAIDs)
   (D) Physical therapy interventions

29. **John, a 55-year-old man, has recently been diagnosed with an encephaloclastic disorder characterized by the progressive loss of brain tissue. He experiences difficulties with movement, coordination, and speech. John's neurologist discusses potential future directions for the management of his condition. Based on John's case, which of the following potential future directions holds promise for managing his encephaloclastic disorder?**

   (A) Deep brain stimulation
   (B) Herbal supplements
   (C) Meditation and mindfulness techniques
   (D) Physical therapy

Answers

1. In this question, we are specifically asking about the genetic factors associated with encephaloclastic disorders. **The correct answer is (D) Genetic mutations.** Many encephaloclastic disorders have a genetic basis, and identifying the specific genes and mutations involved is an important area of research. Mutations in certain genes have been found to contribute to the development and progression of these disorders.

   Option (A) Inflammatory processes: While inflammation and immune dysregulation can play a role in encephaloclastic disorders, it is not a genetic factor.

   Option (B) Excitotoxicity: Excitotoxicity refers to excessive activation of glutamate receptors leading to neuronal damage and is not a genetic factor.

   Option (C) Metabolic abnormalities: Metabolic disturbances, such as mitochondrial dysfunction, can contribute to encephaloclastic disorders. However, metabolic abnormalities are not specifically genetic factors.

2. Option (A) Excessive production of cerebrospinal fluid: Excessive production of cerebrospinal fluid is not a characteristic feature of encephaloclastic disorders. It may be seen in conditions like hydrocephalus, which involve abnormal accumulation of cerebrospinal fluid in the brain.

   Option (B) Progressive degeneration of brain tissue: This is the characteristic feature of encephaloclastic disorders. These conditions involve the progressive degeneration or destruction of brain tissue, leading to neurological symptoms and impairment.

   Option (C) Impaired blood flow to the brain: Impaired blood flow to the brain is not a specific characteristic of encephaloclastic disorders. It can be seen in conditions like ischemic stroke or vascular dementia.

   Option (D) Deficiency of myelin sheath in nerve fibers: The deficiency of myelin sheath in nerve fibers is not a characteristic feature of encephaloclastic disorders. It is typically associated with demyelinating disorders such as multiple sclerosis.

   the correct answer is (B) Progressive degeneration of brain tissue.

3. Option (A) Alzheimer's disease: Alzheimer's disease is a neurodegenerative disorder characterized by the progressive degeneration of brain tissue, particularly in areas responsible for memory and cognitive function. Therefore, Alzheimer's disease is considered an encephaloclastic disorder.

   Option (B) Huntington's disease: Huntington's disease is an inherited neurodegenerative disorder that leads to the progressive degeneration of brain cells, primarily affecting the basal ganglia. Like Alzheimer's disease, Huntington's disease is considered an encephaloclastic disorder.

   Option (C) Cerebral palsy: Cerebral palsy is a group of disorders that affect movement, muscle tone, and posture. It is caused by damage to the developing brain, often before or during birth. However, cerebral palsy is not primarily characterized by the destruction or degeneration of brain tissue. Therefore, cerebral palsy is NOT considered an encephaloclastic disorder.

   Option (D) Traumatic brain injury: Traumatic brain injury refers to brain damage caused by an external force or trauma. Depending on the severity, it can lead to the destruction of brain tissue. Therefore, traumatic brain injury is considered an encephaloclastic disorder.

   Based on the discussion above, the correct answer is (C) Cerebral palsy.

4. Option (A) Rapidly progressive cognitive decline: Rapidly progressive cognitive decline is a common feature in various encephaloclastic disorders, such as Alzheimer's disease and certain types of dementia. The destruction of brain tissue leads to cognitive impairment and decline.

   Option (B) Seizures as the predominant symptom: Seizures can occur in some encephaloclastic disorders, but they are not necessarily the predominant symptom. Seizures can be seen in conditions like epilepsy, which may or may not involve encephaloclastic changes.

   Option (C) Inflammation of the brain tissue: Inflammation of the brain tissue is not a characteristic feature of encephaloclastic disorders. In some other neurological conditions, such as encephalitis or autoimmune disorders, inflammation of the brain tissue may be present.

   Option (D) Preservation of brain volume: Encephaloclastic disorders involve the destruction or degeneration of brain tissue, which leads to a reduction in brain volume. Therefore, preservation of brain volume is not a characteristic feature of encephaloclastic disorders.

   Based on the discussion above, **the correct answer is (D) Preservation of brain volume.**

5. Option (A) Alzheimer's disease: Alzheimer's disease is not characterized by the expansion of CAG trinucleotide repeats. It is a neurodegenerative disorder associated with the accumulation of beta-amyloid plaques and neurofibrillary tangles in the brain.

   Option (B) Huntington's disease: Huntington's disease is the correct answer. It is a genetic encephaloclastic disorder caused by the expansion of CAG trinucleotide repeats in the huntingtin gene. This expansion leads to the production of a mutant huntingtin protein, which causes progressive degeneration of neurons in the brain.

Option (C) Multiple sclerosis: Multiple sclerosis is not characterized by the expansion of CAG trinucleotide repeats. It is an autoimmune disorder where the immune system mistakenly attacks the protective covering of nerve fibers, leading to communication problems between the brain and the rest of the body.

Option (D) Parkinson's disease: Parkinson's disease is not characterized by the expansion of CAG trinucleotide repeats. It is a neurodegenerative disorder associated with the loss of dopamine-producing cells in a region of the brain called the substantia nigra.

Based on the discussion above, **the correct answer is (B) Huntington's disease.**

6. The key findings in this case scenario are progressive cognitive decline, personality changes, choreiform movements, and a positive family history. These features are highly suggestive of a specific encephaloclastic disorder.

   Option (A) Alzheimer's disease: Although Alzheimer's disease can present with progressive cognitive decline, it does not typically manifest with choreiform movements or a positive family history of similar symptoms.

   Option (B) Huntington's disease: Huntington's disease is the correct answer. The clinical manifestations described in the case scenario align with Huntington's disease, including progressive cognitive decline, personality changes, and choreiform movements. The positive family history further supports the diagnosis. Huntington's disease is caused by the expansion of CAG trinucleotide repeats in the huntingtin (HTT) gene.

   Option (C) Multiple sclerosis: Multiple sclerosis does not typically present with choreiform movements or a positive family history of similar symptoms. It is characterized by demyelination of nerve fibers, leading to various neurological symptoms.

   Option (D) Parkinson's disease: Parkinson's disease is characterized by motor symptoms such as tremors, bradykinesia (slowness of movement), and rigidity. It does not typically present with choreiform movements or a positive family history of similar symptoms.

   Based on the information provided, **the most likely diagnosis in this case is (B) Huntington's disease.**

7. Encephalitis (A) refers to inflammation of the brain, usually caused by viral or bacterial infections. It can result in various symptoms, including fever, headache, confusion, and seizures.

   Epilepsy (B) is a neurological disorder characterized by recurrent seizures. It can have various causes, including genetic factors, brain injury, infections, or developmental disorders. However, it does not specifically involve the destruction or degeneration of brain tissue.

   Encephalopathy (D) is a broad term that refers to any brain disorder or disease. It can be caused by various factors, such as metabolic imbalances, toxic substances, infections, or genetic disorders. Encephalopathy may or may not involve tissue destruction, as it encompasses a wide range of conditions affecting brain function.

   The correct answer is (C) Encephalomalacia.

8. Based on the given case scenario, the patient's progressive memory loss, personality changes, ataxia, dysarthria, and the MRI findings of multiple bilateral areas of cavitation in the cerebral hemispheres, the most likely diagnosis is encephaloclastic leukoencephalopathy.

   Alzheimer's disease (A) is a neurodegenerative disorder characterized by progressive memory loss, cognitive decline, and behavioral changes. However, the MRI findings of multiple bilateral areas of cavitation seen in the case scenario are not typical of Alzheimer's disease.

   Multiple sclerosis (B) is an autoimmune disorder that affects the central nervous system, leading to demyelination and the formation of plaques. While multiple sclerosis can cause neurological symptoms, the MRI findings of cavitation seen in this case are not consistent with the characteristic plaques seen in multiple sclerosis.

   Creutzfeldt-Jakob disease (D) is a rare, degenerative brain disorder caused by abnormal prion proteins. It presents with rapidly progressive dementia, motor abnormalities, and characteristic EEG findings. While Creutzfeldt-Jakob disease can cause neurological symptoms, the MRI findings of multiple bilateral areas of cavitation seen in the case scenario are not typical of this condition.

   Encephaloclastic leukoencephalopathy (C) refers to a condition characterized by the destruction and loss of brain tissue, particularly the white matter, leading to cavitation. The clinical presentation of progressive memory loss, personality changes, ataxia, dysarthria, and the MRI findings of multiple bilateral areas of cavitation seen in the case scenario are consistent with encephaloclastic leukoencephalopathy.

   The correct answer is (C) Encephaloclastic leukoencephalopathy.

9. Based on the given case scenario, the patient's sudden weakness on the right side of the body, slurred speech, and confusion, along with the imaging findings of a large area of necrotic brain tissue with surrounding edema on CT scan, suggest encephalomalacia.

   Encephalitis (A) is characterized by inflammation of the brain, often due to viral or bacterial infections. While encephalitis can cause neurological symptoms, the presence of necrotic brain tissue and edema seen on the CT scan is more indicative of encephalomalacia.

   Epilepsy (B) refers to a neurological disorder characterized by recurrent seizures. While seizures can result from brain abnormalities, encephalomalacia specifically refers to the degeneration or softening of brain tissue, as seen in the CT scan findings of necrotic tissue.

   Encephalopathy (D) is a broad term that encompasses various brain disorders, including those resulting from metabolic imbalances, toxic substances, infections, or genetic disorders. While encephalopathy can present with a range of symptoms, the CT scan findings in this case are more consistent with encephalomalacia.

   The correct answer is C) Encephalomalacia.

10. Electrocardiogram (ECG): An electrocardiogram is a test used to record the electrical activity of the heart. While it can be helpful in diagnosing heart-related conditions, it is not directly related to the diagnosis of encephaloclastic disorders. Therefore, ECG is not commonly used in the diagnosis of encephaloclastic disorders.

    Magnetic Resonance Imaging (MRI): Magnetic Resonance Imaging is a diagnostic imaging technique that uses powerful magnets and radio waves to create detailed images of the inside of the body. It is commonly used in the evaluation of brain structure and function, making it an essential investigation for diagnosing encephaloclastic disorders. MRI can help identify areas of brain tissue loss or damage, providing valuable information for diagnosis and treatment planning.

    Complete Blood Count (CBC): A complete blood count is a blood test that provides information about the different components of blood, such as red blood cells, white blood cells, and platelets. While a CBC can help assess general health and detect certain medical conditions, it is not specifically used for diagnosing encephaloclastic disorders. Therefore, CBC is not commonly used in the diagnosis of these disorders.

    Liver Function Test (LFT): Liver function tests are blood tests that assess the liver's health and functionality. These tests measure various liver enzymes and other substances in the blood. LFTs are not directly related to the diagnosis of encephaloclastic disorders and are typically used to evaluate liver diseases. Therefore, LFT is not commonly used in the diagnosis of encephaloclastic disorders.

    The correct Answer: (B) Magnetic Resonance Imaging (MRI).

11. In this case scenario, the patient presents with sudden onset confusion, severe headache, and weakness on the right side of the body, along with right-sided facial droop and hemiparesis. The CT scan of the head reveals an area of hypodensity in the left frontal lobe. Let's discuss each option to determine the most likely diagnosis.

    (A) Ischemic stroke: Ischemic stroke occurs when there is a blockage or narrowing of blood vessels supplying the brain, leading to a lack of blood flow and oxygen to a specific area. While ischemic strokes can present with similar symptoms as described in the case scenario, the presence of an area of hypodensity on the CT scan suggests tissue loss rather than an acute ischemic event. Therefore, ischemic stroke is less likely in this scenario.

    (B) Encephalitis: Encephalitis is inflammation of the brain typically caused by viral infections. It can present with symptoms such as confusion and neurological deficits. However, the CT scan findings of an area of hypodensity are not consistent with the inflammatory changes seen in encephalitis. Therefore, encephalitis is less likely in this scenario.

    (C) Traumatic brain injury: Traumatic brain injury (TBI) occurs due to a sudden physical trauma to the head, leading to brain damage. While TBI can cause similar symptoms as described in the case scenario, the absence of a history of head trauma and the CT scan findings of an area of hypodensity do not support a diagnosis of TBI. Therefore, traumatic brain injury is less likely in this scenario.

Encephaloclastic disorder: Encephaloclastic disorders are characterized by the destruction or loss of brain tissue. In this case scenario, the sudden onset of neurological symptoms, presence of facial droop, hemiparesis, and the CT scan findings of an area of hypodensity in the left frontal lobe are suggestive of an encephaloclastic disorder. The most likely diagnosis in this case is an encephaloclastic disorder.

The correct Answer is (D) Encephaloclastic disorder.

12. In this case scenario, the patient presents with progressive cognitive decline, personality changes, and difficulty with coordination. On examination, bilateral hyperreflexia and a positive Babinski sign (upward extension of the big toe) are noted. Let's discuss each investigation option to determine the most helpful one in confirming the diagnosis of an encephaloclastic disorder.

(A) Electroencephalogram (EEG): An EEG is a test that records the electrical activity of the brain. It is useful in evaluating various neurological conditions, including seizure disorders, encephalopathies, and brain tumors. However, in the case of encephaloclastic disorders, an EEG may not provide specific diagnostic information about the underlying pathology. Therefore, while an EEG can aid in evaluating other neurological conditions, it may not be the most helpful investigation for confirming the diagnosis of an encephaloclastic disorder in this patient.

(B) Magnetic resonance imaging (MRI): MRI is a powerful imaging modality that can provide detailed images of the brain. It is particularly useful in detecting structural abnormalities, such as brain lesions, atrophy, or infarcts. In the case of encephaloclastic disorders, an MRI scan can reveal areas of tissue loss or destruction, which are characteristic findings. Therefore, an MRI is the most helpful investigation in confirming the diagnosis of an encephaloclastic disorder in this patient.

(C) Lumbar puncture: Lumbar puncture, also known as a spinal tap, involves the removal of cerebrospinal fluid (CSF) from the spinal canal for analysis. It is typically performed to evaluate conditions affecting the central nervous system, such as infections or inflammation. However, in the case of encephaloclastic disorders, CSF analysis may not provide specific diagnostic information and is not the most helpful investigation in confirming the diagnosis.

(D) Blood tests: Blood tests are commonly performed to evaluate various medical conditions, including infectious or inflammatory processes. While blood tests can help assess general health, rule out certain systemic causes, and identify potential contributing factors, they may not directly confirm the diagnosis of an encephaloclastic disorder. Therefore, blood tests are not the most helpful investigation for confirming the diagnosis in this scenario.

The correct Answer is (B) Magnetic resonance imaging (MRI).

13. When considering the prognosis of an encephaloclastic disorder, several factors can influence the outcome. Let's discuss each option to determine the most significant predictor of prognosis in this patient.

   (A) Age at onset: The age at which symptoms first appear can provide valuable prognostic information. In general, early-onset encephaloclastic disorders tend to have a worse prognosis compared to those with a later onset. This is because younger individuals have a longer disease duration ahead of them, during which progressive neurological decline can occur. Therefore, age at onset is an important factor to consider but may not be the most significant predictor of prognosis.

   (B) Duration of symptoms: The duration of symptoms, or the length of time the patient has experienced neurological abnormalities, can also impact prognosis. In most cases, a longer duration of symptoms is associated with a more advanced disease stage, which often correlates with a worse prognosis. However, while duration of symptoms is relevant, it may not be the most significant predictor of prognosis.

   (C) Specific etiology: The underlying cause or etiology of an encephaloclastic disorder can significantly influence prognosis. Certain etiologies, such as traumatic brain injury, brain tumors, or genetic conditions, may have distinct prognostic implications. For example, if the underlying cause is a treatable condition, the prognosis may be more favorable compared to an irreversible or progressive disorder. Therefore, the specific etiology is an important consideration but may not always be the most significant predictor of prognosis.

   (D) Treatment response: The response to treatment can provide valuable insights into the prognosis of an encephaloclastic disorder. In some cases, specific interventions or therapies may help slow down disease progression, alleviate symptoms, or improve overall functioning. A positive treatment response is generally associated with a better prognosis. Therefore, treatment response is an essential factor to consider, but it may not always be available or predictable at the time of diagnosis.
   The correct Answer is (C) Specific etiology.

14. Let's discuss each option to determine the most common factor associated with the development of these disorders.

   (A) Genetic predisposition: Genetic factors can play a role in the development of certain encephaloclastic disorders. In some cases, inherited genetic mutations or abnormalities can increase an individual's susceptibility to these conditions. However, it is important to note that encephaloclastic disorders generally have a multifactorial etiology, meaning that both genetic and environmental factors contribute to their development. While genetic predisposition can be a contributing factor, it is not the most common association.

(B) Environmental toxins: Exposure to certain environmental toxins is a well-recognized risk factor for the development of encephaloclastic disorders. Toxins such as lead, mercury, pesticides, and industrial chemicals can have neurotoxic effects, leading to brain damage and the subsequent development of these disorders. Environmental toxin exposure is an important consideration and is often one of the most common associations with encephaloclastic disorders.

(C) Infectious diseases: Some infectious diseases can cause encephaloclastic disorders. Viral infections, such as herpes simplex encephalitis or progressive multifocal leukoencephalopathy, can result in the destruction of brain tissue and subsequent neurological dysfunction. Bacterial infections, such as meningitis or brain abscesses, can also lead to encephaloclastic changes. While infectious diseases can be associated with encephaloclastic disorders, they are not the most common factor.

(D) Traumatic brain injury: Traumatic brain injury (TBI) is a significant risk factor for the development of encephaloclastic disorders. When the brain experiences severe trauma, such as a severe blow or penetrating injury, it can lead to tissue damage and subsequent degeneration. TBI can result from various causes, including motor vehicle accidents, falls, sports injuries, or assaults. Traumatic brain injury is one of the most common associations with encephaloclastic disorders.

The correct Answer is (D) Traumatic brain injury.

15. Let's discuss each option to determine the commonly used treatment modality for these disorders.

(A) Antiviral medications: Antiviral medications are primarily used for the treatment of viral infections that may cause encephaloclastic disorders, such as herpes simplex encephalitis or progressive multifocal leukoencephalopathy. These medications target the viral replication process and help to reduce viral load. However, antiviral medications alone may not be sufficient to treat the underlying encephaloclastic changes in the brain. Therefore, while they may be used in the management of encephaloclastic disorders caused by viral infections, they are not the most commonly used treatment modality.

(B) Surgery: In certain cases, surgical interventions may be necessary for the management of encephaloclastic disorders. This typically applies to situations where there is a focal area of brain tissue damage that can be removed or repaired surgically. For example, in cases of brain abscess or certain types of brain tumors that cause encephaloclastic changes, surgery may be performed to remove the source of infection or tumor. However, surgery is not the most commonly used treatment modality for encephaloclastic disorders as a whole.

(C) Chemotherapy: Chemotherapy is primarily used in the treatment of cancer, including brain tumors that may cause encephaloclastic changes. Chemotherapeutic agents aim to target and destroy cancer cells, thereby reducing tumor size and minimizing the associated encephaloclastic damage. However, not all encephaloclastic disorders are related to cancer, and therefore, chemotherapy is not the most commonly used treatment modality for encephaloclastic disorders in general.

(D) Physical therapy: Physical therapy plays an important role in the management of encephaloclastic disorders. It focuses on improving mobility, strength, coordination, and overall functional abilities in individuals with neurological deficits caused by encephaloclastic changes. Physical therapy techniques, exercises, and interventions can help individuals regain or optimize their physical functioning and enhance their quality of life. Physical therapy is often a key component of multidisciplinary treatment approaches for encephaloclastic disorders and is commonly used in their management.

The correct Answer is (D) Physical therapy.

16. Let's analyze the case scenario to determine the most helpful diagnostic test in confirming the diagnosis of an encephaloclastic disorder in this patient.

(A) Electroencephalography (EEG): Electroencephalography is a non-invasive test that measures electrical activity in the brain. It is useful in evaluating seizure activity and detecting abnormal brain waves. While EEG can provide valuable information about the patient's brain function and help diagnose seizure-related conditions, it may not be specific enough to confirm the diagnosis of an encephaloclastic disorder.

(B) Magnetic Resonance Imaging (MRI): Magnetic Resonance Imaging is a powerful imaging technique that provides detailed images of the brain. It can detect structural abnormalities, such as brain tissue damage, inflammation, or atrophy, which are characteristic of encephaloclastic disorders. Given the sudden onset of symptoms, presence of fever, and neck stiffness, an MRI would be the most appropriate initial imaging modality to evaluate for possible encephaloclastic changes.

(C) Polymerase Chain Reaction (PCR): Polymerase Chain Reaction is a laboratory technique used to amplify and detect specific DNA or RNA sequences. In the context of encephaloclastic disorders, PCR can be helpful in identifying infectious agents, such as viruses or bacteria, that may be causing the brain tissue damage. However, the clinical presentation in this case does not strongly suggest an infectious etiology, making PCR a less likely initial diagnostic test.

(D) Brain Biopsy: Brain biopsy involves the surgical removal of a small piece of brain tissue for microscopic examination. It is an invasive procedure and typically reserved for cases where less invasive tests have been inconclusive. Given the clinical presentation and availability of non-invasive imaging modalities, brain biopsy would not be the most appropriate initial diagnostic test in this scenario.

The correct Answer is (B) Magnetic Resonance Imaging (MRI).

17. Let's analyze the case scenario to determine the most likely diagnosis based on the symptoms and MRI findings.

    (A) Alzheimer's disease: Alzheimer's disease is a neurodegenerative disorder primarily characterized by progressive memory loss, cognitive decline, and behavioral changes. While Alzheimer's disease can lead to brain atrophy, the specific findings of bilateral symmetric caudate nucleus atrophy and movement coordination difficulties make it an unlikely diagnosis in this case.

    (B) Huntington's disease: Huntington's disease is an inherited neurodegenerative disorder caused by an abnormal expansion of CAG repeats in the huntingtin gene. It primarily affects the basal ganglia, including the caudate nucleus. The clinical presentation of progressive cognitive decline, personality changes, movement coordination difficulties, and the characteristic MRI findings of bilateral symmetric caudate nucleus atrophy align with the diagnosis of Huntington's disease. Therefore, Huntington's disease is the most likely condition responsible for these findings.

    (C) Parkinson's disease: Parkinson's disease is a neurodegenerative disorder characterized by bradykinesia, rigidity, tremors, and postural instability. While Parkinson's disease can involve the basal ganglia, including the caudate nucleus, the presence of progressive cognitive decline and bilateral symmetric caudate nucleus atrophy make it less likely in this case.

    (D) Multiple sclerosis: Multiple sclerosis is an autoimmune disorder that primarily affects the central nervous system, leading to demyelination and inflammation. It typically presents with a wide range of symptoms, including motor and sensory disturbances, but is not commonly associated with bilateral symmetric caudate nucleus atrophy. Therefore, multiple sclerosis is an unlikely diagnosis in this case.

    The correct Answer is (B) Huntington's disease.

18. Let's analyze the case scenario to determine the most likely classification of this encephaloclastic disorder.

    (A) Cortical degeneration: Cortical degeneration refers to the degeneration or loss of neurons in the cerebral cortex, which is the outer layer of the brain responsible for higher cognitive functions. The clinical presentation in this case, including progressive memory loss, personality changes, and language difficulties, along with neuroimaging findings of atrophy in the frontal and temporal lobes, suggests cortical involvement. Therefore, cortical degeneration is the most likely classification of this encephaloclastic disorder.

    (B) Subcortical degeneration: Subcortical degeneration involves the degeneration or loss of neurons in the structures beneath the cerebral cortex, such as the basal ganglia or thalamus. However, the clinical presentation and neuroimaging findings in this case are more consistent with cortical involvement rather than subcortical degeneration.

(C) Multifocal encephalopathy: Multifocal encephalopathy refers to the presence of multiple areas of brain damage or dysfunction. However, the case scenario does not indicate the involvement of multiple distinct brain regions. Instead, it suggests predominant atrophy in the frontal and temporal lobes, supporting the classification of cortical degeneration.

(D) Global encephalopathy: Global encephalopathy refers to diffuse brain dysfunction affecting multiple regions of the brain. The case scenario describes specific involvement of the frontal and temporal lobes, rather than widespread involvement throughout the brain. Therefore, global encephalopathy is not the most likely classification in this case.

Answer: (A) Cortical degeneration.

19. Let's discuss the answer choices:

(A) Ischemic infarction: Ischemic infarction refers to the obstruction of blood flow to a specific area of the brain, leading to tissue necrosis. However, the sudden onset of focal neurological deficits and well-defined, circumscribed area of brain tissue necrosis described in the question stem is not typical of ischemic infarction. Ischemic infarction usually presents with more gradual onset and may show a more diffuse pattern of tissue damage.

(B) Traumatic brain injury: Traumatic brain injury (TBI) can lead to tissue necrosis in the brain due to direct injury or secondary mechanisms such as bleeding or edema. While TBI can cause focal neurological deficits, the sudden-onset nature and well-defined, circumscribed area of brain tissue necrosis mentioned in the question stem are not commonly associated with TBI. TBI typically results in more diffuse brain damage rather than a localized necrotic area.

(C) Infectious encephalitis: Infectious encephalitis refers to inflammation of the brain caused by viral, bacterial, or fungal infections. While infectious encephalitis can cause focal neurological deficits, the sudden-onset nature and well-defined, circumscribed area of brain tissue necrosis described in the question stem are not typical of infectious encephalitis. Infectious encephalitis often presents with more diffuse involvement of the brain rather than a localized necrotic area.

(D) Neoplastic infiltration: Neoplastic infiltration refers to the invasion of brain tissue by malignant cells, typically from primary brain tumors or metastatic cancers. The sudden-onset focal neurological deficits and neuroimaging findings of a well-defined, circumscribed area of brain tissue necrosis mentioned in the question stem are consistent with neoplastic infiltration. Brain tumors can cause focal tissue necrosis due to the rapid growth and invasion of tumor cells.

The correct Answer is (D) Neoplastic infiltration.

20. Let's discuss the answer choices:

(A) Surgical resection: Surgical resection involves the removal of the necrotic brain tissue. While surgical intervention may be necessary in some cases of encephaloclastic disorders, such as neoplastic infiltration or certain types of traumatic brain injury, it is not a universally applicable treatment option for all encephaloclastic disorders associated with brain tissue necrosis.

(B) Antibiotic therapy: Antibiotic therapy is primarily used in the treatment of infectious encephalitis, which may present with brain tissue necrosis. However, not all encephaloclastic disorders are caused by infections. Therefore, antibiotic therapy may not be the most commonly used treatment approach for encephaloclastic disorders as a whole.

(C) Radiation therapy: Radiation therapy is commonly used in the treatment of certain types of brain tumors, including those associated with neoplastic infiltration. It aims to target and destroy cancer cells. However, radiation therapy is not a standard treatment approach for all encephaloclastic disorders associated with brain tissue necrosis.

(D) Supportive care: Supportive care involves providing symptomatic treatment and ensuring the patient's comfort and well-being. It is a crucial aspect of managing encephaloclastic disorders, regardless of the underlying cause. Supportive care may include measures such as pain management, physical therapy, rehabilitation, and psychological support. It is the most commonly used treatment approach for encephaloclastic disorders associated with brain tissue necrosis, as it focuses on optimizing the patient's quality of life.

The correct Answer is (D) Supportive care.

21. Let's discuss the answer choices:

(A) 1 in 1000 individuals: This prevalence rate suggests that encephaloclastic disorders are relatively common, affecting approximately 1 in every 1000 individuals. However, this rate may be higher than the actual prevalence of encephaloclastic disorders.

(B) 1 in 10,000 individuals: This prevalence rate suggests that encephaloclastic disorders are less common, affecting approximately 1 in every 10,000 individuals. This rate is more plausible, considering the nature of encephaloclastic disorders and their relatively lower occurrence.

(C) 1 in 100,000 individuals: This prevalence rate suggests that encephaloclastic disorders are even rarer, affecting approximately 1 in every 100,000 individuals. While encephaloclastic disorders are not as common as some other neurological conditions, they may still occur more frequently than this rate suggests.

(D) 1 in 1000,000 individuals: This prevalence rate suggests that encephaloclastic disorders are extremely rare, affecting approximately 1 in every 1000,000 individuals. While encephaloclastic disorders are not as prevalent as some other neurological disorders, they are still more common than this rate suggests.

The correct Answer is (B) 1 in 10,000 individuals.

22. Let's discuss the answer choices:

   (A) Hemiparesis: This refers to weakness or paralysis affecting one side of the body. In the given case scenario, the patient presents with left-sided weakness, indicating hemiparesis. Hemiparesis is a common clinical manifestation of encephaloclastic disorders, particularly when caused by ischemic stroke.

   (B) Ataxia: Ataxia refers to uncoordinated movements and lack of muscle control. It is not a typical manifestation of encephaloclastic disorders like ischemic stroke. Therefore, it is unlikely to be the correct answer in this case.

   (C) Visual disturbances: While visual disturbances can occur with certain brain disorders, they are not a characteristic feature of encephaloclastic disorders like ischemic stroke. Therefore, this is an unlikely choice for the clinical manifestation in this case.

   (D) Memory loss: Memory loss is not a common immediate manifestation of encephaloclastic disorders like ischemic stroke. While it may occur in the later stages or as a consequence of stroke, it is not the primary clinical feature seen in the given case scenario.

   The correct Answer is (A) Hemiparesis.

23. Let's discuss the answer choices:

   (A) Age of the patient: Age can be an important factor in determining the prognosis of encephaloclastic disorders, such as ischemic stroke. Older patients may have a higher risk of complications and poorer outcomes. However, in this case, the most significant factor influencing the prognosis is likely to be something more specific to the treatment and management of the condition.

   (B) Past medical history: While the patient's past medical history, including conditions like atrial fibrillation and hypertension, can contribute to the risk of developing stroke, it is not the most significant factor influencing the prognosis of the encephaloclastic disorder in this case. The focus should be on factors more directly related to the acute event and its management.

   (C) Timeliness of treatment: The timeliness of treatment is a crucial factor in determining the prognosis of encephaloclastic disorders like ischemic stroke. The administration of thrombolytic therapy within the recommended time window can help restore blood flow to the affected area and improve outcomes. Early intervention is associated with better prognosis and reduced risk of disability.

   (D) Severity of neurological deficits: The severity of neurological deficits, such as the extent of weakness and speech difficulties, can provide insights into the initial impact of the encephaloclastic disorder. While it is an important consideration, it may not be the most significant factor influencing the prognosis. The response to treatment and rehabilitation efforts can also play a role in determining the long-term outcome.

   The correct Answer is (C) Timeliness of treatment.

24. Let's discuss the answer choices:

(A) Nerve Conduction Studies (NCS): NCS is a test that measures the speed and strength of electrical signals as they travel through the nerves. It is primarily used to evaluate peripheral nerve function and can help diagnose conditions such as peripheral neuropathy or nerve compression. In this case, where the suspected pathology is located within the central nervous system (CNS), NCS may not be the most appropriate electrophysiological test.

(B) Electromyography (EMG): EMG is a test that evaluates the electrical activity of muscles and the associated nerve function. It can help diagnose conditions affecting the muscles or the nerve-muscle junction. While EMG can provide valuable information in certain cases, it may not be the most appropriate electrophysiological test for evaluating encephaloclastic disorders.

(C) Electroencephalogram (EEG): EEG is a non-invasive test that records electrical activity in the brain. It is commonly used to evaluate brain function and detect abnormal patterns associated with various neurological conditions, including encephaloclastic disorders. However, in this case, where the primary concern is muscle weakness and falls, a different electrophysiological test may be more appropriate.

(D) Visual Evoked Potential (VEP): VEP is an electrophysiological test that assesses the electrical responses generated in the visual cortex in response to visual stimuli. It is primarily used to evaluate the integrity and function of the optic nerve and the visual pathways within the brain. While VEP can be informative in certain cases, it may not be the most suitable test for evaluating the muscle weakness and falls seen in this patient.

The correct Answer is (A) Nerve Conduction Studies (NCS).

25. Let's discuss the answer choices:

(A) Complete Blood Count (CBC): A CBC is a routine blood test that provides information about the different components of blood, including red blood cells, white blood cells, and platelets. While a CBC is a valuable screening test, it may not directly aid in the diagnosis of an encephaloclastic disorder.

(B) Liver Function Tests (LFTs): LFTs evaluate the function of the liver by measuring various enzymes, proteins, and substances in the blood. While liver dysfunction can sometimes lead to neurological symptoms, it is not the most specific initial blood test for evaluating encephaloclastic disorders.

(C) Creatine Kinase (CK) levels: CK is an enzyme found in muscles and other tissues. Elevated CK levels can indicate muscle damage or breakdown, which may be relevant in certain encephaloclastic disorders associated with muscle involvement. However, it may not be the most useful initial blood test in the evaluation of all encephaloclastic disorders.

(D) Genetic Testing: Genetic testing involves analyzing an individual's DNA to identify changes or mutations that may be associated with specific diseases, including encephaloclastic disorders. Genetic testing can be a valuable tool in the diagnosis and classification of these disorders, especially in cases where there is a suspected genetic basis or family history. However, it may not be the most appropriate initial blood test for all patients.

The correct Answer is (D) Genetic Testing.

26. Let's discuss the answer choices:

    (A) Encephaloclastic disorders are more common in children than in adults: This statement is generally incorrect. While some encephaloclastic disorders, such as certain forms of leukodystrophies, may manifest early in childhood, there are also numerous types that can affect individuals of all ages, including adults.

    (B) Encephaloclastic disorders have a higher prevalence in males than in females: This statement is not universally true. The prevalence of encephaloclastic disorders can vary depending on the specific condition. In some cases, there may be a slight male predominance, while in others, there is no significant gender difference.

    (C) Genetic factors play a minimal role in the development of encephaloclastic disorders: This statement is generally incorrect. Many encephaloclastic disorders have a genetic component, either as inherited conditions or due to de novo mutations. Genetic factors can play a significant role in the pathogenesis of these disorders.

    (D) Encephaloclastic disorders are primarily caused by infectious agents: This statement is generally incorrect. While some encephaloclastic disorders can be triggered by infectious agents, such as certain viral infections, it is not the primary cause for most cases. Encephaloclastic disorders can have diverse etiologies, including genetic, metabolic, autoimmune, toxic, and vascular causes.

    The correct Answer is None of the above.

27. Let's discuss the answer choices:

    (A) Visual disturbances: While visual disturbances can occur in some encephaloclastic disorders, they are not typically associated with lesions in the left frontal lobe. Visual impairments are more commonly observed when the occipital lobe or the pathways responsible for visual processing are affected.

    (B) Memory loss and confusion: Memory loss and confusion are not the most likely clinical manifestations in this case. While cognitive impairments can occur in encephaloclastic disorders, they are typically associated with lesions in other areas of the brain, such as the temporal lobe or the hippocampus.

    (C) Hemiparesis and aphasia: Hemiparesis (weakness on one side of the body) and aphasia (difficulty with speech and language) are commonly observed in individuals with brain tissue destruction in the frontal lobe. The left frontal lobe is specifically responsible for controlling movements on the right side of the body and language processing. Therefore, these clinical manifestations are most likely in this case.

(D) Sleep disturbances and excessive daytime sleepiness: Sleep disturbances and excessive daytime sleepiness are not typically associated with encephaloclastic disorders, especially when there is a focal lesion in a specific area of the brain like the left frontal lobe.

The correct Answer is (C) Hemiparesis and aphasia.

28. Let's discuss the answer choices:

(A) Antipsychotic medications: While antipsychotic medications are commonly used to manage certain behavioral symptoms associated with encephaloclastic disorders, they are not the primary treatment for the underlying condition. In this case, the patient's symptoms are likely due to the progressive loss of brain tissue in the temporal lobes, which requires a different approach.

(B) Antibiotics: Antibiotics are not the appropriate treatment for encephaloclastic disorders. Encephaloclastic disorders involve the destruction of brain tissue and are not caused by infectious agents that would require antibiotic therapy.

(C) Surgical resection of the affected brain tissue: Surgical resection of brain tissue is not typically performed in encephaloclastic disorders. These disorders involve widespread degeneration or destruction of brain tissue, making surgical intervention impractical and potentially harmful.

(D) Symptomatic management and supportive care: Symptomatic management and supportive care are the mainstay of treatment for encephaloclastic disorders. This approach focuses on addressing the patient's symptoms, improving quality of life, and providing support to the patient and their caregivers. This may include interventions such as cognitive rehabilitation, behavioral interventions, and supportive services.

The correct Answer is (D) Symptomatic management and supportive care.

The most appropriate treatment option for managing the patient's condition, characterized by progressive cognitive decline, memory loss, and behavioral changes with bilateral atrophy and significant loss of brain tissue in the temporal lobes, is symptomatic management and supportive care. Since encephaloclastic disorders involve irreversible damage to brain tissue, the primary goal of treatment is to alleviate symptoms and provide supportive measures to enhance the patient's well-being.

29. Let's discuss the answer choices:

(A) Stem cell therapy: Stem cell therapy holds promise as a potential future direction for the management of encephaloclastic disorders. Stem cells have the ability to differentiate into various cell types, including neurons, and may have the potential to replace damaged or lost brain tissue. Ongoing research is being conducted to explore the safety and efficacy of stem cell therapy in treating neurological disorders.

(B) Psychotherapy: Psychotherapy, while valuable in addressing psychological and emotional aspects of encephaloclastic disorders, is not specifically a future direction for the management of the condition. Psychotherapy can be beneficial in helping patients and their families cope with the challenges associated with the disease, but it does not target the underlying neurodegenerative process.

(C) Nonsteroidal anti-inflammatory drugs (NSAIDs): While inflammation is thought to play a role in certain neurodegenerative disorders, including encephaloclastic disorders, the use of NSAIDs as a future direction for management is not well-established. There is ongoing research exploring the potential benefits of anti-inflammatory agents in neurodegenerative diseases, but further studies are needed to determine their efficacy and safety.

(D) Physical therapy interventions: Physical therapy interventions are beneficial in managing the functional impairments associated with encephaloclastic disorders, such as mobility and balance issues. However, they are not specifically a future direction for the management of the condition, as physical therapy is already an established part of the comprehensive care approach for these disorders.

The correct Answer is (A) Stem cell therapy.

Stem cell therapy represents a potential future direction for the management of encephaloclastic disorders. The ability of stem cells to differentiate into various cell types, including neurons, offers the possibility of replacing damaged or lost brain tissue. While research in this field is ongoing, it is important to note that stem cell therapy is still in the experimental stage and requires further investigation to determine its safety, efficacy, and long-term outcomes.

30. Let's discuss the answer choices:

(A) Deep brain stimulation: Deep brain stimulation (DBS) is a potential future direction for the management of encephaloclastic disorders. It involves the implantation of electrodes in specific regions of the brain to deliver electrical impulses. DBS has shown promise in managing symptoms related to movement disorders, such as Parkinson's disease. While its effectiveness in encephaloclastic disorders is still being explored, it holds potential for mitigating motor symptoms and improving overall quality of life. However, further research and clinical trials are needed to establish its efficacy and safety specifically for encephaloclastic disorders.

(B) Herbal supplements: While herbal supplements may have potential benefits for overall health and well-being, they are not specifically a future direction for managing encephaloclastic disorders. The degeneration of brain tissue in encephaloclastic disorders requires more targeted and evidence-based interventions. It is important to consult with healthcare professionals before considering any herbal supplements, as they may interact with other medications or have unintended side effects.

(C) Meditation and mindfulness techniques: While meditation and mindfulness techniques can be valuable in managing stress, promoting relaxation, and improving mental well-being, they are not specifically a future direction for the management of encephaloclastic disorders. These techniques may help individuals cope with the impact of the disorder on their daily lives, but they do not address the underlying neurodegenerative process.

(D) Physical therapy: Physical therapy is an important component of comprehensive care for individuals with encephaloclastic disorders. It focuses on improving mobility, strength, balance, and coordination through targeted exercises and interventions. While physical therapy is already an established approach, ongoing advancements in technology and techniques may further enhance its effectiveness in the future.

The correct Answer is (A) Deep brain stimulation.

Deep brain stimulation holds promise as a potential future direction for managing encephaloclastic disorders. By delivering electrical impulses to specific regions of the brain, DBS aims to modulate abnormal neuronal activity and alleviate motor symptoms. While its efficacy for encephaloclastic disorders is still being investigated, early studies and case reports suggest potential benefits. However, it is essential to recognize that DBS is a complex procedure that requires careful patient selection and ongoing monitoring.

References

1. Teasdale G. Claude Bernard and encephalomalacia. J Neurol Neurosurg Psychiatry. 2000;69(5):573.

Chapter 19
Cerebral Palsy

**Qasim Mehmood, Hafiza Qurat ul ain, Muhammad Zeeshan,
and Ahsan Rashid Rana**

Test your learning and check your understanding of this book's contents: use
the "Springer Nature Flashcards" app to access questions using ▶ https://
sn.pub/YnQHwS
To use the app, please follow the instructions in Chapter 1.

19.1 Introduction

Cerebral palsy is a neuromotor disorder that primarily affects motor system, muscle
tone, and postural development of the body of a child. The underlying pathophysiology is not well-known but damage to the developing brain during the prenatal to
neonatal period is seen in majority of the cases. Although early neuropathological
lesions are not progressive, over time children with CP can develop a variety of
secondary deficits that can differentially affect their functional abilities [1].

Based on international consensus, the generally agreed definition of cerebral
palsy is "It represents a group of persistent movement and postural disorders leading to activity limitation that are thought to be nonprogressive disorders and arise in
the developing fetus or immature brain". Movement disorders in cerebral palsy are
often accompanied by sensory, perceptual, cognitive, communicative and behavioral deficits, epilepsy, and secondary musculoskeletal problems [2].

Q. Mehmood (✉) · M. Zeeshan
King Edward Medical University, Lahore, Pakistan

H. Qurat ul ain · A. R. Rana
CMH Multan Institute of Medical Sciences, Multan, Pakistan

© The Author(s), under exclusive license to Springer Nature
Switzerland AG 2024
K. F. AlAli, H. T. Hashim (eds.), *Congenital Brain Malformations*,
https://doi.org/10.1007/978-3-031-58630-9_19

There are three main types of cerebral palsy: spastic (70–80%), dyskinetic (10–20%), ataxic (5–10%), or a combination of the three [1]. Some children develop other disabilities such as seizures, intellectual disability, difficulty learning to chew, swallow and speak, communication difficulties, vision and hearing problems, cognitive impairment, growth problems, sleep disorders, dental problems, slow learning, and challenging behavior [2]. The precise needs of this heterogeneous group vary widely. Every child is unique with varying degrees of impairment. Classification is important in understanding the individual child's disability, and for coordinating the control of care. However, treatment should be adapted to every child's needs [2].

19.2 Classification of Cerebral Palsy

19.2.1 According to Severity

Cerebral Palsy is often classified by the level of severity as mild, moderate and severe.

- **Mild Cerebral Palsy:** It means that the child can move without help; his or her everyday activity is not limited [2].
- **Moderate Cerebral Palsy:** It means that the child will require braces, medications, and adaptive technology to do daily activities [2].
- **Severe Cerebral Palsy:** It means that the child would need a wheelchair and would have significant challenges in the accomplishment of daily activities and would require support [2].

19.2.2 Topographical Classification

Topographical classification describes the parts of body that are affected.

- **Monoplegia:** Means only one limb is affected. It is considered that this may be a type of hemiplegia/hemiparesis where one limb is notably impaired.
- **Diplegia:** It usually indicates that the legs are more susceptible to damage than the arms. It mainly affects the lower body.
- **Hemiplegia:** Indicates arms and legs are affected on one side of the body.
- **Triplegia:** Indicates that three limbs are affected. This can be both arms and one leg, or both legs and one arm, or it can refer to the upper and lower extremities and the face.
- **Double hemiplegia:** Indicates that all four limbs are affected, but one side of the body is more affected than the other.
- **Quadriplegia:** It means that all four limbs are involved [2].

19.2.3   Classification Based on Muscle Tone

Based on muscle tone, cerebral palsy can be divided into hypertonic and hypotonic cerebral palsy. Hypertonia means increased muscle tone and is associated with spastic cerebral palsy. Hypotonia means decreased muscle tone and is associated with non spastic cerebral palsy [2].

19.2.4   Functional Classification

There are three systems by which cerebral palsy can be classified functionally [2].

1. Gross motor system
2. Manual ability system
3. Communication system

19.3   Risk Factors of Cerebral Palsy

The risk factors fall into the following categories: pre-conception; concerning the broadly defined health and living conditions of the mother, prenatal; which are related to the course of pregnancy, and perinatal; as well as risk factors in the neonatal and infant period [3].

One of the most important risk factors for developing cerebral palsy is prematurity. The frequency and severity of neurodevelopmental disorders correlate with gestational age, with shorter gestational age being more severe. Low birth weight in preterm infants is another major risk factor [4].

19.4   Clinical Presentation of Cerebral Palsy

Cerebral palsy affects children in many physical and neurological ways. The severity of the condition and the degree of associated motor impairment depend on the type of brain injury the child experiences. There are the various symptoms and signs of cerebral palsy. Symptoms of cerebral palsy in infants may include abnormal muscle tone, crossed or stiffened legs whilst being picked up, delay in sitting, crawling, rolling over, and walking, difficulty grasping the objects or clapping their hands, excessive drooling, inability to elevate their own head, overextended back and/or neck when being picked up, and stiffness of joints and/or muscles (spasticity) [5].

Cerebral palsy in toddlers may present as abnormal posture, crawling in a lop-sided manner, difficulty with fine motor skills like eating, brushing teeth, or coloring, hearing loss or blindness, hopping on their knees when trying to walk, inability to stand, uncontrollable muscle movement, scooting around on their buttocks, speech problems, and stiff muscles, joints, or tendons [5]. Furthermore, there are various neurological problems associated with cerebral palsy like autism, attention deficit hyperactivity disorder (ADHD), behavioral problems, epilepsy (seizure disorder), intellectual disabilities, learning disabilities, speech and language issues (dysarthria), sensory impairments, and visual/hearing impairment [5].

19.4.1 Spastic Cerebral Palsy

Common symptoms of spastic cerebral palsy include abnormal walking, awkward reflexes, muscle stiffness of one side of the body, and permanently tightened muscles or joints [5].

19.4.2 Ataxic Cerebral Palsy

Ataxic cerebral palsy may manifest as coordination issues, depth perception problems, difficulty with speech, shakiness and tremors, and spreading feet apart when walking [5].

19.4.3 Athetoid Cerebral Palsy

Common symptoms of athetoid cerebral palsy include feeding issues, floppy limbs, problems with posture, and stiff or rigid body [5].

19.4.4 Hypotonic Cerebral Palsy

Clinical presentation of hypotonic cerebral palsy may include flexible joints and ligaments, floppy or loose muscles, lack of head control, and poor balance and stability [5].

19.5 Diagnosis and Screening

There isn't a single particular test which can diagnose cerebral palsy with higher sensitivity and specificity, so health care providers use a combine clinical and radiological approach, during first few months of infancy in high-risk children, to define it.

19.5.1 Clinical Assessment

Studies had shown that complete history and physical examination along with neuromuscular system examination may help us in identifying features (e.g., persistent primitive reflexes, Moro reflex etc.) and movements abnormalities (e.g., truncal hypotonia, distal limb spasticity etc.) over the period of time, which can help in making the final diagnosis. Clinicians may use these following assessment methods.

Prechtl Qualitative Assessment of General Movements (GMs)

GMs focus on the commonly occurring movements during the first 3 months of life which are "fidgety movements pattern". These are fluent muscle movement and their occurrence confirm reorganization of motor cortex. Absence or any abnormality in this pattern are highly predictive of cerebral palsy, which has to be identified during clinical assessment [6].

Hammersmith Infant Neurological Examination (HINE)

This tool can easily be performed even with un experienced staff. It tells us not only about the children at risk but also about the extent and severity of CP the child would develop, by using "global HINE score" that ranges from 0 to 78. HINE basically elaborate five domains of neurological examination (cranial nerves function, posture quality, quantity of movements, muscle tone, reflexes). Therefore, a child with the score of less than 40 will have severe motor impairment, 40-60 will have moderate motor impairment and more than 60 will have normal motor outcomes [7].

Others Assessment methods are

- Albert infant motor scale (AIMS)
- Developmental assessment of young infant (DAYC) [6]

19.5.2   Radiological Assessment

Radiological assessment is combined with clinical examination to increase sensitivity index for better diagnosis of cerebral. It includes.

Brain MRI

It is the best and most effective neuroimaging to predict CP in high-risk children. It demonstrates any brain lesion in white matter, impaired myelination of posterior limb of Internal capsule [6], basal ganglia, cortical lesions with sensitivity 83% and specificity 95%. Brain MRI is much better than Cranial US for diagnostic purpose but cost effective [8].

Cranial Ultrasound

Mostly it used in premature infants in first month of their life. It could be used in combination with MRI or separately where MRI isn't feasible, but has less diagnostic value as compared to MRI. US can be used along bedside and for Screening purposes as it is portable, no radiational effect less expensive, easily operated than MRI. It detects any intracranial hemorrhage or hypoxic Injury occurred during birth which may lead to CP [9].

Brain CT

Computed tomography (CT) scan has more value in older children as can locate the extend of lesion but not be used in early infancy because of radiational effect on the developing brain. It may detect cortical atrophy in older children [10].

CNN Image Segmentation

It is a new way which combine 3D brain MRI under deep leaning technology, that could assist in better diagnosis of CP [11].

19.6   Treatment of Cerebral Palsy

Child with cerebral palsy need comprehensive approach by physiotherapy, medical and surgical interventions to normalize life activities along with prevention and rehabilitation of complication that develops as a result of illness.

19.6.1 Non-pharmacological Measures

- **Physical therapy:** It helps to improve motor movements, reflexes and muscle coordination to have proper gait and strength during daily life activities. It prevents further disuse atrophy in effected limb. Physiotherapist uses combined approach of electrical stimulation, swimming and walking equipment to improve joints mobility [1, 12].
- **Constrain Induce Movement therapy:** It emphasize on the use of paralyzed limb and reduce movement activity in normal limb under observed protocol to prevent disuse atrophy in normal limb [12].
- **Goal Directed Training:** Specified directed movements will help the child to improve working speed [13].
- **Speech therapy:** Focus on word pronunciation for better communication skills [1].
- **Occupation therapy:** Provide child with Learning environment and equipment to build on better cognitive ability [1].
- **Assistive Aids:** Facilitate the child with elevator, wheelchairs, and electric stairs to prevent him from inferiority complex [1].
- **Parental Training:** To encourage the child in his/her daily life activities to improve self-confidence [1].
- **Psychological support:** To parents and child during regular follow-up sessions [1].

19.6.2 Medical Treatment

It basically aimed to improve symptomatic treatment of disease and reduce movement limitations. It includes drugs for.

- **Spasticity and Dystonia:** Muscle relaxant and anticholinergic drugs that will relieve spasticity. These are baclofen, diazepam, dantrolene, and benzodiazepines and more invasive drugs like botulinum toxins, intrathecal baclofen [1].
- **Epilepsy:** Anti-epileptic drugs like phenytoin, clonazepam, phenobarbital, and carbamazepine, are used for symptomatic relive and prevent progression of seizure [1]. In resistive situations, ketogenic diet [4] and invasive options are adopted.
- **Stem cell Replacement:** This method of treatment is still under trials and will help in full recovery of brain cells from traumatic injuries [14].

19.6.3   Surgical Treatment

This method of treatment plays important role if medical therapy failed. It facilities movement by correcting postural and structural abnormalities by lengthening the tendon and muscle that will prevents further complications by reliving contractures and muscle stiffness [15].

19.7   Prevention of Cerebral Palsy

Risk of Cerebral Palsy can be prevented by following measures

- By infection screening on regular follow-up [16]
- Proper pre-natal and obstetric care [1, 16]
- By providing best possible care to newborn during early age
- Stop smoking, alcohol, and other sedative drugs during pregnancy [1, 16]
- Proper vaccination during pregnancy [1]
- Child vaccination according to EPI [1]
- Preterm delivery combined with magnesium sulfate [16]
- Pre-eclampsia treatment [16]
- Steroid treatment in preterm infants [16]
- Hypothermic therapy in risky children [16]
- Antioxidant therapy during first trimester [17]

Exercise

Q 1. Cerebral palsy is a

(a) Neuromotor disorder
(b) Psychiatric disorder
(c) Infection
(d) Toxin

Q 2. The most significant risk factor of cerebral palsy is

(a) Diabetes
(b) Hypertension
(c) Prematurity
(d) None

Q 3. Types of cerebral palsy include

(a) Spastic
(b) Hypotonic
(c) Ataxic
(d) All of these

Q 4. Treatment of cerebral palsy is

(a) Pharmacological
(b) Non-pharmacological
(c) Surgical
(d) Any of these

Q 5. Non-pharmacological measures of managing cerebral palsy is

(a) Physical therapy
(b) Speech therapy
(c) Behavioural therapy
(d) All of these

Q 6. Assisted devices for cerebral palsy patients include

(a) Dancing chairs
(b) Wheel chairs
(c) Electric guitar
(d) None of these

Q 7. In order to prevent cerebral palsy, child should be

(a) Vaccinated according to EPI
(b) Not vaccinated
(c) Vaccinated according to EMI
(d) All of these

Q 8. Monoplegia involves

(a) Both legs
(b) Both arms
(c) Only one limb
(d) One leg and arm

Q 9. Best test to predict cerebral palsy in a child

(a) T test
(b) Brain MRI
(c) Chest X ray
(d) None of these

Q 10. Non-pharmacological measures to treat cerebral palsy are

(a) Physical therapy
(b) Speech therapy
(c) Psychological support
(d) All of them

References

1. Patel DR, Neelakantan M, Pandher K, Merrick J. Cerebral palsy in children: a clinical overview. Transl Pediatr. 2020;9(Suppl 1):S125.
2. Classification of Cerebral Palsy https://www.physio-pedia.com/Classification_of_Cerebral_Palsy Accessed 26 Jan 2023.
3. Compagnone E, Maniglio J, Camposeo S, Vespino T, Losito L, De Rinaldis M, Gennaro L, Trabacca A. Functional classifications for cerebral palsy: correlations between the gross motor function classification system (GMFCS), the manual ability classification system (MACS) and the communication function classification system (CFCS). Res Dev Disabil. 2014;35(11):2651–7.
4. Sadowska M, Sarecka-Hujar B, Kopyta I. Cerebral palsy: current opinions on definition, epidemiology, risk factors, classification and treatment options. Neuropsychiatr Dis Treat. 2020;12:1505–18.
5. Cerebral palsy symptoms https://www.cerebralpalsyguide.com/cerebral-palsy/symptoms/ Accessed 26 Jan 2023.
6. Haataja L. Early diagnosis of cerebral palsy. Pediatr Med. 2020;3:9.
7. Romeo DM, Ricci D, Brogna C, Mecuri E. Use of hammersmith infant neurological examination in infant with cerebral palsy: a critical review of literature. Dev Med Child Neurol. 2015; https://doi.org/10.1111/dmcn.1278.
8. Arabella RK, Mahmudul HAI, Sarah M, Catherine M, Gulam K, Nadia B, Atul M. Early diagnosis of cerebral palsy in low-and middle income countries. Brain Sci. 2022;12(5):539. https://doi.org/10.3390/brainsci12050539.
9. De Vries LS, van Haastert IC, Rademaker KJ, Koopman C, Groenendaal F. Ultrasound abnormalities preceding cerebral palsy in high-risk preterm infants. J Pediatr. 2004;144:815–20.
10. Kundu GK, Ahmed S, Akhter S, Islam S. Neuro-imaging changes in cerebral palsy: a cross sectional study. Mymensingh Med J. 2020;29(1):121–8. PMID: 31915347.9
11. Rui Y, Haoran Z, Shusheng H, Xiaoping Z, Qian Z. Computer-aided diagnosis of children with cerebral palsy under deep learning convolutional neural network image segmentation model combined with three-dimensional cranial magnetic resonance imaging. J Healthc Eng. 2021;2021 https://doi.org/10.1155/2021/1822776.
12. Monik CD, Alexandera LT. Constrain-induce movement therapy for infant with or at risk for cerebral palsy: a scoping review. Am J Occup Ther. 2022;76:2. https://doi.org/10.5014/ajot.2022.047894.
13. Sakti PD, Shankar G. Evidence-based approach to physical therapy in cerebral palsy. Indian J Orthop. 2019;53:20–34. https://doi.org/10.4103/ortho.Ijortho_241_17.
14. Aanhita K, Nasrin L, Jafar A. The role of stem cells in the treatment of cerebral palsy: a review. Mol Neurobiol. 2017:4963–72. https://doi.org/10.1007/s12035-016-0030-0.
15. Abigail K, Lynn MD, Michael T, Henry GMD. Surgical management of spasticity inn persons with cerebral palsy. ScienceDirect. 2009;1(9):834–8. https://doi.org/10.1016/j.pmrj.2009.07.01616.
16. Michael O'shea T. Diagnosis, treatment, and prevention of cerbral palsy in near-term/term infant. Clin Obstet Gynecol. 2008;51(4):816–28. https://doi.org/10.1097/GRF.0bo13e3181870ba7.
17. Alan DS. Prevention of cerebral palsy, autism spectrum disorder, and attention deficit-hyperactivity disorder. Med Hypotheses. 2014;82(5):522–8. https://doi.org/10.1016/j.mehy.2014.02.003.

Chapter 20
Congenital Brain Malformation in the Arab World

May Saad Al-Jorani and Moatamn Skuk (iD)

Test your learning and check your understanding of this book's contents: use the "Springer Nature Flashcards" app to access questions using ▶ https://sn.pub/YnQHwS
To use the app, please follow the instructions in Chapter 1.

20.1 Introduction

Inherited diseases genetically or in the acquired form will eventually alter the morphological pattern of an organ or particular part of the body. These types of malformations are caused without previous etiological factors "de-novo" or transmitted from parents, in both cases, the congenital anomaly will exist from the beginning of embryo life. On the other hand, disruptive anomalies are gained due to external factors such as infections, bleeding, and reduced blood flow, in which, the body's nature is developed normally but once affected by these factors, the affected part will be disrupted. Although the risk of recurrence for inherited disorders is different based on the mutations of the genes, it is very low in disruptive anomalies. [1].

The exemplary conditions of the disruptive anomalies are hydran- and hemihydranencephaly [2], disruption of fetal brain FBD-like-phenotype [3], disruptive sequence of the twin [4]

M. S. Al-Jorani (✉)
College of Medicine, Mustansiriyah University, Baghdad, Iraq

M. Skuk
al-Kindi medical college, Baghdad, Iraq

K. F. AlAli, H. T. Hashim (eds.), *Congenital Brain Malformations*,
https://doi.org/10.1007/978-3-031-58630-9_20

The obscurity of the cerebral hemisphere can be seen in hydranencephaly [2]. Also, the disruption of the fetal brain FBD-like-phenotype is inherited microcephaly in which the skull is small and collapsed, while the rugae of the scalp are eminent with brain devastation in the supra-tentorium region [3]. The infections and disruptive lesions can lead to these long-term sequential effects in the prenatal period. Upon this, the cerebellum has many related anomalies such as agenesis, cleft, hypoplasia on one side and global-type, and vanishing condition [5–8].

The microangiopathy results from the dominant-type alteration in the COL4A1 gene. This condition is characterized by defects in the capillaries of the brain, which in turn, may cause bleeding or reduced blood flow. This brain disorder will eventually produce porencephaly or hypoplasia in one side of the cerebellum [9, 10].

Microcephaly is caused by homozygous alteration of the NED-1 gene, this gene can lead to other various disorders of the corpus callosum and the scalp like agenesis and rugae, respectively [11] (Table 20.1).

Table 20.1 Various brain malformations in the Arab world (isolated congenital anomalies)

Malformation	Number of cases and % of subtotal congenital brain/ CNS anomalies	Country	Period of the study	Reference
1. Corpus callosum hypoplasia	14 (23.3%)	Khartoum State _Sudan	6 months (September 2016–March 2017)	[12]
2. Corpus Collosum agenesis	15 (18.75%)	Tehran_ Iran	September 2009 and September 2010	[13]
3. Microcephaly	27 (25.7%)	Khartoum State _Sudan	6 months (September 2016–March 2017)	[12]
	777 (21.31%)	Cairo_Egypt	(1995–2009)	[14]
	28 (2.4%)	Riyadh_ Saudi Arabia	3 years	[15]
	2 (11.1%)	UAE	January 1992 to January 1994	[16]
	2 (2.5%)	Iran	September 2009 and September 2010	[13]
4. Primary microcephaly	2 (16.6%)	Al_Jahra_ Kuwait	January 2000 to December 2001	[17]
5. Macrocephaly	18 (17.1%)	Khartoum State _Sudan	6 months (September 2016–March 2017)	[12]
6. Megalencephaly	4 (5%)	Iran	September 2009 and September 2010	[13]

Table 20.1 (continued)

Malformation	Number of cases and % of subtotal congenital brain/CNS anomalies	Country	Period of the study	Reference
7. Hemi-megalencephaly	2 (2.5%)	Iran	September 2009 and September 2010	[13]
8. Polymicrogyria	5 (6.25%)	Iran	September 2009 and September 2010	[13]
9. Congenital hydrocephalus	8 (13.4%)	Khartoum State _Sudan	6 months (September 2016–March 2017)	[12]
	677 (18.57%)	Cairo_Egypt	(1995–2009)	[14]
	82 (0.092%)	Hashemite Kingdom of Jordan	2004-2005 and 2008-2011	[18]
	25 (2.1%)	Riyadh_ Saudi Arabia	3 years	[15]
	1 (8.3%)	Al-Jahra_ Kuwait	January 2000 to December 2001	[17]
10. Encephalocele	11 (0.9%)	Riyadh_ Saudi Arabia	3 years	[15]
	1 (0.5%)	Setif_ Algeria	3 years	[19]
11. Colpocephaly	8 (13.4%)	Khartoum State _Sudan	6 months (September 2016–March 2017)	[12]
12. Schizencephaly	8 (13.4%)	Khartoum State _Sudan	6 months (September 2016–March 2017)	[12]
	7 (8.75%)	Iran	September 2009 and September 2010	[13]
13. Dandy-Walker variant	5 (8.3%)	Khartoum State _Sudan	6 months (September 2016–March 2017)	[12]
	4 (5%)	Iran	September 2009 and September 2010	[13]
	2 (11.1%)	UAE	January 1992 to January 1994.	[16]

(continued)

Table 20.1 (continued)

Malformation	Number of cases and % of subtotal congenital brain/CNS anomalies	Country	Period of the study	Reference
14. Heterotopia	4 (6.6%)	Khartoum State _Sudan	6 months (September 2016–March 2017)	[12]
15. Periventricular Heterotopia	1 (1.25%)	Iran	September 2009 and September 2010 September 2009 and September 2010	[13]
16. Corpus callosum and cerebellar vermis hypoplasia	4 (3.8%)	Khartoum State _Sudan	6 months (September 2016–March 2017)	[12]
17. Cerebellar vermis hypoplasia	1 (1.25%)	Iran	September 2009 and September 2010	[13]
18. Cerebellar Hypoplasia	9 (11.25%)	Iran	September 2009 and September 2010	[13]
19. Pachygyria and absence of corpus callosum	3 (2.9%)	Khartoum State _Sudan	6 months (September 2016–March 2017)	[12]
20. Pachygyria Complex	11 (13.75%)	Iran	September 2009 and September 2010	[13]
21. Chiari type 1 malformation	1 (1.25%)	Iran	September 2009 and September 2010	[13]
22. lissencephaly and pachygyria	2 (1.9%)	Khartoum State _Sudan	6 months (September 2016–March 2017)	[12]
23. lissencephaly	9 (11.25%)	Iran	September 2009 and September 2010	[13]
24. cerebrocerebellar Lissencephaly and agenesis of corpus callosum	1 (5.5%)	UAE	January 1992 to January 1994	[16]
25. congenital hydrocephalus and pachygyria	2 (1.9%)	Khartoum State _Sudan	6 months (September 2016–March 2017)	[12]

Table 20.1 (continued)

Malformation	Number of cases and % of subtotal congenital brain/CNS anomalies	Country	Period of the study	Reference
26. Neural tube defect	1078 (29.57%)	Cairo_ Egypt	(1995–2009)	[14]
	54 (4.6%)	Riyadh_ Saudi Arabia	3 years	[15]
27. Cranial cerebrovascular anomalies	430 (11.79%)	Cairo_ Egypt	(1995–2009)	[14]
28. Cranial anomalies	284 (7.79%)	Cairo_ Egypt	(1995–2009)	[14]
29. Cerebral defects	281 (7.71%)	Cairo_ Egypt	(1995–2009)	[14]
30. Neuroectodermal anomalies	119 (3.26%)	Cairo_ Egypt	(1995–2009)	[14]
31. holoprosencephaly	7 (8.75%)	Iran	September 2009 and September 2010	[13]
	1 (8.3%)	Al-Jahra_ Kuwait	January 2000 to December 2001	[17]
32. polymicrogyria	5 (6.25%)	Iran	September 2009 and September 2010	[13]
33. Joubert syndrome	2 (2.5%)	Iran	September 2009 and September 2010	[13]
34. Anencephalus	26 (2.2%)	Riyadh_ Saudi Arabia	3 years	[15]
	3 (25%)	AL-Jahra_ Kuwait	January 2000 to December 2001	[17]
	69 (32.1%)	Setif_ Algeria	3 years	[19]
	7 (38.8%)	UAE	January 1992 to January 1994	[16]
35. Spina bifida	17 (1.4%)	Riyadh_ Saudi Arabia	3 years	[15]
	122 (56.7%)	Setif_ Algeria	3 years	[19]
36. Spina bifida and Anencephaly	23 (10.7%)	Setif_ Algeria	3 years	[19]
37. Meningomyelocele	2 (16.6%)	Riyadh_ Saudi Arabia	3 years	[15]
	5 (27.7%)	UAE	January 1992 to January 1994	[16]
38. Meckel–Gruber syndrome	3 (25%)	AL-Jahra_ Kuwait	January 2000 to December 2001	[17]
39. Polymicrogyria, hypoplasia of cerebellum and brain stem, and agenesis of the corpus callosum	1 (5.5%)	UAE	January 1992 to January 1994	[16]

20.2   Gender Differences in Congenital Brain Anomalies in Different Countries (F<M Underlines)

In Egypt [14], the proportion of males = 8831 was more than females = 4712 which equals 1.8:1.

In Morocco [20], the proportion of males is 57.9% which is higher than the proportion of females 40.5%.

In Tunisia, Males = 2266, females = 2094.

Male 156 (41.3%) females 222 (58.7%) in Iraq

Algeria males 88 (40.9%), females 126 (58.6%)

Iran: males = 38 (48%), females = 42 (52%)

Hashemite kingdom of Jordan: congenital hydrocephalus: Females = 33 (40.2%) males = 49 (59.8%)

UAE: (55% females, 45% males)

Libya: Major Congenital anomalies males 61, females 57

In general, the proportion of congenital anomalies in males is more than in females in the countries of the highest anomalies proportions (Egypt and Tunisia) or at a close percentage in some countries. Sex-related congenital anomalies are recognizable in countries with the highest proportion of genetic anomalies. Hence, inherited risk factors could affect the future proportion of chromosomal alterations in the absence of prenatal genetic counseling (Table 20.2).

Table 20.2 The total proportion of congenital brain malformations among different countries

Number of congenital Brain/ CNS malformations	Number of total congenital malformation	Number of total patients/ total birth	% of congenital brain malformation/ total births	% of congenital brain malformation/total congenital malformations	Period of the study	Country	Reference
1. 105	??	2114 patients	4.9%	?	6 months (September 2016–March 2017)	Khartoum State _Sudan	[12]
2. 3646	13543	660 280 patients	0.5%	26.9%	(1995-2009)	Cairo_ Egypt	[14]
3. 80	?	405 patients	19.7%	?	September 2009 and September 2010	Tehran_ Iran	[13]
4. 137	706	68 704 Births	0.19%	19.4%	January 2011 to December 2014	Rabat_ Morocco	[20]
5. 1929	4498	9678 autopsied fetuses	19.9%	42.8%	February 1991 to December 2011	Tunis_ Tunisia	[21]
6. 161	1179	28 646 births	0.56%	13.6%	1 July 2010 through 30 June 2013	Riyadh_ Saudi Arabia	[15]
7. 120	378	9653 births	1.2%	31.7%	2005 to 2008	Al-Najaf_ Iraq	[22]
8. 12	97	7739 births	0.15	12.3%	January 2000 to December 2001	Al-jahra region_n Kuwait	[17]
9. **0.95/1000** **2.7~3**	2876	117498		~ 0.10%	1980-1990	Bahrain	[23]

(continued)

Table 20.2 (continued)

Number of congenital Brain/ CNS malformations	Number of total congenital malformation	Number of total patients/ total birth	% of congenital brain malformation/ total births	% of congenital brain malformation/total congenital malformations	Period of the study	Country	Reference
10. 215	?	28500	0.75	?	3-years period	Sétif_ Algeria	[19]
11. ?	1678	101160	?	?	?	Doha_ Qatar	[24]
12. 18	173	16 419	0.10%	10.4%	January 1992 to January 1994	United Arab Emirate	[16]
13. **1.6/1000 0.28~ 0.3**	130	39 501 births	?	0.2%	September 1996 to December 2002	Sana_ Yemen	[25]
14. 22% **12.1~12**	55	4,027	0.2%	21.8%	5 months in 2010	Gaza_ Palestine	[26]
15. 79	541	21 988	0.35%	14.6%	January 1993 through December 2002	Sultanate of Oman	[27]
16. 36	161	16186	0.22%	22.3%	1995	Benghazi_ Libya	[28]
17. **11.21% 7.1~7**	64	3865	0.18%	10.9%	2/1/1991 and 7/31/1993	South of Beirut	[29]

20.3 Family History and Consanguinity in Congenital Brain Anomaly Among Countries

There are many risk factors that contributed to increasing the incidence of congenital anomalies in general and brain malformations specifically. Here, we will mention the common factors and their available data that are present in different Arab countries to highlight the most important ones.

In Sudan [12], more than half of the parents were relatives 67.2%, 15.2% of the patients had a congenital anomaly in their family history, and 22.9% & 6.7% of mothers had a history of miscarriage and fetal death, respectively. Metabolic screening, genetic counseling & testing & diagnosis, and advanced neuroimaging studies are not available nor always feasible in the health care system regarding their importance in the early detection of congenital anomalies. Also, epilepsy and the impairment of the nervous system growth, which need neuroimaging studies for their assessment, were the most common conditions in this study. Even the available neuroimaging studies such as the 1.5 Tesla magnetic resonance imaging scan may miss some congenital malformations due to their low resolution. Family counseling is also very important to discuss the situation with the family. All these important factors are not always offered or available in developed countries and it has a major impact on these conditions.

In Egypt [14], the proportion of consanguineous marriage is 45.8%, the family history of congenital anomaly is 16.69%, drug history of unknown type was present in 36.32% of the mothers of babies with congenital anomalies, and 55.44% of mothers were smokers. Living near or exposed to pollution and factories was observed in 58.57% of this study. Pesticide uses in Egypt are not regulated regarding their correct type and amount. Educated families whose fathers have professional occupation is observed in 14.72% of this study, indicating that congenital malformations are present in high proportion in low-socioeconomic populations. Other factors such as birth weight >2.5 kg have been noted in 71.04% of children with congenital anomalies, pre-eclampsia in 39.43% of mothers, and common cold and fever in 16.69%. multiparity was observed in 54% of this study. 54% is the proportion of multiparity, 59.96% is the mother's age older than 35, and 7.28% is the DM proportion in mothers. On the other hand, antenatal care and multivitamins/folic acid were given to 31.8% &27.5% of mothers, respectively, and 68.2% didn't have antenatal care (Fig. 20.1).

The link between all these risk factors and their long-term effects has a cornerstone in association with genetic counseling, environmental, biological risk etiologies will reduce the proportion of birth defects and neurodevelopmental delay.

In Iran [13], 20% & 8.7% of mothers had a history of incomplete course of folic acid administration and a history of congenital brain malformation previously. Their data indicated that folate and genetic counseling, especially for women with a previous history of congenital malformation can be effective in protecting the next child from unpredicted risks (Fig. 20.2).

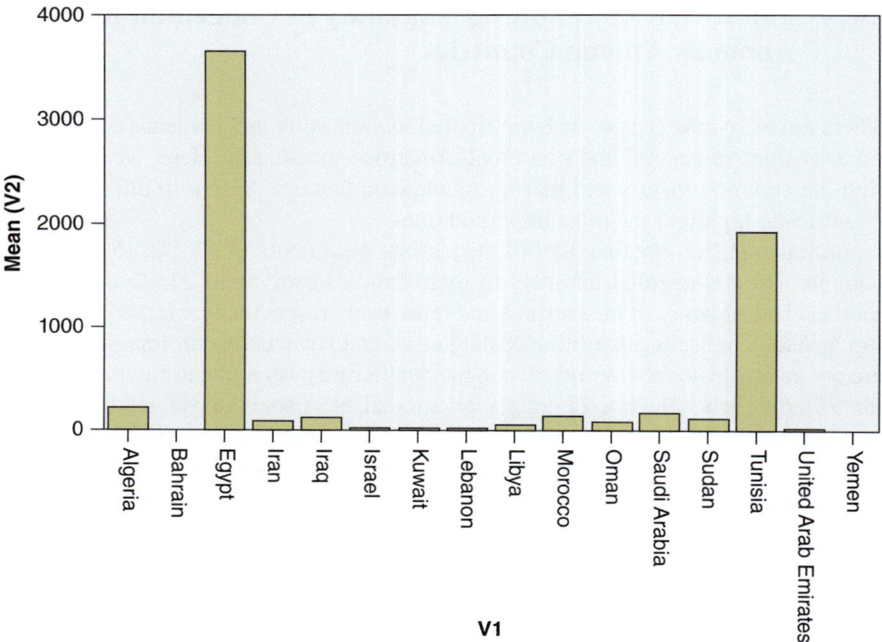

Fig. 20.1 The mean of the cases per countries

In Morocco [20], 13.3% of mothers had a miscarriage, 118 (17.3%) of babies are stillbirth, and 12.3% is the proportion of chromosomal abnormalities. There is a deficit in testing stillborn, dead infants who are delivered at the house, inadequate follow-up after delivery, and unavailability of genetic tests are the major reasons for lacking complete information regarding the true prevalence of babies with congenital anomalies in the study area. On the contrary, advanced methods for fetal examination, and genetic and chromosomal testing will enhance the early diagnosis of congenital malformations and reduce the high incidence of inherited disorders in developing countries.

In Tunisia [21], consanguinity marriage was detected among 1743 (30.19%) mothers in the study, while parental consanguinity is considered related to a higher proportion of congenital anomalies. In the study, although there was no correlation between maternal age, low birth weight, and the origin of the mothers with birth defects, there was a remarkable association between consanguinity, especially parental type, with birth defect rates. The socio-economic status of the mothers who are not residents in the country was lower than residents, hence the culture and the social conditions are important factors in the assessment roles for future births. In general, some differences can be seen in this study when compared with other studies where genetics and origin of the patients were not the visual factors that contribute to these results, but here, consanguinity was of important consequence.

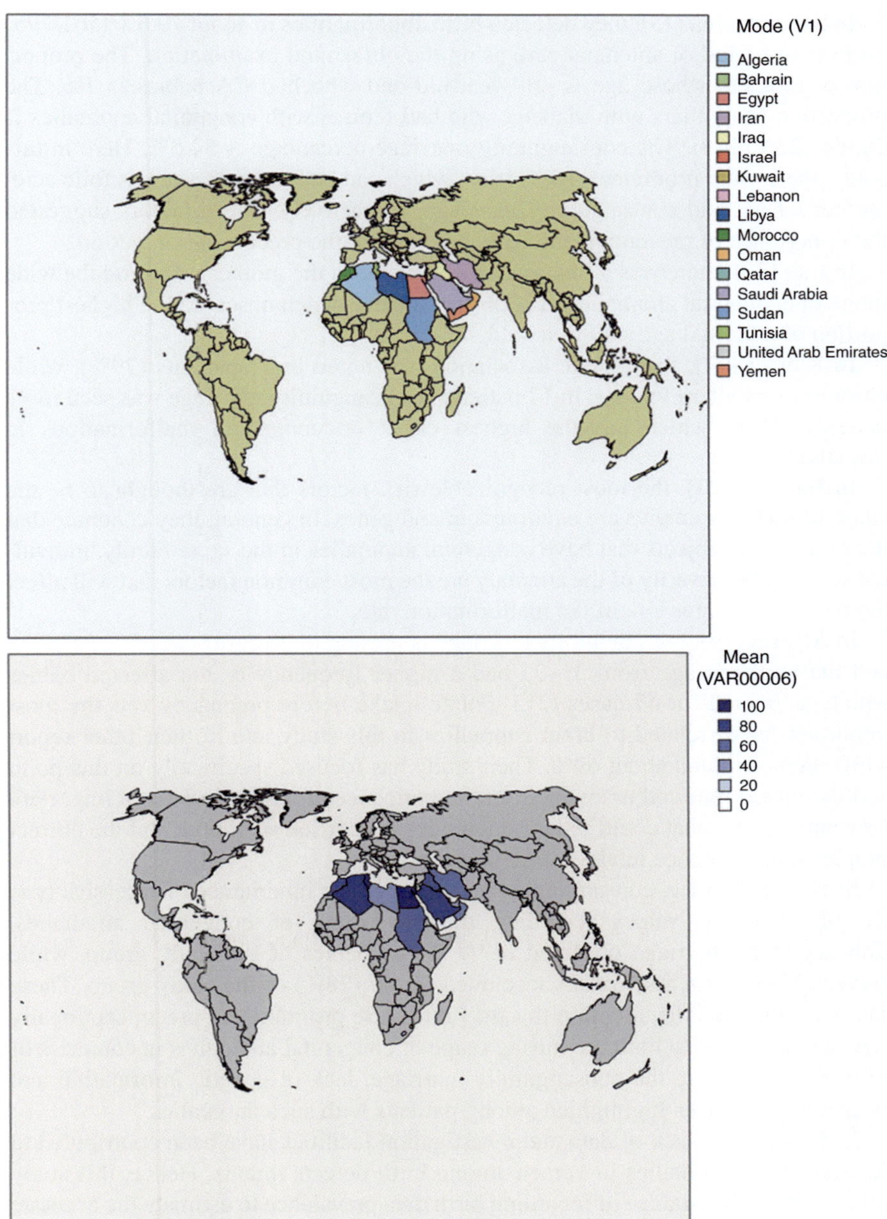

Fig. 20.2 The distribution of the percentages per countries

In Saudi Arabia [15], they detected birth abnormalities in about 70.6% (561/795) during the period of antenatal care using the ultrasound examination. The proportion of mothers whose age is <40-year-old and who had CA babies is 7%. The proportion of mothers with diabetes who had fetuses with congenital anomalies is 18.9% (223/1179). The consanguinity marriage percentage is 54.5%. Here in this study, there were prominent risk factors, which can be modified, such as folic acid, mother's DM, and consanguinity marriage, respectively. These factors suggested the importance of prevention and early care during the preconception period.

In Iraq [22], there was a link association between the mother's age and the wide range of congenital anomalies in 2006 specifically which observed the highest proportion of maternal age <40 years old.

In Kuwait [17], the genetic association was noted in 77 patients (79%), while chromosomal alteration was in 17 patients. Consanguinity marriage was seen in 47 patients (59%) which has the highest effect on congenital malformations in this study.

In Bahrain [23], the most recognizable risk factors that are thought to be the cause of these anomalies are environment and genes. In general, they conclude that the number of subjects that have congenital anomalies in the same family, individual sex, and the severity of the anomaly are the most common factors that will affect the recurrence status risk of the malformation rate.

In Algeria [19], consanguinity marriage is present in 28 cases out of 215 (13%), and the mother's age from 31–35 had a higher frequency of the affected babies which accounted for 47 cases /215. Folate intake before pregnancy was the most important factor related to brain anomalies in this study and in their other report which demonstrated about 69%. Their study has focused specifically on this point and its related required assessment in the periconceptional period as an important preventive factor that could reduce anomalies proportion with time and the correct supplements reference intake before pregnancy.

In UAE [16], race, consanguinity, and rare genetic inheritance of recessive type are of important values regarding the proportion of congenital anomalies. Consanguinity marriage observed in 99 (57%) babies of the study group, while preventable genetic association accounted for 49 (28%) of the study group. These data have directed the attention toward future care program and preconceptionally counseling service to limit the raising range of congenital anomalies in countries of Arab Muslim where the consanguinity marriage, lack of genetic information and awareness have been highlighted among patients with such anomalies.

In Yemen [25], lack of data and investigation facilities have been contributed to the congenital anomalies in Yemen among birth defects infants. Hence, this study suggested the importance of recording birth data prevalence to estimate the accurate proportions and to assess the risk factors correctly.

In Palestine [26], there was a remarkable correlation between birth defects and the exposure of couples to elements derived from the war and the present attacks of the country. On the contrary to other Arab studies, consanguinity marriage was not associated with high rate of congenital anomalies, but the genetic mutation has an impact on the recurrence of birth defects. However, duet to the special circumstances in Palestine, many data are not available and many birth defects have been diagnosed clinically at birth. Recurrence of the anomalies has occurred in the same family without affecting their collaterals, whether same or different anomaly. The only correlation observed in these families is the parents' exposure to white phosphorus and other types of bombing elements.

In the Sultanate of Oman [27], the consanguinity of marriage among parents of the affected children was 76%. High rates of rare syndromes were observed among consanguineous parents in this study. Since they mention the unavailability of abortion due to fetal reasons among Arab countries due to legal and ethical causes, they emphasize the importance of genetic counseling and the technical facilities to enhance the preventive methods for future medical and technical development.

In Libya [28], the low birth weight, maternal age < 40 years-old and cesarian section delivery were associated with a high rate of major malformations when compared with normal babies. Consanguinity marriage rate was not detected in this study, but congenital anomalies in Libya were I a moderate rate when compared with global incidence. In this study, they observed the correlation between chromosomal alteration and age-related fertility manner.

In Lebanon [29], high proportion of congenital malformations was associated with consanguinity marriage of the first cousin and with low-birth-weight infants.

20.4 Diagnostic Approach to Congenital Brain Anomalies

In pregnancy, the first line of imaging study is the Ultrasonography "US". It can be implemented at different times during the first, second, and third trimesters. The main limitations in the US are acoustic shadow, artifactual shadow, and depth due to the mother's abdomen, gases or bones, and depth infiltration, respectively. Viability of the fetus, growth, site of the placenta, amniotic fluid, and the main fetal defects are all can be assessed during screening level one at any trimester. The survey, which is a level two assessment, can be performed in the 2ndtrimester to assess the anatomy and growth of the fetus. The third level is the advanced assessment of the fetal complex situations in detailed form [30, 31].

When these limitations are observed in addition to factors such as the position of the fetus, a small volume of amniotic fluid, the mother's body habits, and others, the second step will be the Magnetic Resonance Imaging of the fetus which can be in the 2nd trimester. MRI indications for the fetal brain are infarctions, brain masses, hemorrhage, vascular anomalies, and any suspected congenital conditions. [32]

The type of imaging technique in addition to the patient character and the experience of the radiologist is the key element for the accurate diagnosis of fetal anomalies, thus, multidisciplinary factors are involved to establish the maximum benefits of genetic evaluation and the parental and family counseling [33, 34].

20.5 Genetic Tests to Evaluate Various Malformations in the Antenatal and Neonatal Time

There are many types of genetic tests such as single gene, Narrow, cytogenetic, and karyotyping tests, and lastly the Chromosomal microarray analysis "CMA". Once these steps can't reveal the results, the next method will be the sequencing of the whole genome or whole exome using the next-generation sequence [35–37].

When a suspected specific syndrome or genetic familial malformation is expected to implement and rarely in situations like brain anomalies, single gene testing is performed. Narrow testing has various ranges of accuracy and coverage and it is the panel for genetic brain anomalies. Numerical and structural assessment for chromosomal abnormalities such as aneuploidy "numerical" and structural alteration such as duplication or deletion or others, is performed by cytogenic testing. During metaphase, the leading test to visualize chromosomes using the Giemsa banding stain is the Karyotyping method [35]. The CMA method, which is sensitive to alterations such as deletion or duplications, needs no culture and can be applied to raw materials [36].

In Western countries, about 88 per 1000 cerebral palsy cases are reported to have congenital brain anomalies [38]. However, In the Arab world, little data is known to be available to compare the results with different global regions. In a study of UAE newborns with congenital anomalies, about 13.8% of them had central nervous system malformations. In their study, a 38.7% consanguinity rate was observed in newborns having CNS malformations [39]. On the contrary, some Arab countries have a very high rate of consanguinity marriage among children with congenital anomalies in general and brain malformations specifically. Regarding that rate, in a study conducted in Sudan [12], the consanguineous rate was 76.2% and the family history rate was 15.2% among them.

20.6 Conclusion

Egypt and Tunisia have the highest mean of congenital brain anomalies among all other countries. The lowest number of brain congenital anomalies was observed in Yemen and Bahrain. Although the economic status of the country is an important factor to count in the process of early detection of congenital anomalies in general or brain malformations specifically, our results have directed the light over some modifiable risk factors where their absence can reduce the proportion of the genetic alterations. One of the most important factors is the consanguinity marriage and the other factor is family history. Families with these anomalies' history should be observed under a regular program through prenatal, natal, and post-natal care or clinical counseling if genetic investigations are not available. Consanguinity and family history are correlated and the education of the families with alterations in their medical history is critical.

References

1. Hennekam RC, Biesecker LG, Allanson JE, Hall JG, Opitz JM, Temple IK, et al. Elements of morphology: general terms for congenital anomalies. Am J Med Genet A. 2013;161A(11):2726–33. [Internet]. [cited 2022 Aug 19] Available from: https://pubmed.ncbi.nlm.nih.gov/24124000/

2. Cecchetto G, Milanese L, Giordano R, Viero A, Suma V, Manara R. Looking at the missing brain: hydranencephaly case series and literature review. Pediatr Neurol. 2013;48(2):152–8. [cited 2022 Aug 22] [Internet] Available from: https://pubmed.ncbi.nlm.nih.gov/23337012/

3. Moore CA, Weaver DD, Bull MJ. Fetal brain disruption sequence. J Pediatr. 1990;116(3):383–6. [Internet]. [cited 2022 Aug 22] Available from: https://pubmed.ncbi.nlm.nih.gov/2308027/

4. Zankl A, Brooks D, Boltshauser E, Largo R, Schinzel A. Natural history of twin disruption sequence. Am J Med Genet A. 2004;127A(2):133–8. [Internet]. Jun 1 [cited 2022 Aug 22] Available from: https://onlinelibrary.wiley.com/doi/full/10.1002/ajmg.a.20680

5. Boltshauser E, Schneider J, Kollias S, Waibel P, Weissert M. Vanishing cerebellum in myelomeningocele. Eur J Paediatr Neurol. 2002;6(2):109–13. [Internet]. [cited 2022 Aug 22] Available from: https://pubmed.ncbi.nlm.nih.gov/11995957/

6. Poretti A, Leventer RJ, Cowan FM, Rutherford MA, Steinlin M, Klein A, et al. Cerebellar cleft: a form of prenatal cerebellar disruption. Neuropediatrics. 2008;39(2):106–12. Apr [cited 2022 Aug 22]; [Internet] Available from: https://pubmed.ncbi.nlm.nih.gov/18671186/

7. Poretti A, Huisman TAGM, Cowan FM, del Giudice E, Jeannet PY, Prayer D, et al. Cerebellar cleft: confirmation of the neuroimaging pattern. Neuropediatrics. 2009;40(5):228–33. [Internet]. [cited 2022 Aug 22] Available from: https://pubmed.ncbi.nlm.nih.gov/20221959/

8. Poretti A, Limperopoulos C, Roulet-Perez E, Wolf NI, Rauscher C, Prayer D, et al. Outcome of severe unilateral cerebellar hypoplasia. Dev Med Child Neurol. 2010;52(8):718–24. [Internet]. Aug [cited 2022 Aug 22]; Available from: https://pubmed.ncbi.nlm.nih.gov/19863638/

9. Vermeulen RJ, Peeters-Scholte C, van Vught JJMG, Barkhof F, Rizzu P, van der Schoor SRD, et al. Fetal origin of brain damage in 2 infants with a COL4A1 mutation: fetal and neonatal MRI. Neuropediatrics. 2011;42(1):1–3. [Internet] [cited 2022 Aug 22] Available from: https://pubmed.ncbi.nlm.nih.gov/21500141/

10. Yoneda Y, Haginoya K, Kato M, Osaka H, Yokochi K, Arai H, et al. Phenotypic spectrum of COL4A1 mutations: porencephaly to schizencephaly. Ann Neurol. 2013;73(1):48–57. [Internet]. [cited 2022 Aug 22] Available from: https://pubmed.ncbi.nlm.nih.gov/23225343/

11. Paciorkowski AR, Keppler-Noreuil K, Robinson L, Sullivan C, Sajan S, Christian SL, et al. Deletion 16p13.11 uncovers NDE1 mutations on the non-deleted homolog and extends the spectrum of severe microcephaly to include fetal brain disruption. Am J Med Genet A. 2013;161A(7):1523–30. [Internet] [cited 2022 Aug 22] Available from: https://pubmed.ncbi.nlm.nih.gov/23704059/

12. Mohammed IN, Suliman SA, Elseed MA, Hamed AA, Babiker MO, Taha SO. Congenital brain malformations in Sudanese children: an outpatient-based study. Sudan J Paediatr. 2018;18(1):48. [Internet]. [cited 2022 Aug 22] Available from: /pmc/articles/PMC6113775/

13. Zamani GR, Shervin-Badv R, Niksirat A, Alizadeh H. CNS structural anomalies in Iranian children with global developmental delay. Iran J Child Neurol. 2013;7(1):25. [Internet] [cited 2022 Aug 23] Available from: /pmc/articles/PMC3943080/

14. Shawky RM, Sadik DI. Congenital malformations prevalent among Egyptian children and associated risk factors. Egypt J Med Hum Genet. 2011;12(1):69–78.

15. Kurdi AM, Majeed-Saidan MA, al Rakaf MS, Alhashem AM, Botto LD, Baaqeel HS, et al. Congenital anomalies and associated risk factors in a Saudi population: a cohort study from pregnancy to age 2 years. BMJ Open. 2019;9:9. [Internet]. [cited 2022 Aug 24] Available from: https://pubmed.ncbi.nlm.nih.gov/31492776/

16. Al-Gazali LI, Dawodu AH, Sabarinathan K, Varghese M. The profile of major congenital abnormalities in the United Arab Emirates (UAE) population. J Med Genet. 1995;32(1):7. [cited 2022 Aug 25] [Internet] Available from: /pmc/articles/PMC1050171/?report=abstract

17. Madi SA, Al-Naggar RL, Al-Awadi SA, Bastaki LA. Profile of major congenital malformations in neonates in Al-Jahra Region of Kuwait. East Mediterr Health J. 2005;11:4.

18. Alebous HDA, Hasan AA. Prevalence of congenital hydrocephalus in the Hashemite kingdom of Jordan: a hospital-based study. Nat Sci (Irvine). 2012;04(10):789–91.

19. Houcher B, Begag S, Egin Y, Akar N. Neural tube defects in Algeria. Neural tube defects—role of folate, prevention strategies and genetics. 2012.

20. Elghanmi A, Razine R, Jou M, Berrada R. Congenital malformations among newborns in Morocco: a retrospective study. Pediatr Rep. 2020;12(1):3–6. [Internet] Feb 2 [cited 2022 Aug 23] Available from: /pmc/articles/PMC7160859/

21. Aloui M, Nasri K, ben Jemaa N, ben Hamida AM, Masmoudi A, Gaïgi SS, et al. Congenital anomalies in Tunisia: Frequency and risk factors. J Gynecol Obstet Hum Reprod. 2017;46(8):651–5.

22. Sallal A, Kadhim Ibadi A, Abdulrazzaq yassin Abdullah and. Survey of malformations at birth in Al-najaf Al-ashraf province. 2011.

23. Epidemiology of congenital abnormalities in Bahrain [Internet]. [cited 2022 Aug 24]. Available from: https://apps.who.int/iris/handle/10665/118706

24. Salameh K, Rahman S. 625 major birth defects among baby, S Borns in Qatar. Arch Dis Child. 2012;97(Suppl 2):A181.

25. Ali Sallam AK, Eissa EM, al Solwi AH. Birth Defect Rates Requiring Emergency Surgery at Al-Sabeen Hospital, Sana'a, Yemen. Ann Saudi Med. 2004;24(4):303. [Internet] [cited 2022 Aug 28] Available from: /pmc/articles/PMC6148115/

26. Naim A, al Dalies H, el Balawi M, Salem E, al Meziny K, al Shawwa R, et al. Birth defects in Gaza: prevalence, types, familiarity and correlation with environmental factors. Int J Environ Res Public Health. 2012;9(5):1732. [Internet]. [cited 2022 Aug 28] Available from: /pmc/articles/PMC3386584/

27. Sawardekar KP. Profile of major congenital malformations at Nizwa Hospital, Oman: 10-Year review. J Paediatr Child Health. 2005;41(7):323–30.

28. Singh R, Al-Sudani O. Major congenital anomalies at birth in Benghazi, Libyan Arab Jamahiriya, 1995. East Mediterr Health J. 2000;6(1):65–75. [Internet]. [cited 2022 Aug 28] Available from: https://www.researchgate.net/publication/11968579_Major_Congenital_Anomalies_at_birth_in_Benghazi_Libyan_Arab_Jamahiriya_1995

29. Major congenital malformations presenting in the first 24 hours of life in 3865 consecutive births in south of Beirut. Incidence and pattern—PubMed [Internet]. [cited 2022 Aug 28]. Available from: https://pubmed.ncbi.nlm.nih.gov/10349259/

30. Filly RA. Level 1, level 2, level 3 obstetric sonography: I'll see your level and raise you one. Radiology. 1989;172(2):312. [Internet] [cited 2022 Sep 12] Available from: https://www.researchgate.net/publication/20491082_Level_1_level_2_level_3_obstetric_sonography_I'll_see_your_level_and_raise_you_one

31. AIUM-ACR-ACOG-SMFM-SRU practice parameter for the performance of standard diagnostic obstetric ultrasound examinations. J Ultrasound Med. 2018;37(11):E13–24. [Internet] [cited 2022 Sep 12] Available from: https://pubmed.ncbi.nlm.nih.gov/30308091/

32. PRACTICE PARAMETER 2 Fetal MRI.

33. Oegema R, Barakat TS, Wilke M, Stouffs K, Amrom D, Aronica E, et al. International consensus recommendations on the diagnostic work-up for malformations of cortical development. Nat Rev Neurol. 2020;16(11):618–35. [Internet]. [cited 2022 Sep 12] Available from: https://pubmed.ncbi.nlm.nih.gov/32895508/

34. Aldinger KA, Timms AE, Thomson Z, Mirzaa GM, Bennett JT, Rosenberg AB, et al. Redefining the etiologic landscape of cerebellar malformations. Am J Hum Genet. 2019;105(3):606–15. [Internet] [cited 2022 Sep 12] Available from: https://pubmed.ncbi.nlm.nih.gov/31474318/

35. Hay SB, Sahoo T, Travis MK, Hovanes K, Dzidic N, Doherty C, et al. ACOG and SMFM guidelines for prenatal diagnosis: Is karyotyping really sufficient? Prenat Diagn. 2018;38(3):184–9. [Internet] [cited 2022 Sep 12] Available from: https://pubmed.ncbi.nlm.nih.gov/29315677/

36. Committee Opinion No. 581. The use of chromosomal microarray analysis in prenatal diagnosis. Obstet Gynecol. 2013;122(6):1374–7. [Internet] [cited 2022 Sep 12] Available from: https://pubmed.ncbi.nlm.nih.gov/24264715/
37. Committee Opinion No. 682. Microarrays and next-generation sequencing technology: the use of advanced genetic diagnostic tools in obstetrics and gynecology. Obstet Gynecol. 2016;128(6):e262–e8. [Internet] [cited 2022 Sep 12] Available from: https://pubmed.ncbi.nlm.nih.gov/27875474/
38. Retterer K, Juusola J, Cho MT, Vitazka P, Millan F, Gibellini F, et al. Clinical application of whole-exome sequencing across clinical indications. Genet Med. 2016;18(7):696–704. [Internet] [cited 2022 Oct 2] Available from: https://pubmed.ncbi.nlm.nih.gov/26633542/
39. Al-Gazali L, Sztriha L, Dawodu A, Bakir M, Varghese M, Varady E, et al. Pattern of central nervous system anomalies in a population with a high rate of consanguineous marriages. Clin Genet. 1999;55(2):95–102. [Internet]. [cited 2022 Oct 2] Available from: https://pubmed.ncbi.nlm.nih.gov/10189086/

Index